AF646031

The Science and Art
Microincision Cataract Surgery
(BIMICS & COMICS)

System requirement:

- **Operating System – Windows XP or above**
- **Web Browser – Internet Explorer 8 or above, Google Chrome, Mozilla Firefox and Safari**
- **Essential plugins – Java & Flash player**
  - Facing problems in viewing content it may be your system does not have java enabled.
  - If Videos don't show up – it may be the system requires Flash player or need to manage flash setting
  - You can test java and flash by using the links from the troubleshoot section of the CD/DVD.
  - Learn more about flash setting from the link in the troubleshoot section.

Accompanying CD/DVD ROM is playable only in Computer and not in DVD player.

CD/DVD has Autorun function – it may take few seconds to load on your computer. If it does not work for you then follow the steps below to access the contents manually:

- Click on my computer
- Select the **CD/DVD drive** and click open/explore – this will show list of files in the **CD/DVD**
- Find and double click file – **"launch.html"**

DVD Contents

1. 1.5 mm COMICS. Fernando Aguilera-Zarate
   [Video corresponding to Chapter 3].
2. Extreme Hard Nucleus with Intrepid OZil [Part 1]. Khiun F Tjia.
   [Video corresponding to Chapter 4].
3. Extreme Hard Nucleus with Intrepid OZil [Part 2]. Khiun F Tjia.
   [Video corresponding to Chapter 4].
4. 0.9 mini-Tip for hard Nucleus. Khiun F Tjia.
   [Video corresponding to Chapter 4].
5. Multiple Fracture Technique. COMICS. Alejandro Cruz-Hernández.
   [Video corresponding to Chapter 5].
6. 1.6 mm COMICS. Francisco Sánchez-León.
   [Video corresponding to Chapter 6].
7. COMICS in Radial Keratotomy Eye. Francisco Sánchez-León.
   [Video corresponding to Chapter 6].
8. Femtosecond Laser for MICS. Jorge L Alió.
   [Video corresponding to Chapter 8].
9. Challenging Cases with BIMICS. I Howard Fine.
   [Video corresponding to Chapter 19].
10. Exchange of Accomodative IOL. Luis Felipe Vejarano-Restrepo.
    [Video corresponding to Chapter 20].
11. Management of Congenital Lens Agenesia. Luis Felipe Vejarano-Restrepo.
    [Video corresponding to Chapter 20].

The Science and Art
Microincision Cataract Surgery
(BIMICS & COMICS)

Editor-in-Chief

Arturo Pérez-Arteaga MD

Medical Director and Founder
Ophthalmic Center of Ambulatory Surgery
Centro Oftalmológico Tlalnepantla, Mexico
Head Professor
Neurosciences Department, School of Medicine
Facultad de Estudios Superiores Iztacala
National University of Mexico (UNAM), Mexico

Co-Editor

Luis Felipe Vejarano-Restrepo MD

Medical Director
Fundación Oftalmológica Vejarano
Popayán, Colombia
Head Professor
Surgical Sciences Department
Universidad del Cauca, Colombia

Foreword

Ashok Garg

JAYPEE - HIGHLIGHTS
MEDICAL PUBLISHERS, INC.

Jaypee Brothers Medical Publishers (P) Ltd.

Headquarter
Jaypee Brothers Medical Publishers (P) Ltd
4838/24, Ansari Road, Daryaganj
New Delhi 110 002, India
Phone: +91-11-43574357
Fax: +91-11-43574314
Email: jaypee@jaypeebrothers.com

Overseas Offices

J.P. Medical Ltd.
83 Victoria Street London
SW1H 0HW (UK)
Phone: +44-2031708910
Fax: +02-03-0086180
Email: info@jpmedpub.com

Jaypee-Highlights Medical Publishers Inc.
City of Knowledge, Bld. 237, Clayton
Panama City, Panama
Phone: +507-317-0496
Fax: +507-301-0499
Email: cservice@jphmedical.com

Jaypee Brothers Medical Publishers (P) Ltd
17/1-B Babar Road, Block-B, Shaymali
Mohammadpur, Dhaka-1207
Bangladesh
Mobile: +08801912003485
Email: jaypeedhaka@gmail.com

Jaypee Brothers Medical Publishers (P) Ltd
Shorakhute, Kathmandu
Nepal
Phone: +00977-9841528578
Email: jaypee.nepal@gmail.com

Website: www.jaypeebrothers.com
Website: www.jaypeedigital.com

© 2013, Jaypee Brothers Medical Publishers

All rights reserved. No part of this book and DVD ROM may be reproduced in any form or by any means without the prior permission of the publisher.

Inquiries for bulk sales may be solicited at: jaypee@jaypeebrothers.com

This book has been published in good faith that the contents provided by the contributors contained herein are original, and is intended for educational purposes only. While every effort is made to ensure the accuracy of information, the publisher and the editors specifically disclaim any damage, liability, or loss incurred, directly or indirectly, from the use or application of any of the contents of this work. If not specifically stated, all figures and tables are courtesy of the editors. Where appropriate, the readers should consult with a specialist or contact the manufacturer of the drug or device.

The Science and Art: Microincision Cataract Surgery (BIMICS & COMICS)

First Edition: 2013

ISBN 978-93-5025-919-1

Printed at: Ajanta Offset & Packagings Ltd., New Delhi

DEDICATIONS

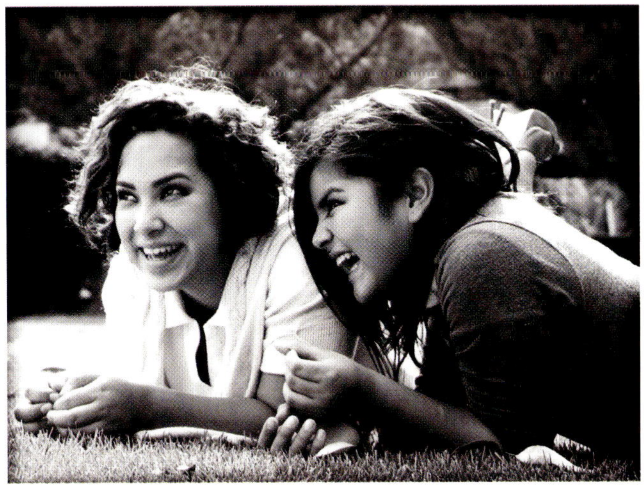

This book is dedicated to my beloved genetic and non-genetic legacy (sons and daughters) and to my medical students at the university; those lovely growing kids and young doctors, reaching at high speed the way to adulthood, with the hope and deep desire of their happiness.

I hope that you can be able to understand and live under the premise that 'to know' is better and more valuable for the human, than living under the premise of 'to have'. I hope that you can comprehend that the only thing that we can truly possess is the knowledge. That the knowledge gives a never-ending peaceful state; 'to know' is a real pleasure. That no one really can obtain anything without giving what he knows to others. That a learned concept becomes sterile if it has not the ability to find a goodness application in the society that surrounds and involves us.

Vision, mission and knowledge conform the way to freedom.

Arturo Pérez-Arteaga

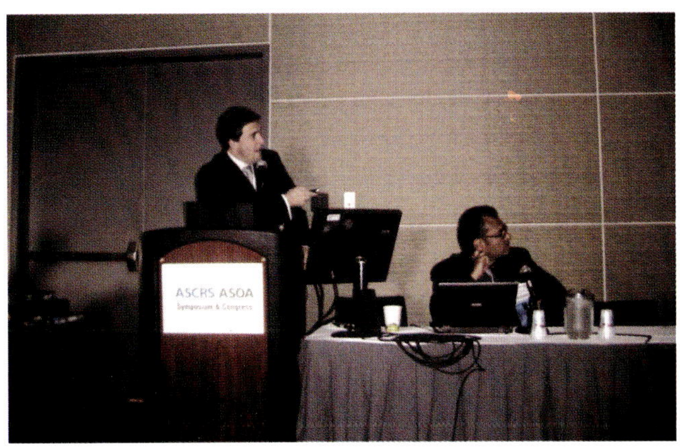

I want to dedicate my chapters to my family; my wife Mary and only son Pablo who always had to hold so many nights alone because of my dedication to Ophthalmology, to prepare my lectures and write chapters. I know that the life goes so fast but even I give my life for them. I also love my career and I have to take some of their time to it, even though they always give me their support and understanding and thanks of that I really feel and totally realize.

A very special dedication to my very good friend Arturo Pérez-Arteaga, and to the existing friendship between us. This surgical relation began with the Microincision Cataract Surgery since 2004 and thanks to our surgical techniques, our friendship became stronger. I want to thank him for the confidence that he had given in all our instructional courses and also in many books that we had written together; this is also true in this new outstanding book project of MICS surgery (Biaxial and Coaxial in one book). Even that I contributed with my knowledge, the big developer and executer was Arturo and I truly believe that this publication will be a success in the Ophthalmology world. Thanks my friend for your pure friendship and your confidence. I hope that the time that you spend working in this project, your family can be able to understand and forgive you. You are thirsty of new ideas. We need you…

Luis Felipe Vejarano-Restrepo

Contributors

Arturo Pérez-Arteaga MD
Medical Director and Founder
Ophthalmic Center of Ambulatory Surgery
Centro Oftalmológico Tlalnepantla,
Mexico
Head Professor
Neurosciences Department, School of Medicine
Facultad de Estudios Superiores Iztacala
National University of Mexico (UNAM), Mexico

Luis Felipe Vejarano-Restrepo MD
Medical Director
Fundación Oftalmológica Vejarano
Popayán, Colombia
Head Professor
Surgical Sciences Department
Universidad del Cauca, Colombia

Fernando Aguilera-Zárate MD
Medical Director
Instituto de Ojos, Mexicali, Baja California
Mexico

Khiun F Tjia MD
Co-chief Medical Editor
Cataract & Refractive Surgery Today Europe
Review Member
AAO Cataract Subcommittee
Board Member
NIOIC (Dutch Cataract Society)

Alejandro Cruz-Hernandez MD
Head Cataract Surgeon
Ambulatory Ophthalmic Surgery Clinic
Laser Ocular Lómas, Mexico

Francisco Sánchez-León MD
Medical Director
Ambulatory Ophthalmic Surgery Center
Novavision Laser Center.
Estado de México, Mexico

Mark Packer MD FACS CPI
Clinical Associate Professor of Ophthalmology
Oregon Health & Science University
Drs Fine, Hoffman & Packer
Eugene, Oregon, USA

Jorge L Alio MD Phd
Professor and Chairman of Ophthalmology
Miguel Hernandez University, Alicante, Spain
Medical Director
Vissum Corporation, Spain

George HH Beiko BM BCh FRCS(C)
Assistant Professor
McMaster University
Lecturer
University of Toronto, Canada

Amar Agarwal MS FRCS FRC(Ophth)
Chairman & Managing Director
Agarwal Eye Institute
Chennai, India

Robert J Weinstock MD
Director
Cataract & Refractive Surgery
The Eye Institute of West Florida
Largo, Florida, USA

Jérôme Jean-Philippe Bovet MD
Visiting Professor
JJ Hospital
Consultant Ophthalmic Surgeon FMH
Medical Director
OnO SA
Onex, Switzerland.

Cyres K Mehta MD
Surgical Director and Chief
The International Eye Centre
Mumbai, India

Keiki R Mehta MD
Surgical Director and Chief
The Mehta International Eye Institute
Mumbai, India

I Howard Fine MD
Clinical Professor of Ophthalmology
Oregon Health and Science University
Portland, OR
Drs Fine, Hoffman & Packer
Eugene, Oregon, USA

Richard S Hoffman MD
Clinical Professor of Ophthalmology
Oregon Health and Science University
Portland, OR
Drs Fine, Hoffman and Packer
Eugene, Oregon, USA

Foreword

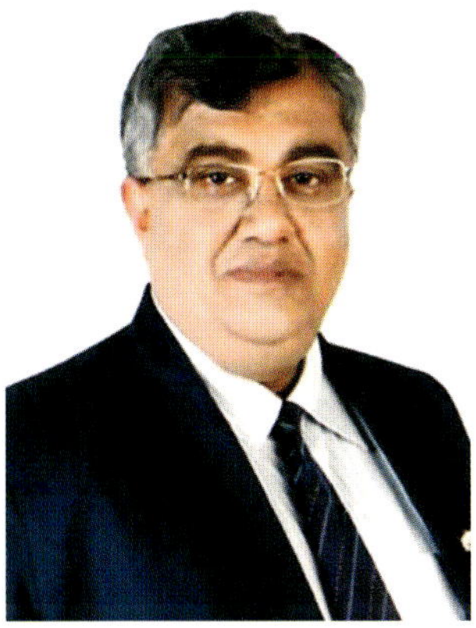

Cataract Removal Technology has undergone rapid advancements and innovations especially in the last two decades. From modest and conventional surgical techniques in the early 80s, now it has become high-tech customized visual enhancement outdoor surgery with excellent visual outcomes. New Microsurgical techniques, foldable advanced aberration free lens implants, gel technology, refractive lenses and futuristic pharmacokinetics have completely changed the cataract scenario in the 21st century. With the advent of new MICS Techniques especially COMICS & BIMICS and foldable lenses, there is more speedy recovery, reduced risk of postoperative astigmatism and return to improved vision in a very short time. Individual eye tailored cataract surgery is now customized to eliminate dependence on glasses for distance, near and intermediate vision.

In this new book *The Science and Art: MICS (BIMICS & COMICS)* my dear friend Dr Arturo Pérez-Arteaga, in collaboration with Dr Luis Felipe Vejarano-Restrepo, has assembled an impressive collection of chapters divided in four sections to cover all aspects of MICS beautifully. Special feature is their line-up of famous international contributors who have shared their experiences regarding pearls and strategies of MICS techniques.

Section – I of this book is devoted to all important history and background of MICS.

Section – II deals with coaxial microincision cataract surgery, phacodynamics and surgical techniques step by step in a lucid manner.

Section – III includes biaxial microincision cataract surgery innovative techniques, phaco machine dynamics and special techniques like microphakonit by Prof Amar Agarwal and Tri MICS by Dr Jerome Jean-Philippe Bovet.

Section – IV is quite interesting covering newer techniques in COMICS and BIMICS by international masters along with management of complicated cases and futuristic innovations in MICS.

Dr Arturo Pérez-Arteaga and Dr Felipe Vejarano-Restrepo deserve to be congratulated for their stupendous efforts and excellent book on MICS. I hope this comprehensive book on MICS shall provide cutting edge knowledge about COMICS and BIMICS to ophthalmologists worldwide. I am sure this book shall undoubtedly benefit cataract surgeons to sharpen their surgical skills and knowledge. Finally, my kudos to editors, international contributors and publishers M/s Jaypee Highlights Inc. for bringing such a beautiful and well-timed volume on MICS.

Ashok Garg MS PhD FIAO FRSM FAIMS ADM
Chairman and Medical Director
Garg Eye Institute and Research Centre,
Hisar, India
Brand Ambassador of Ophthalmology, WHO
Deputy Director General (Asia Office)
IBC Cambridge (UK)
Incoming President
Indian Intraocular Implant &
Refractive Society (IIRSI)

Preface

As many concepts in a lot of fields of medicine are changing, so is cataract surgery also constantly changing. Recently, innovations performed by important researches have moved this particular technique through new trends based upon decreasing the incision size. Microincision Cataract Surgery (MICS) is a new concept developed during the last decade.

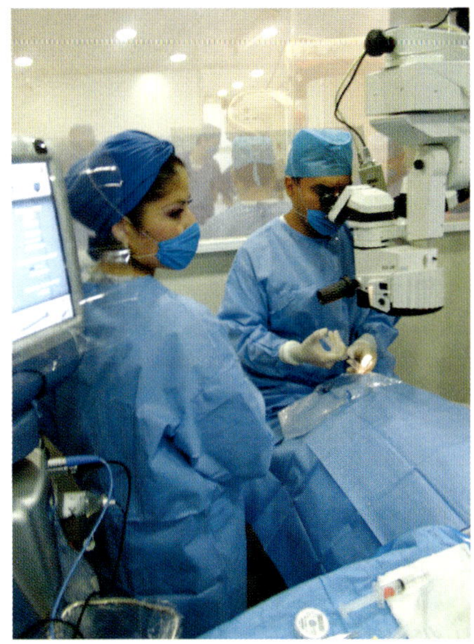

If well, the concept talks by itself regarding the reduction of the incision size. The term MICS has been used by some researches for many purposes and to name to various individual techniques, either coaxial or biaxial, during the time of evolution of these new trends. Some authors have utilized this term according to some particular measures of the incision size, while some others have utilized the term to some other kind of approach (e.g. biaxial). Currently, the term MICS is talking about incision size either in the biaxial or in the coaxial approach. Some terms, like Phakonit or Bimanual Cataract Surgery took importance when the techniques were created by the authors, have been reunited with the term MICS and are divided in coaxial or biaxial (COMICS or BIMICS), according to particular approach that the surgeon is using. In the coaxial approach, the irrigation is placed in the same handpiece that is in the aspiration, while in the biaxial approach, the irrigation and the aspiration are in different devices and so performed through different axis.

Interestingly, the most important discoveries of this movement of cataract surgery in the research of the smaller and smaller incisions occurred not in the incision size itself. During the process of decreasing the incision size, the most important developments happened in the field of the performance of phacoemulsification process itself. New trends appeared in the fields like instrumentation, phaco power modulations, phacoemulsification modalities and, in particular, the big improvement in the management of fluidics; since our particular point of view (and as you will see while reading this book, since the point of view of many authors) the key in MICS has been the changes in fluidics performance. While at the beginning of the process, the surgeons created a new way of fluidics management; with the increased number of surgeons performing MICS, the industry understood and new machines with improved fluidics were created. The main advantage of this process is located in the point of less tissue damage and so the decrease in the inflammatory response. The correct performance of MICS leads to the decrease of the postoperative inflammation; the decreased inflammation reduces postoperative complications and improves the visual recovery in time and degree.

If all is well, MICS keeps constant concepts, because these techniques have been developed by many authors worldwide, sometimes differences exist between the physicians in the performance of the surgery. When the surgeon finds that a particular technique is able to give good results in his/her patients, he/she keeps the changes, leading this way to a customized technique. That is why, currently, there are many ways to perform MICS; either coaxial or biaxial, the technique can be very different from one surgeon to another. There are differences in machines, instrumentation, settings, approaches, maneuvers, tools and ideas; even called MICS, two surgeons can perform the surgery in a very different way. The transition is continuous. The transition is something that we experienced and we are still experiencing.

The objective of this book is to demonstrate to the reader by many different ways to perform MICS by some of the most important surgeons in the world, and some applications of this technique to other fields also rather than cataract surgery (e.g. refractive lens exchange). We have tremendous honor to have leaders and pioneers as the contributors of this book in the creation and development of MICS. The ophthalmic community recognizes their work and their knowledge. The reader will be able to notice the differences from one surgeon to another and will be able to decide the particular concepts that might incorporate to his/her surgical practice. The reader will be able to take again some forgotten ideas and mix them with the new ones in performing so a customized and useful technique for the benefit of his/her patients. It is not the objective of this book to find a final technique or a final conclusion in MICS; you will see that what is useful for one author may be useless for the other. In this book, the authors contributed concepts, ideas, knowledge and surgical experience for the goodness of our cataract patients; joining most of the current concepts in MICS.

The idea of working in a project like this was born during the years since we have been performing Instructional Courses at meetings like the American Academy of Ophthalmology (AAO), the American Society of Cataract and Refractive Surgery (ASCRS) and the European Society of Cataract and Refractive Surgery (ESCRS). We have seen through this "window" how MICS was born and how MICS has been evolving during the last decade. We have had the honor that most of the contributors to this have been instructors in our courses. We have been professors but also we have learned from other professors, the audience and from each other. For this reason, we can qualify this project as a description of personal techniques. This book has not a specific sequence; the reader is able to go directly to the information through a particular author or through a particular technique. The concepts are reinforced with pictures and in the case of some authors with surgical videos that demonstrate the written concepts.

This book goes from basic concepts described many years ago until recent applications in MICS, like the very new Femto MICS technique. Definitively, this is not the end in MICS. This book is just describing what is happening now and the basic concepts that gave life to "what is happening now". New concepts will be in the arena of the cataract surgery during incoming meetings and articles this year, maybe at the same time when this book is being presented. This is the history of the human knowledge, the addition of new concepts to what we have previously learned. But we believe that sometimes, in a particular moment, we have to stop and take some time to obtain a clear view to see where we are standing.

That was our idea…

Arturo Pérez-Arteaga
Luis Felipe Vejarano-Restrepo

Section 1

History & Background

1 How MICS was Born? Where are We Now?

Arturo Pérez-Arteaga (Mexico),
Luis Felipe Vejarano-Restrepo (Colombia)

Evolution of Surgical Techniques

Cataract surgery has been evolving at a very rapid way during the last decades, passing from extracapsular extraction to ultrasonic phacoemulsification, which has become progressively the standard method for cataract surgery around the world, because it affords less astigmatism induction, rapid astigmatism stabilization, less postoperative inflammation and less possibility of postoperative complications than extracapsular cataract extraction.

One of the latest crucial breakthroughs in phacoemulsification has been to perform the phacoemulsification surgery through a microincision with a bimanual approach, using a sleeveless phaco tip. Co-axial MICS, as we know today, did not evolve directly from standard phacoemulsification, even that phacoemulsification was described since the early years as a coaxial procedure. Bi-axial technique was born from the idea of performing a less invasive technique in comparison to standard phacoemulsification; this idea leads to the creation of bimanual techniques, currently known as Bi-axial techniques. From this evolution of techniques leading by Biaxial procedures, the idea of performing the same through coaxial was started. Co-MICS is currently a byproduct of Bi-MICS, in particular for those surgeons that did not want to pass through the change process from coaxial to biaxial phaco, it means, the learning curve.

The idea of removing the crystalline lens through two microincisions has been proposed since 1985 by Dr. Steven Shearing, MD in Las Vegas USA, as he propounded the separation of ultrasound/aspiration and the irrigation hand piece; it means like the pars plana vitrectomy procedures.[1,2] However, it was not until that independently Agarwal in India and Tsuneoka in Japan began that technique in 1998 and 1999, respectively, that it gained popularity. Although it is still practiced by a small percentage of the world's surgeons, authors hope that its benefits can be slowly understood.[3,4]

Agarwal coined the term "Phakonit" (as you will see in the chapter written by him in this textbook), which initially stood for phacoemulsification (phaco) performed with a needle opening (N) via an ultra small incision (I) with the sleeveless ultrasound tip (T). Originally, Agarwal described an incision as small as 0.9 mm, using a standard sleeveless Microtip. Although initially the theoretical possibility of a possible thermal burn was a concern, this fear was dispelled by several studies. Tsuneoka showed experimentally in a porcine eye that using a sleeveless ultrasound tip, the temperature of the cornea at the incision elevated only 8.4°C without developing thermal burns. In other experiments, Olson et al. demonstrated that clinically unusual parameters were necessary to produce a wound burn in bimanual phaco and moreover, when using "cold phaco" with a bare 19-gauge aspiration needle in human cadaver eyes, a wound burn could not be produced at the highest energy settings unless all flow into the eye and all aspiration were occluded. These settings are well beyond clinically applicable conditions.[5-7] The authors' explanation is that it is difficult to completely occlude a linear stab incision with a metal circular instrument, unlike the situation in standard coaxial phaco, where a flexible irrigation sleeve fills the wound and reduces the flow around the sleeve, particularly in a tight wound.

The sleeveless phaco needle has been a terrible fear for many surgeons to move from coaxial to biaxial phacoemulsification.

The combinations of a tight wound, filled by a flexible irrigation sleeve, and complete occlusion of aspiration, and therefore complete blockage of irrigation results in a wound burn. So in fact, the risk of thermal burn may be less in phakonit than in coaxial phaco.

Agarwal initially reported 305 eyes that underwent the technique successfully.[3,6,7,9] He had the assistant continuously pouring cooled balanced salt solution (BSS®) over the phaco needle. The original incision had to be enlarged in order to implant the intraocular lens (IOL). No one case of thermal wound occurred. Tsuneoka and coauthors also initially reported 637 cases that underwent cataract surgery through a 1.4 mm incision without a case of thermal burn.[4] Likewise the authors of this chapter, working in different surgical centers and for almost a decade of performing all our cataract surgeries under this basis, have not found any single case of corneal wound burn in our patients.

Around the world several other surgeons, including the author of this chapter, have reported their results using bimanual microincision surgery with different phaco machines.

Jorge Alió coined the term Microincision Cataract Surgery (MICS), as you will be able to see in this textbook in the chapter written by him. At that time he reported good visual performance of two available IOLs, which may be implanted through microincisions. In a prospective randomized consecutive case series, he reported that microincision cataract surgery significantly lowered mean phacoemulsification time, mean total phacoemulsification percent, mean effective phaco time and surgically induced astigmatism when compared with coaxial phacoemulsification. Howard Fine has highlighted the advantages of maintaining a more stable intraocular environment during lens removal,[1] as you also will be able to read in the chapter written by him in this textbook. This advantage may be especially important in high myopia, patients who are at a greater risk for retinal detachment following lens extraction or high hyperopes with shallow anterior chamber, decreasing the possibility of an expulsive hemorrhage.

In 2002, Olson was the first to use a 0.8 mm phaco needle and a 21-gauge irrigating chopper in bimanual cataract surgery and called this technique microphaco.

These techniques of performing phacoemulsification through incisions around 1.0–1.5 mm have been spreading around the world. Other names given to these techniques are bimanual phacoemulsification and sleeveless phaco.[2,5,8] Recently, Agarwal reported the microphakonit, a similar technique, but using a 0.7 mm needle and a 0.7 mm irrigating chopper through a sub 1 mm incision. Many chapters in this textbook, including one written by Agarwal himself, talk about the performance of 700 micron cataract surgery, currently the smaller possible incision size for lens removal.

Currently definitions describe that standard coaxial phacoemulsification can be performed through a 2.8–3.2 mm incision. Other techniques that use smaller incisions include micro-coaxial phacoemulsification, which uses a 1.8–2.2 mm incision, and biaxial MICS, which uses a 1.2–1.4 mm incision. In micro-coaxial phacoemulsification, irrigation, aspiration and phacoemulsification are performed with the same instrument (phaco handpiece), used in standard coaxial phacoemulsification. The only difference between the two techniques is the smaller main incision in micro-coaxial phacoemulsification, which is the result of the development of the phaco tip sleeves. In biaxial MICS, however, the irrigation and phacoemulsification aspiration steps are separate; an irrigation chopper is used for irrigation and a sleeveless phaco tip for aspiration and phacoemulsification. Micro-biaxial (or bimanual microphacoemulsification) is named to biaxial techniques performed through 700 micron instrumentation.

Going from a 0.9 mm phaco needle to a 0.7 mm needle diminished the aspiration flow rate, the holding power and in general the efficiency of the tip. So in order to have a feasible procedure, a modified 30 degree tip was developed by MicroSurgical Technology Inc. (MST) Redmond, USA, with thinner walls, allowing for an increased inner diameter thereby increasing efficiency close to that of a 0.9 mm tip. Agarwal uses his end-opening sharp irrigating chopper and gas forced infusion, initially he employed an external air pump[9] and then the anterior vented gas forced infusion (AVGFI) system of the Alcon's Accurus equipment,[8] with the infusion pump preset to 100 mm Hg. Authors have already published results with a phakonit technique through 1.2–1.5 mm, using the 20 gauge Microtip, or 19 gauge Standard or MicroFlow® tips. Now Surgeons have available a specially designed 0.7 mm Nanotip (MST), which allows them to perform the surgery through 0.8 mm incision. Because of the good results of these techniques, authors are using it in all their adult and pediatric cataract patients.

When microincisional techniques were born in a biaxial approach, some kind of skepticism by the side of the coaxial surgeons, the fear of corneal thermal burns and the need to avoid the learning curve from coaxial to biaxial, encouraged the industry to the micro-coaxial techniques, leading the creation of smaller phaco tips and smaller phaco sleeves. It has become part of the history of cataract surgery the communication (an electronic mail) from Prof. A Akahoshi from Japan, to the Alcon engineers, asking for new micro-coaxial instrumentation (tips and sleeves) based upon the growing enthusiasm of the cataract surgeons over biaxial techniques; the idea was to make smaller incisions in the very well known, 'coaxial mode'. Formany surgeons this way microcoaxial technique was born. So all the new instrumentations, the new softwares, the new machines, the new methods of IOL implantation and the new models of IOLs that were born for micro-coaxial (and that are described in this textbook) were born from this inquiry of the coaxial surgeons based upon the new biaxial techniques. This is why authors can say that Co-MICS is a byproduct of Bi-MICS, created by a group of surgeons and the industry, for those surgeons that do not desire to go upon the hill of the learning curve of biaxial.

Current Terminology

For the purposes of this book, the authors are going to standardize in a didactic mode all the names given to these cataract removal technologies. It is currently a hard work to match all the names that these techniques have received through the years and for many authors. Authors of this chapter are not pretending to establish a worldwide accepted terminology; this is what practitioners were able to find and the way they are going to understand each other during the lecture of this book. Maybe new terminology in the future can help us to establish better criteria and an improvement in our knowledge of these techniques.

Authors are agreeing with the reports of Arshinoff and Grabow,[10,11] regarding the term biaxial and coaxial to describe the differences between both methods of phacoemulsification performed at this time, according to the axis of the incoming fluid to the eye. Arshinoff wrote these words in the article of Journal of Cataract & Refractive Surgery (Volume 31, Issue 4, Page 646, April 2005) as follows:

"The point is that all these terms are meaningless, except that they may sound good, unless you think about it. None of them differentiates the procedure under discussion from coaxial phaco. However "biaxial phaco" clearly refers to the fundamental difference in the procedure separating it from coaxial phaco. Biaxial makes no specific reference to incision size, which undoubtedly changes over time; does not imply lack of dexterity of coaxial surgeons; and is not a mixed, obscure acronym. Biaxial is simply what is different from coaxial in biaxial phaco. The rest is left to innovators of the future."

1. **Coaxial Cataract Surgery (CACS):** Cataract surgery performed with three functions in one hand; irrigation, aspiration and some additional form of energy to remove the lens [e.g. ultrasonic power (linear or torsional), water force (AquaLase®), laser power...]. An additional side port incision can be used in some cases.
2. **Micro-coaxial Cataract Surgery (MCACS):** Variation of the CACS performed through one incision of less than 2.2 mm. An additional side port incision can be used in some cases.
3. **Biaxial Cataract Surgery (BACS):** Cataract surgery performed through two incisions with a division of functions between right and left hands. Irrigation and aspiration are used separately with instruments that are able to allow surgical manipulation inside the eye through incisions of 1.5 mm or less. The additional source of energy to remove the lens is used in the same hand that the aspiration.
4. **Micro-biaxial Cataract Surgery (MBACS):** Variation of BACS where the incisions are lesser than 1.0 mm.
5. **Passive Infusion (PI):** Irrigation inside the eye during the cataract surgery obtained only by the force of gravity.
6. **Forced Infusion (FI):** Irrigation inside the eye during the cataract surgery created in an active mode by an air pump.
7. **Internal Forced Infusion (IFI):** Variation of FI where the air pump is integrated to the machine that the surgeon is working with for the cataract extraction.
8. **External Forced Infusion (EFI):** Variation of FI where the air pump is a separate equipment of the machine that the surgeon is working with for the cataract extraction.
9. **Coaxial Phacoaspiration:** Variation of CACS where the only energy for lens extraction is aspiration (vacuum).
10. **Biaxial Phacoaspiration:** Variation of BACS where the only energy for lens extraction is aspiration (vacuum).
11. **Micro-coaxial Phacoaspiration:** Variation of MCACS where the only energy for lens extraction is aspiration (vacuum).
12. **Micro-biaxial Phacoaspiration:** Variation of MBACS where the only energy for lens extraction is aspiration (vacuum).
13. **Biaxial Refractive Lens Exchange:** Clear lens extraction for refractive purposes performed with BACS techniques.
14. **Micro-biaxial Refractive Lens Exchange:** Clear lens extraction for refractive purposes performed with MBACS techniques.
15. **Microincision:** For coaxial techniques, cataract surgery performed through an incision smaller than

2.2 mm. For biaxial techniques, cataract surgery performed through two incisions smaller than 1.5 mm.

16. **Bimanual:** Term apply to the use of both hands for cataract extraction. Once BACS was named Bimanual Cataract Surgery, but a bimanual approach can be seen in CACS and in BACS.
17. **Sleeveless:** Term applies to a cataract surgery performed with a nude phaco tip. It has the same application when the sleeve is cut; in both ways the sleeve is not going through the incision.
18. **Phakonit:** Term coined by Amar Agarwal where the cataract surgery is in a biaxial mode and the incisions are smaller than that required by coaxial phacoemulsification by eliminating the sleeve that covers the phaco needle (or by cutting it). Thus the wound size in phakonit reduces to 0.9 mm.
19. **Microphakonit:** Term coined by Amar Agarwal, and consists of a phakonit performed with instrumentation of 0.7 mm (irrigating cannulas, irrigating choppers, aspiration cannulas and phaco needle). It is the smaller size of lens extraction until the writing of this book.
20. **Microincision Cataract Surgery (MICS):** Term coined by Jorge Alió that consists in the cataract surgery (lens removal) through sub 2 mm incisions aiming to reduce surgical trauma, surgical induced astigmatism and corneal aberrations.
21. **Bimanual Microincisional Surgery:** Term applied sometimes for BACS.
22. **Microphaco:** Term applied sometimes for BACS.
23. **Bimanual Phacoemulsification:** Term applied sometimes to BACS.
24. **Bimanual Microincision Phaco:** Term applied sometimes to BACS.
25. **Ultra small-incision Phaco:** Term applied sometimes to BACS.

References

1. Fine IH, Hoffman RS, Packer M. Optimizing refractive lens exchange with bimanual microincision phacoemulsification. J Cataract Refract Surg. 2004;30(3):550-4.
2. Cavallini GM, Campi L, Masini C, et al. Bimanual microphacoemulsification versus coaxial miniphacoemulsification: prospective study. J Cataract Refract Surg. 2007;33(3):387-92.
3. Agarwal A. Bimanual Phaco. Mastering the Phakonit/MICS Technique. New Jersey: Slack Inc.; 2004.
4. Tsuneoka H, Hayama A, Takahama M. Ultrasmall-incision bimanual phacoemulsification and AcrySof SA30AL Implantation through a 2.2 mm Incision. J Cataract Refract Surg. 2003;29(6):1070-6.
5. Kurz S, Krummenauer F, Gabriel P, et al. Biaxial microincision versus coaxial small-incision clear cornea cataract surgery. Ophthalmology. 2006;113(10):1818-26.
6. Agarwal A. Microphakonit surgery performed with 0.7-mm tip. Ocular Surgery News Europe/Asia-Pacific Edition; 2005.
7. Prakash DP. Cutting phaco sleeve permits ultra-small incision surgery. Ocular Surgery News Europe/Asia-Pacific Edition; 2003.
8. Arturo Pérez-Arteaga. Accurus forced infusion good for MICS, surgeon says. Ocular Surgery News U.S. Edition; 2003.
9. Amar Agarwal. Gas-forced infusion: A solution for surge. Ocular Surgery News U.S. Edition; 2006.
10. Arshinoff SA. Biaxial phacoemulsification. J Cataract Refract Surg. 2005;31(4):646.
11. Grabow HB. Biaxial phacoemulsification. J Cataract Refract Surg. 2006;32(4):547-8.

2 Forced Infusion

Arturo Pérez-Arteaga (Mexico)

Introduction, History and Background

When phacoemulsification was conceived, Prof Charles Kelman determined the need of fluid going inside the eye with the objective to maintain an open anterior chamber, and avoid the collapse of the globe, while performing phacoemulsification and aspiration. All the techniques of phacoemulsification and aspiration performed since then utilize an irrigation system for these purposes.

Phacoemulsification was conceived as a coaxial procedure, not as biaxial ones The fear for many surgeons in the early years was the corneal thermal burn in phacoemulsification; so the sleeve surrounding the phaco tip was born. So many kind and diameters of sleeves have been designed since then, surrounding the phaco needle to allow the incoming fluid to reach the anterior chamber by this way and preventing so the thermal burn. The amount of fluid [balanced salt solution (BSS)] has been determined for decades by the bottle height and the diameter of the sleeve that surrounds the phaco needle. As much the bottle height, more fluid incoming through the sleeve and as the height decreases, less fluid is incoming to the eye. During those years many phaco machines were designed with control of the bottle height (either mechanical or automated) with the objective to control the desired amount of fluid incoming. All the systems that work with the force of gravity to obtain a desired amount of fluid were called passive infusion irrigation systems.

While some surgeons and investigators were working in the development of phacoemulsification for cataract surgery, almost at the same years, another group was working in the developing of vitreoretinal surgery. When pars plana vitrectomy (PPV) was conceived, it was described as a biaxial procedure. The investigators developed a system where a handpiece is performing cutting and aspiration in one hand and another hand is performing irrigation. So in PPV, the irrigation is in a device independent of the aspiration.

This was the mode how the techniques were conceived: while PPV was conceived as a biaxial procedure, phacoemulsification was conceived as a coaxial procedure. Phacoemulsification has been developed by the industry, performed by the surgeons and learned at the residence training programs as a coaxial procedure under the basis of passive infusion for decades.

During the clinical performance of PPV, the posterior segment surgeons recognized the need of controlling the intraocular pressure, in particular during the interchange of fluids and/or air inside the vitreous cavity. The need of pressurizing the globe in some steps of the vitreoretinal surgery pushed for the creation of infusion pumps, with the objective to control the pressure of fluid incoming the eye. This was the born of the infusion pumps (Fig. 1).

The infusion pump is an air pump, not a fluid pump (Fig. 2). It was integrated to the vitrectomy machines [like the Accurus from Alcon (Fig. 1) or the Millennium from Bausch & Lomb (Fig. 3)]. The pump takes air from the environment and pushes it in a positive way into a glass bottle that contains fluid. The air cushion created by the pump inside the bottle, pushes actively the fluid contained also into the bottle; when an exit is offered to this fluid

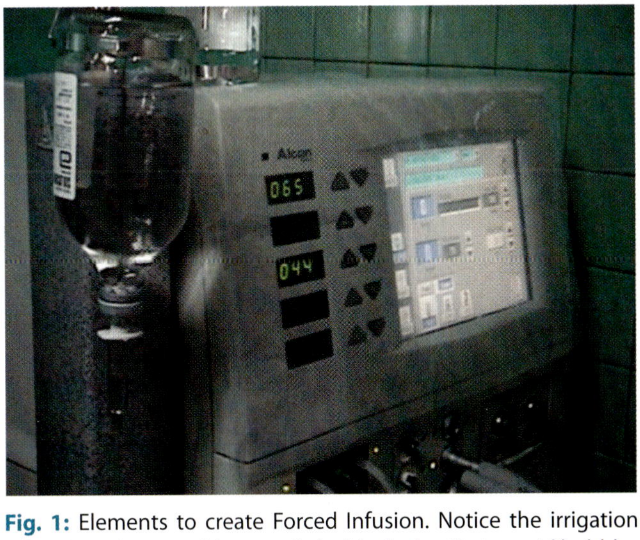

Fig. 1: Elements to create Forced Infusion. Notice the irrigation administration set with a needle inside the bottle to avoid bubbles

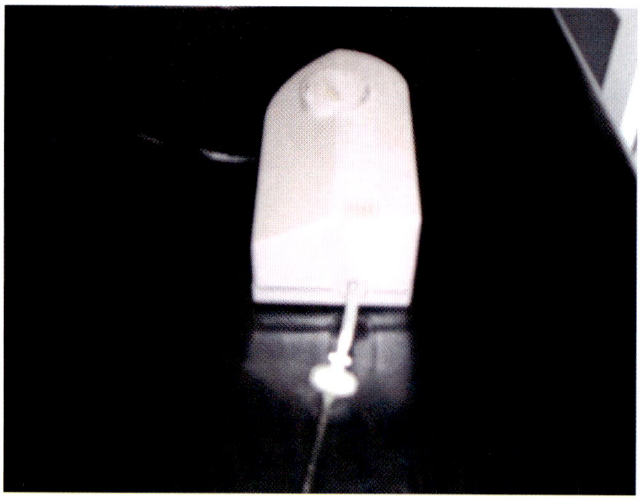

Fig. 2: External air pump with an air filter connected

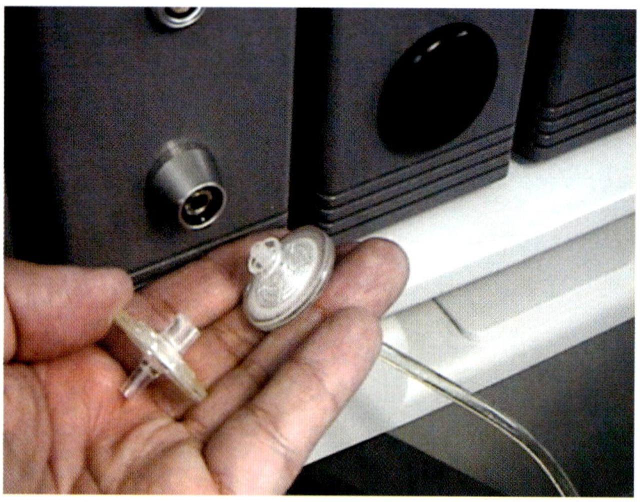

Fig. 3: Air pump of the Millennium Surgical System

(through a tube, cannula or other device), the fluid is pushed by the air at the desired pressure (Fig. 4). The amount of fluid is determined by the air pressure, by the diameter of the device that liberates the fluid and in less part, by the gravity force. This was called active infusion irrigation system (or air pressure system) by the posterior segment surgeons, who were the pioneers in its utilization.[1-6]

When biaxial phacoemulsification was first conceived by Shearing, the system not only progress in part for the fear of thermal burns to the cornea with a phaco needle without sleeve but also because of the lack of a safe infusion system.

When Amar Agarwal developed phakonit, same fears were manifested by the ophthalmic community. Surge was a terrible problem to solve when biaxial cataract surgery started, because the diameter of the irrigation devices was less in size in comparison to the coaxial systems that utilize an irrigation sleeve (that has more diameter). Sunita Agarwal developed the use of an external air pump to actively push the fluid inside the eye, increasing this way the amount of fluid incoming through (Fig. 2). This external air pump was described as an aquarium air pump connected through an air filter and then to a tube to the glass bottle that contains the intraocular solution. The air produced by the air pump creates a cushion (Fig. 4) that actively pushes the air through a tube, and so through a small-diameter irrigation device (cannula or chopper), obtaining this way the desired amount of fluid (as the infusion pump for vitreoretinal surgery). Active infusion systems started for cataract surgery with this invention of Sunita.[7-11]

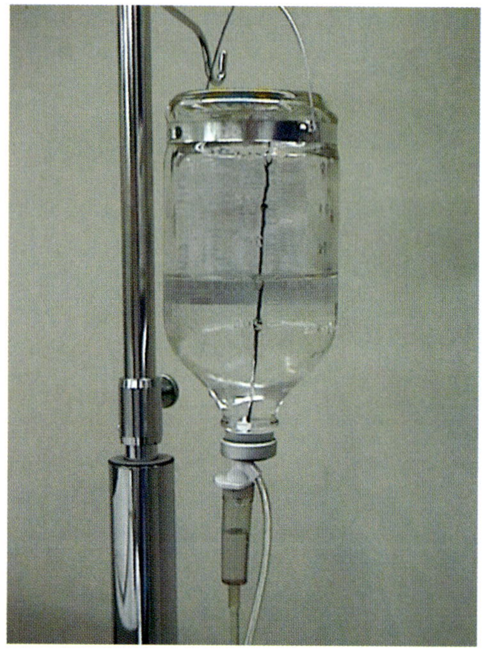

Fig. 4: The air cushion inside the bottle enters through a needle and actively pushes the fluid through the administration set

At that time author realized that the aquarium air pump described was functioning under the same principle that the air pumps developed for vitreoretinal surgery. So author started to work with the hybrid machines, it means those that possess phacoemulsification and vitrectomy systems (e.g. Accurus, Millennium) with the objective to create the active infusion for cataract surgery with the air pump integrated in the same phaco machine. The idea worked really fine, and author described the parameters for setting the air pump integrated in the phaco machines for phakonit. The use of the air pump integrated in the machine for controlling the amount of fluid incoming the eye in cataract surgery was named internal forced infusion by Amar Agarwal and author himself (Figs 3 and 5).[6,12-15]

Section 2

Coaxial Microincision Cataract Surgery

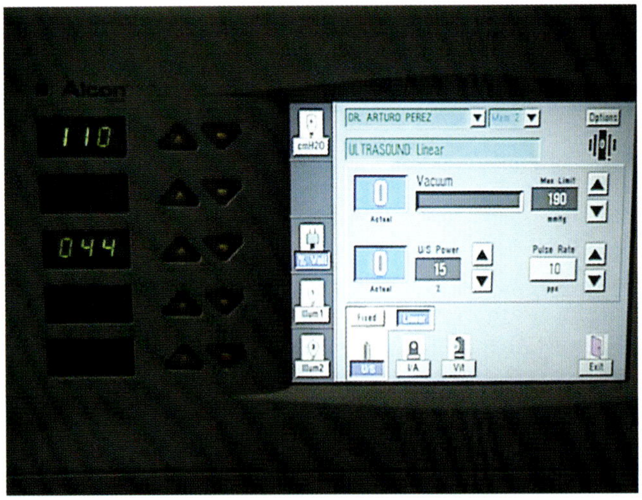

Fig. 5: Control panel of the infusion pump of the Accurus machine. Notice the anterior vented gas forced infusion (AVGFI) set at 100 cm H_2O

This internal infusion system was much more comfortable for the surgeons, because there was no need to add an external pump to the machine; the same preexisting pump (for PPV purposes) in the phaco machine can be presetting controlling this way the intraocular pressure and avoiding the surge during cataract surgery (Figs 3 and 5).

There have been taken many years for cataract surgeons worldwide to understand the advantages of forced infusion in cataract surgery. Many fears preexisting like lesion to the intraocular tissues (corneal endothelium, posterior capsule or even optic nerve) because of the forced infusion, delayed the widespread of this technological tool; nevertheless the advantages of avoiding collapses of the globe (surge), while performing phacoemulsification through small irrigating devices, were understood with the time and many surgeons started to learn the management of the infusion pump, it means the internal forced infusion.[1-6]

The main disadvantage of the internal forced infusion was the fact that the air pump was not incorporated in the standard phaco machines; at that time this air pump was found only within the hybrid phaco machines, those who performed phacoemulsification and posterior vitrectomy. We can understand according to the evolution of eye surgery, that the air pump was conceived for posterior segment surgery; so at this moment if the cataract surgeon was working with an equipment exclusively developed for phacoemulsification surgery (e.g. Legacy, Infinity), the creation of internal forced infusion was impossible, because the lack of an air pump in those kind of phaco systems, and then the need to incorporate an external air pump, making more difficult the learning curve to MICS.

Recently Bausch & Lomb developed the Stellaris Phaco System, understanding the benefits of the internal forced infusion, incorporating an air pump in a machine developed only for phacoemulsification procedures. This is the first phaco machine without capability to perform PPV with an air pump incorporated. It has been a triumph for the microincision cataract surgeons to be understood by the industry and author feels very happy for this. Nevertheless, later on the posterior vitrectomy system was incorporated to the Stellaris machine, which also becomes a hybrid machine. Nevertheless, if you want to have the Stellaris with only the phacoemulsification function, it will include the air pump.

As a part of the evolution of biaxial surgery, smaller diameters of instrumentation were developed. Currently, the smaller system for cataract extraction existing is 700 micron. As the irrigation diameter becoming smaller, the need of forced infusion was increasing. Nevertheless, author has admitted that some surgeons worldwide, who work perfectly with the 700 micron system, are capable to operate without the use of forced infusion, trusting only in the bottle height to avoid surge.[1,2,6,10,12] People like Agarwal, Vejarano and author himself find more safer to work the 700 micron phaco system with forced infusion, either external or internal, according to the phaco machine they are using.[6]

Because of the development of micro-biaxial systems for lens extraction, a new wave of thinking started to work with micro-coaxial systems. So, coaxial cataract surgery also became smaller. The industry developed new micro-sleeves and micro-tips, trying to reduce at maximum the incision size. Because the irrigation sleeve is made of soft material, in comparison with the irrigation devices for biaxial surgery (they are made of metal), the micro-coaxial surgery found its limits; the micro-sleeve is compressed by the tissues, decreasing this way the amount of irrigation, thus compromising the stability of the anterior chamber. One solution has been of course the development of new materials for the sleeve, which is more resistant to compression, but another solution is the use of forced infusion. The increase in the force of infusion is capable to overcome the compression created over the sleeve by the tissues at the incision site in micro-coaxial cataract surgery. Forced infusion is a powerful tool either for micro-coaxial or micro-biaxial phacoemulsification systems.[1,2,4-6]

Author strongly believes that the incision size must not be determined by the intraocular lens (IOL); many surgeons worldwide think that they should not change to the challenge of smaller and smaller incisions because at the end of the day there is currently no IOL capable to be implanted through a microincision (e.g. 700 micron incision); so even that the lens extraction can be performed

through really small incisions, there is the need to increase the size of the incision (or the creation of a third incision) for the IOL implantation. Author strongly believes that, either coaxial or biaxial, the good fluidics performance is the key factor to determine the instrumentation size. When the fluidics work perfectly inside the eye, the inflammatory process of the tissues is reduced at minimum; when the eye is in aphakia it is not important the incision size for the IOL implantation (either increased or a new one); the inflammatory response is determined mainly by the technique performed for lens extraction. The surgeon must keep in mind that the main inflammatory response of the tissues is not created during the IOL implantation procedures; it is really created during the lens extraction process. So author believes that the cataract surgeon is using either micro-coaxial or micro-biaxial systems for lens extraction, and even the kind of IOLs of preference, the forced infusion system, now easily to manage because is incorporated in many phaco machines, is a powerful tool that should be utilized to improve the fluidics performance of the microincisional cataract surgery. As Sunita Agarwal pointed, "One moment of surge during surgery means one month of corneal edema at the postoperative period, two surges means two months, and so on…".[3,4]

At this point of the history coaxial and biaxial systems have a frontier, and this frontier is not determined by the infusion force. It is very difficult to phacoemulsificate a hard cataract with a 700 micron phaco needle, and not because of the ultrasonic power transmission; it is because the hard cataract pieces create a tampon inside the phaco tip. This situation is not found in medium or soft cataracts, but it is a fact during the phacoemulsification of hard cataract with the 700 micron system. The solution for this is to withdraw the tip from the eye and clean it with a smaller diameter device (avoiding the withdrawing of the irrigation, in micro-biaxial surgery). If well, there is a solution for this situation, it is not the ideal fact, in particular in hard cataracts. So maybe because of this, author has found in 700 micron, the current limitation, when talking about size incision for cataract surgery. The limitation is at the aspirating system and not in the infusion system. Maybe in the future surgeons can overcome this technical and physical limitation; what do you think about it? One current solution is to perform irrigation through a 0.7 cannula (or chopper) and phacoemulsification through a phaco needle of 0.9; nevertheless the diameter of the aspirating system (the phaco needle) is wider in comparison to the diameter of the irrigation device, the surge can be avoided with the use of forced infusion, and so there is no risk of tamponade of the phaco tip, like it occurs in the 0.7 phaco tip in cases of hard cataracts.

The forced infusion has completely solved the trouble of surge; to demonstrate this, author and his colleagues have used even a 900 micron aspirating cannula and a 25 G irrigating cannula (viscoelastic cannula) at the same time for biaxial cortical aspiration or for cleansing the posterior capsule, and no surge is present, because of the act of the forced infusion. Remember that this is only feasible when surgeons have closed tight incisions and no leakage is present; otherwise surge will be the rule.[6] So author encouraged surgeons to work with forced infusion, either external or internal. It has become a kind of insurance for the surgeon, a safe tool for their skills and a nice improvement for their patient.

Preparation, Development and Use of Forced Infusion in Operating Room

Fluidics

As it has seen in the previous concepts, the diameter of the irrigating chopper (or cannula) and the bottle height will determine the amount of fluid going inside the eye (passive infusion). Macro irrigators allow enough fluid to perform an entire cataract procedure without the need of change the parameters that the learning surgeon is accustomed to use for coaxial procedures.

While decreasing the diameter of the irrigating cannulas and choppers, less fluid is outgoing through the line and so inside the eye; maybe this amount of fluid will be enough to fill the anterior chamber, but when aspiration starts, the fluid outgoing through the aspiration line will be more than the fluid incoming through the irrigation device, creating this way surge and instability of the anterior chamber.

The only way to maintain a stable anterior chamber is to increase the fluid incoming inside the eye; the fluid incoming must always be superior to the fluid outgoing; this is a golden rule. If the surgeon does not want to depend on external variables when he/she is transitioning to diameters less that 1 mm in biaxial cataract surgery, then forced infusion becomes an extraordinary tool that will allow the surgeon to keep with the "golden rule alive" to avoid surge and increase the anterior chamber stability; this allows the surgeon to trust in a reliable technique.

Surgeons want to move to smaller diameters, either coaxial or biaxial. When surgeons ask themselves about the reasons of this movement, they go through different responses until they find the right one:

The answer is not the IOL; there is not still an available IOL that can go inside a 700 mm incision

- The answer is not the astigmatism: studies have confirmed that there is not a statistical difference of the astigmatism induced by 1.1 mm incisions in comparison to 0.9 mm or even 0.7 mm
- The answer is not the status: the selfishness position of being doing something different to others
- The answer is in the fluidics: as less diameter of the irrigating instrumentation, less amount of fluid will be needed for the entire procedure. As less fluid is needed for a procedure, more benefit obtained for the corneal endothelial cells. As fewer traumas to the endothelial cells, better corneas will be seen at the next day, the visual recovery for the patient is faster and so the direct object of this utility is in the patients.[3,4]

Maybe it is a paradigm difficult to understand that while surgeons are increasing the irrigation force (with the use of forced infusion) they are able to perform a cataract surgery with less amount of intraocular solution. This is possible because of the less diameter of the irrigator and also because the closed environment at the anterior chamber allowed by microincisions and micro-instrumentation. This is the key of fluidics improvement in MICS, which increased with the use of forced infusion.[12]

It will be very nice, at less in theory, that surgeons can be somehow able to maintain a wide open anterior chamber with positive pressure that help them to perform an entire cataract surgery (it means to aspirate all the lens material) without the need to irrigate inside the eye; surgeons will obtain complete clear corneas the next day. Until this day it is impossible, but what is a complete reality is that surgeons are able to decrease, in a substantial way, the fluid incoming inside the eye. They can obtain this only by decreasing the irrigation diameter of the instrumentation, but they will be able to obtain the stability of the anterior chamber, while irrigating through ultra-small cannulas, through ultra-small incisions, with the friendly help of the forced infusion.

Many surgeons think that increasing the fluid in an active mode (forced infusion) the intraocular pressure will increase to dangerous levels and a lot of fluid will be spending. This is not true; when surgeons use forced infusion they are only creating the necessary amount of fluid to compensate the fluid outgoing through the aspiration line, but when no aspiration is acting, there is a complete balance of pressures between the air cushion inside the bottle, the column of BSS and the anterior chamber of the eye with no fluid incoming to the anterior chamber (even if the foot pedal is in position one) and no fluid outgoing (it means leakage) because of well constructed incisions. Currently, surgeons can work an entire cataract case with the 700 micron diameter instrumentation with only 40–50 cc of BSS.[6]

Definitions

Passive Infusion

It is the amount of fluid going inside the eye using only the gravity as the force that pushes it. It depends only of the altitude of the BSS bottle and is influenced by some environmental and surgical conditions. As the passive infusion depends only on the gravity force, the final amount of fluid incoming to the eye is influenced by many factors, some of them as minimal like the material containing the solution (glass, plastic, rigid, solid). The main factor to determine the amount of fluid coming to the eye in passive infusion is the bottle height, but because in MICS we are working with irrigation devices of smaller diameters than traditional phaco, there is a physical limitation to increase more and more the bottle level, to reach the desired positive pressure, like the extension in the elevation arm or the height of the operating room´s ceiling. Some other factors influencing the amount of fluid coming inside the eye are the quantity of fluid remaining inside the bottle, the diameter of the irrigation line and irrigation cannula, level above the sea where the surgeon is working (atmospheric pressure), density of the solution and the amount of vacuum utilized in different steps of the phacoemulsification procedure.

Active or Forced Infusion

It is the amount of fluid going inside the eye using and active pump that creates air cushion as the force that pushes the fluid. It depends on other influencing factors in less amount in comparison to either passive infusion, like atmospheric pressure, density of the fluid, diameter of the irrigation line and also the altitude of the bottle being the main influence that creates the irrigation the active created column of air inside the BSS bottle, decreasing so the importance of other influencing factors.

The Forced Infusion can be divided also in two different modes:

(a) **Internal Forced Infusion:** In this mode the column of air inside the bottle is created by an air pump incorporated in the same phaco machine that the surgeon is using to perform phacoemulsification (Figs 3 and 5).

(b) **External Forced Infusion:** In this mode the column of air inside the bottle is created by an air pump independent of the phaco machine that the surgeon is using to perform phacoemulsification. As was described by Amar Agarwal and Sunita Agarwal, even an air pump for a fish aquarium is enough to create this air cushion. With the time surgeons learned

to use air pumps with a regulator, it means they can push more or less air according to their needs, and the control is in their hands (like the air pumps of the phaco machines). It is very useful to have in particular when the surgeon has not a phaco machine with air pump. Please notice that if surgeons' phaco machine possesses a particular sensor to recognize the amount of fluid incoming, they can place it in a separate line (Fig. 2).

Creating Forced Infusion

The surgical equipments that contain an air pump are traditionally those with the capability to perform both anterior and posterior segment surgery. The air pump is included in these systems for the fluid interchange in vitreoretinal surgery. It is used to pressurize the eye in posterior segment surgery. This air pump is the main element to create internal forced infusion. If surgeon's equipment does not have an air pump, then he/she can incorporate an external air pump utilizing the same principles described here. The only phaco machine (non for vitreoretinal surgery) that has an air pump currently is Stellaris from Bausch & Lomb.

The control of the air pump system is in the panel or in the digital controls of the phaco system (Fig. 5), so the surgeon can turn on/off the pump and increase or decrease the amount of desired air as the surgery starts and is ongoing. If an external is in use, be aware to choose one air pump that includes a regulator, otherwise surgeons will have a fixed pressure and they will not be able to do the changes in the parameters, situation of particular importance for some steps of the surgery (Fig. 2).

The elements to create internal forced infusion are as follows (Fig. 1):

1. The air pump external or of the phaco system functioning.
2. The line to connect the air pump to the drip chamber of the irrigation administration set: This line is provided by each manufacturer; in the end that is connected to the air pump this line must have an air filter (to be sure the air is clean) and in the another end the adapter to the drip chamber. It is also possible to create this line if it is not available with the manufacturer, only is needed to adapt the air filter to one compatible with the air pump of each phaco system. If using an external air pump be sure to make compatible the air exit with any model of air filter; never inject air to your bottle without a filter because of possible contamination (Figs 1 to 4).
3. The bottle of intraocular solution (Fig. 4): To create always a standard positive pressure author's suggestion is to use always a 500 cc glass bottle; the height of the bottle now has minimal importance. Once the active column of air has reached the drip chamber, the air will go over the water inside the bottle through the metal needle, avoiding the creation of bubbles. The system will create the positive pressure needed within the bottle; this is the reason why a plastic bottle or a bag containing the intraocular solution are not a good option; if surgeons have a material with low compliance, like glass, they can be sure to obtain the desired pressure. The Anterior Vented Gas Forced Infusion (AVGFI) from Alcon contains this metal needle to reach the air cushion over the water level, which avoiding bubbles.
4. The irrigation administration set: It will connect the pressurized bottle to the irrigating chopper or cannula, but also is able to keep pressure inside, because it has to go through a roller clamp (in some systems outside and in others inside the cassette) that will be controlled by the foot switch; so when the roller clamp is closed the pressure is keeping inside but when it is open by the foot of the surgeon the predetermined pressure is liberated and the forced infusion reaches the eye (Fig. 6).
5. The control panel: It will be different in each surgical system but it is very easy to find if the surgeons know that it is the part of the system that controls the amount of air outgoing the internal air pump. If the surgeon is using an external air pump, then the "control panel" is the regulator of the air outgoing; be aware to calibrate

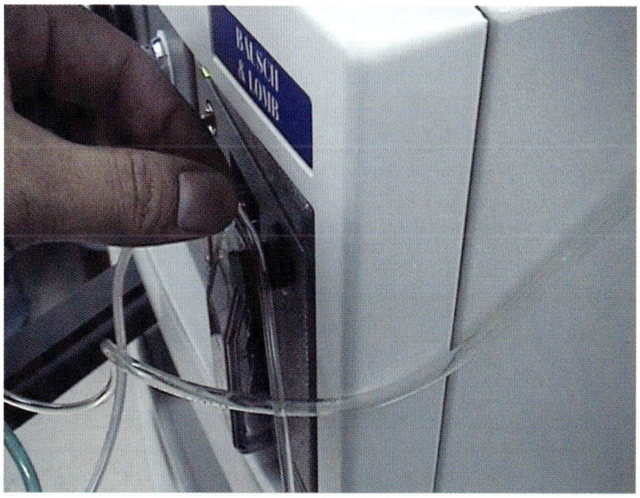

Fig. 6: External roller clamp in the Millennium Surgical System

it making a comparison at least one time with the control panel of a machine with an incorporated air pump, in order to avoid excessive pressure. Surgeons should perform their marks of levels of pressure in the external regulator; be sure that it is preset according to the instrumentation (Figs 1 & 5).

Anterior Vented Gas Forced Infusion Tubing System of the Accurus Surgical System and Pressurized Infusion Control of the Constellation Surgical System

The anterior vented gas forced infusion tubing of the Accurus and the pressurized infusion control of the Constellation Surgical Systems are air pumps with a regulator integrated inside the machine designed by the Alcon engineers to pressurize the infusion line for anterior and posterior segment surgery. The main application, until now, has been in vitreoretinal surgery for the interchange between air and fluid and control of transoperative intraocular pressure. They have not been too much used in anterior segment surgery, because the passive infusion has been enough to perform a coaxial and biaxial phacoemulsification. But now in coaxial microincision cataract surgery (COMICS) and biaxial microincision cataract surgery (BIMICS), for the users of these machines, these internal infusion systems have found a precise application. The pressurized infusion control on the new Constellation Surgical System is exactly the same air pump digitally controlled (AVGFI) of the Accurus machine. There are some small differences in programming between both machines, in particular in the pre-setting parameters (as has been widely accepted by Alcon itself), the physical and fluidic basis are the same. The main difference is because the distance of the patient´s eye to the cassette connectors and it is noticed much more in vitreoretinal surgery.

This air pump found in both systems contains all the elements described to create internal forced infusion for BIMICS and COMICS and the surgeon can have them directly from the manufacturer. These elements are the filtered line pre-connected to the drip chamber with a needle (to avoid bubbles) and the irrigation administration set that will be connected to the cassette. Both systems contain an internal clamp that is controlled by the surgeon through the foot switch or via panel (Fig 1).

The control of both systems is in the digital panel and once it is on the display will show 65 cm H_2O of positive pressure as a basal measure. Now the surgeon can increase or decrease the desired pressure as needed; also the surgeon can preset two different values of pressure at the foot switch and reach them easily anytime during the surgery by a simple movement of the foot. The display can also be in the scale of millimeters of mercury (mm Hg) if the surgeon wants to use this measure.

The adequate positive pressure for phakonit with outflow diameters between 0.7 mm and 0.9 mm is at the range from 80 cm H_2O to 140 cm H_2O; the variation will depend upon the diameter of the irrigation line and the kind of irrigating chopper in use, the behavior of the anterior chamber during the procedure (factors influencing like the incision size) and the above mentioned factors that can decrease or increase the outgoing fluid. Author starts with the preset in both machines with 110 cm H_2O of positive pressure, 20–30% of ultrasonic power and 180 mm Hg of vacuum for micro-tips (0.9 mm) and 120 mm Hg for high rate tips (like angled Kelman); from this point the surgeon can move up and down depending on the individual case; for irrigation/aspiration the forced infusion remains the same and the vacuum can be at 400 mm Hg.

Bottle Infusion Tool of the Millennium Microsurgical System

This system is also an air pump integrated in the posterior segment module of this surgical system. It was designed for the interchange air/fluid and the pressurization of the eye during vitreoretinal surgery. Not all Millennium machines contain this posterior segment surgery module, so the surgeon must be sure that it is integrated in the machine he or she is working with (Figs 6 to 9).

The surgeon will obtain from Bausch & Lomb only the air line ready to connect at the air filter by one side to the air pump module and by the other to the drip chamber; it is not pre-connected like the AVGFI system and also has not a needle to go inside the bottle, so the surgeon must have an independent irrigation administration set to make this system work. Also, do not forget to change to a compatible air filter. The line is connected to the drip chamber, the drip chamber of the irrigation administration set is connected to the bottle and this irrigation administration set must go through the roller clamp (this system uses an external clamp) and so now the surgeon can control the forced infusion with the foot switch. Finally the irrigating chopper or cannula is connected to the end of the irrigation line (Figs 6 to 9).

The bottle infusion tool control is in the panel of the Millennium system; the surgeon must press first "Tools"

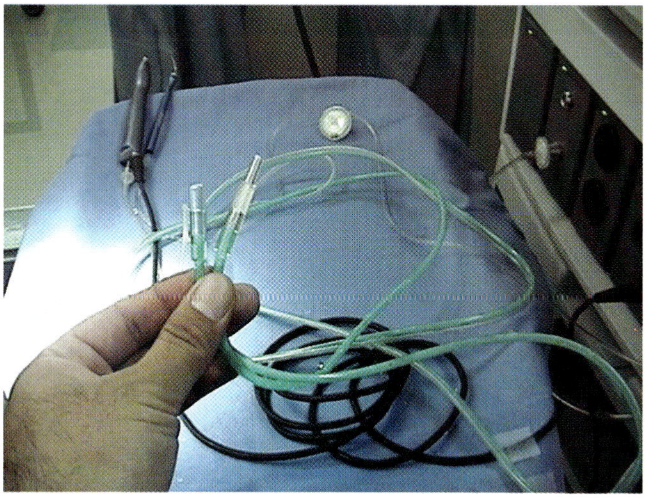

Fig. 7: Change at the green line provided by Millennium, to the anterior vented gas forced infusion (AVGFI) line provided by Alcon

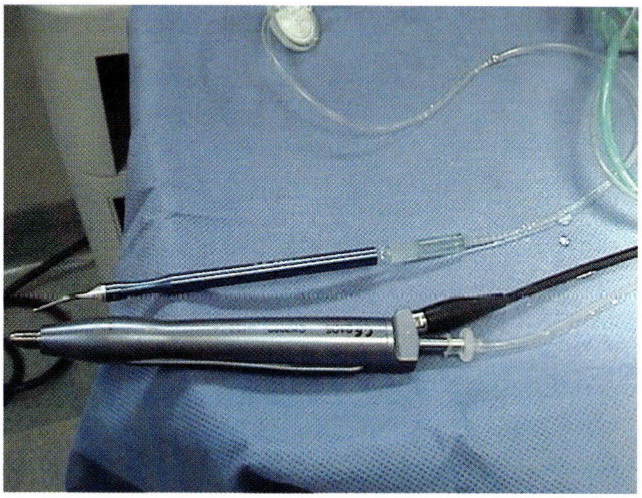

Fig. 9: Irrigating chopper connected to the line with active infusion

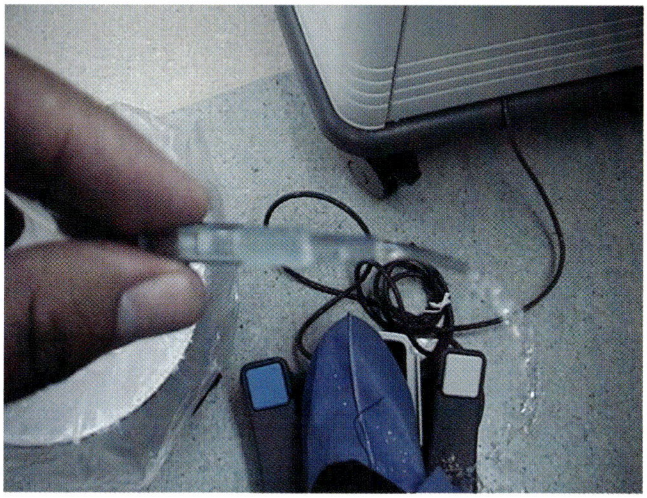

Fig. 8: Infusion control in the foot pedal after passing the line through the roller clamp

and then choose "Bottle Infusion"; when it is on, the air will start to flow through the air pump; the measure in this machine is display in mm Hg. Our settings in the Millennium are 80 mm Hg of positive pressure, 15–30% of phaco power and 130–150 mm Hg of vacuum.

During the surgery the surgeon can increase or decrease the forced infusion according to the case conditions and instrumentation used. In this system, the surgeon cannot program different positive pressures in the foot switch, like in the Accurus machine, so each change required during the surgery must be done in the panel.

Remember that in this system there is no rigid line to connect the drip chamber with the bottom of the bottle (needle), so bubbles within the solution are common. If the surgeon doesn't want bubbles, a sterile AVGFI system can be used and only the air filter must be changed because is not compatible with the exit of the Millennium´s air pump (Fig 4).

The Stellaris Surgical System

Since the Stellaris was introduced in 2007, those of us who perform phaco surgery have benefited from the optimized phaco power, separate control of ultrasound and vacuum, excellent control of fluidics, the dual linear foot pedal, and of course, the 1.8 mm microincision. With microincision cataract surgery (MICS), the system provides a self-sealing incision that results in fewer traumas to the eye during surgery and faster healing postoperatively. For sometime, Bausch & Lomb developed the vitreoretinal surgery component for the Stellaris, and the result was the Stellaris PC. The Stellaris PC is by itself an elegantly engineered system with multiple features to improve posterior segment surgeries, including but not limited to an ultra-high pneumatic vitreous cutter, advanced illumination, and an easy-to-use interface.

Nevertheless the pressurized infusion system is available in the "only cataract" Stellaris Surgical System.

This function can be found in the panel as "pressurized infusion option" and can be managed in the Stellaris exactly with the same lectures and features that the previous released (and described here) Millenium Surgical System. The pack delivered by the company is called the Pressurized Infusion Pack and contains the connection port, the filter

and the BSS bottle spike. The purpose of this pressurized infusion system, as the company describes, is to provide an appropriate pressure to the accessory bottle, with the objective to obtain the desired infusion rate according to the needs of the particular case. This system is activated by the surgeon. It is the first time ever a pressurized system is incorporated into a phacoemulsification machine that has no functions of posterior segment surgery. The fluidics is managed by a double-pump system, which is interchangeable during surgery, through EQ fluidics technology. EQ stands for 'equalizing', which means that infusion and aspiration work in mutual equilibrium. This equilibrium can be obtained either with passive or forced infusion; the system is able to work with both. The forced infusion is pre-programmed by the surgeon with the same features described in the Millennium Surgical System.

External Forced Infusion and Internal Forced Infusion with Other Machines

All the phaco machines capable to perform phacoemusification and posterior vitrectomy are good to develop internal forced infusion for MICS. The surgeon must follow these steps:[13-15]

1. Find the air pump in the phaco system or use one external with the regulator calibrated in mm Hg or cm H_2O.
2. Find the tool to control the air pump at the panel (on/off and increase or decrease the fluid). If an external is in use this is the regulator.
3. Connect a line with an air filter to the air pump and the extreme to the drip chamber to the irrigation administration set (with or without needle).
4. Connect the irrigation administration set to the 500 cc. glass bottle and pass the line through the internal (in the cassette) or external clamp of the phaco machine managed with the foot switch.
5. Start with a positive pressure between 70 mm Hg and 90 mm Hg, or 100 cm H_2O and 120 cm H_2O (according to the machine measures) and increase or decrease depending on the case.
6. If the surgeon doesn't want to have bubbles in the bottle an AVGFI system can be used; just look for a compatible air filter and switch it if needed.

The air incoming inside the bottle actively pushes the fluid into the eye at the desired pressure. As the irrigation fluid is consuming, the air cushion inside the bottle is increasing and the compliance inside the system is also increasing, so a good recommendation for the surgeon is to remember to change to a new bottle when approximately 150 cc of solution is remaining inside it. This precaution has two reasons:

- As the air column grows the capacity of response of the system becomes slow.
- It avoids creating forced infusion of "air" inside the eye when the bottle gets empty.

Conclusions

The advantages of the air pump system for MICS are:

- It actively pushes fluid into the eye so the system is independent of gravity forces and/or bottle height
- The amount of fluid controlled with the air force of the air pump
- The amount of fluid that reaches the eye can have varieties depending upon the irrigating chopper's flow-rate the surgeon is using, so it can be regulated
- The increase of fluid avoids surge and its surgical consequences
- The continuous maintenance of the anterior chamber allows the surgeon to freely manipulate the instruments and tissues inside the eye, making easy the surgery
- The positive pressure creates a tense zonnula and so a firm capsular bag facilitating the chop maneuvers
- The endothelium is pushed forward while the posterior capsule is pushed back, protecting both structures
- The continuous irrigation outgoing through the phaco tip incision cools continuously the tip and the cornea, decreasing the thermal burns

In the case of the internal forced infusion the surgeon uses the air pump contained in the same phaco machine he/she is using.

The advantages of the internal forced infusion over the external are:

- The surgeon doesn't have to incorporate an external air pump to the surgical system to obtain the advantages of the forced infusion. The creation of the irrigation force is inside the same machine
- The surgeon can control all the parameters (forced infusion rate, ultrasonic power modulations and vacuum settings) in the panel of the same surgical system
- The forced infusion rate can be actively and digitally controlled during the surgery, adjusting so the parameters to the conditions and/or the surgical steps of the surgery
- The surgeon increases the confidence to the surgical system he or she is working with.

The disadvantage of the internal forced infusion is that not all the phaco machines have an air pump inside.

References

1. Chang, David. High Vacuum Bimanual Phaco attainable with STAAR Cruise Control. Ocular Surgery News. 2003.
2. Prakash DP. Cutting phaco sleeve permits ultra-small incision surgery. Ocular Surgery News. 2003.
3. Agarwal A, et al. Bimanual Phaco. Mastering the Phakonit/MICS Technique. New Jersey: Slack Inc.; 2004.
4. Agarwal A. Microphakonit Surgery performed with 0.7-mm Tip. Ocular Surgery News. Europe/Asia Pacific edition. 2005.
5. Vejarano LF, Tello A, Vejarano A. Phakonit Incisions and use of a pressurized inflow system. J Cataract Refract Surg. 2004;30(5):939.
6. Pére-Arteaga A. Step by Step to Biaxial Lens Surgery. New Delhi: Jaypee Brothers Medical Publishers; 2008.
7. Agarwal A, Agarwal A, et al. Phakonit phacoemulsification through a 0.9 mm corneal incision. J Cataract Refract. Surg. 2001;27:1548-52.
8. Agarwal A, Agarwal A, et al. Phakonit: Lens removal through a 0.9 mm incision. J Cataract Refract Surg. 2001;27:1531-2.
9. Agarwal A, Agarwal S, Agarwal A. Phakonit and laser phakonit: lens removal through a 0.9-mm incision. Phacoemulsification, Laser Cataract Surgery and Foldable IOLs. New Delhi: Jaypee Brothers Medical Publishers; 2000. pp. 204-16.
10. Tsuneoka H, Shiba T. Feasibility of ultrasound cataract surgery through a 1.4 mm incision. J Cataract Refract Surg. 2001,27:934-40.
11. Agarwal A. Bimanual 0.9 mm approach to phaco promises astigmatic neutral cataract surgery and faster rehabilitation. Eurotimes. 2003.
12. Alió, Jorge. MICS ready to go. Ocular Surgery News. 2003.
13. Pérez-Arteaga A. Accurus Forced Infusión good for MICS. Ocular Surgery News. 2003.
14. Pérez-Arteaga A. Bottle Infusión tool of the Millennium Surgical System for Phakonit. Ocular Surgery News. 2003.
15. Pérez-Arteaga A. Anterior vented gas forced infusion of the Accurus surgical system for phakonit. J Cataract Refract Surg. 2004;30(4):933-5.

3

Coaxial Microincision Phacoemulsification of Cataracts

Fernando Aguilera-Zarate (Mexico)

As cataract surgery has evolved, great advances in techniques and instrumentation have been developed. One of these improvements is the reduction of size of cataract incision to less than 2 mm (microincision).[1-6]

Advantages of C-MICS (1.6 mm) Surgery

Why should surgeons go further decreasing the size of the phaco incision to less than 2.0 mm? Are there really advantages of this approach? Is it worthwhile the effort to learn new surgical techniques and spend in new instrumentation?

Coaxial Microincision Cataract Surgery (C-MICS) is different from biaxial microincision cataract surgery (B-MICS); in that the irrigation inflow is coaxial with the ultrasound needle, so the learning curve of C-MICS is shorter, and it translates in no need to develop somewhat difficult new surgical skills, and no special instrumentation is needed. The reason why coaxial microincisional phacoemulsification was prone for complications was the lack of proper instrumentation that gave solution to the problems when performing coaxial phaco through a sub 2 mm incision.[4-7]

There are few misconceptions with C-MICS because of the reduction of the incision size.[5,6,11]

The Emulsification Power in Microincision is Reduced

This is false. The delivered ultrasound power depends basically on the diameter of the tip of the phaco needle. The larger the surface of contact with the cataract material, the more emulsification effect surgeon gets. New specially designed phaco tips for 1.6 mm incisions with broader tip surfaces and more bevel angle (53 degrees) give more emulsification power than standard 2.8 incision phaco needles with 30 degree bevel (146% vs. 100%) (Fig. 1).

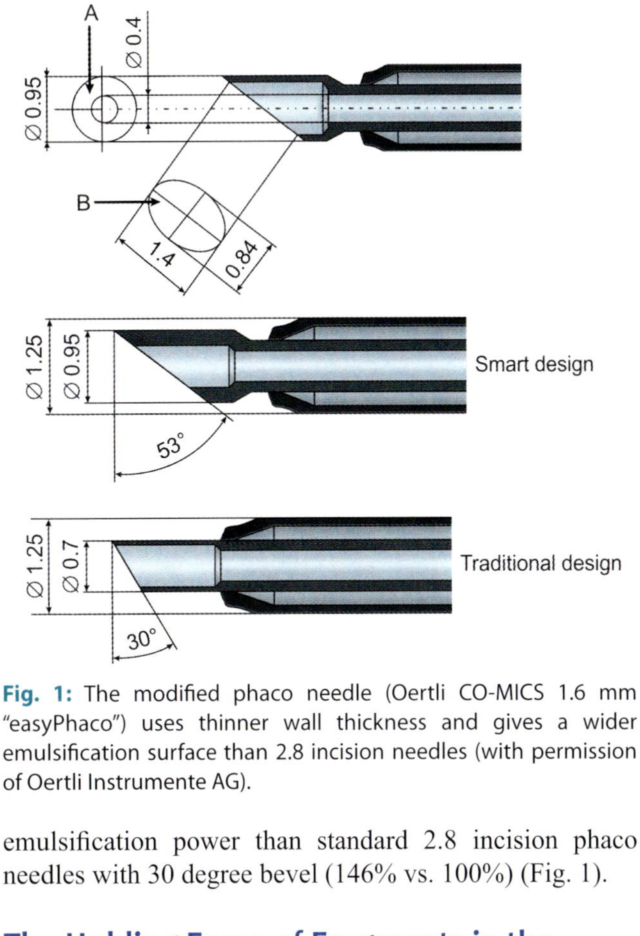

Fig. 1: The modified phaco needle (Oertli CO-MICS 1.6 mm "easyPhaco") uses thinner wall thickness and gives a wider emulsification surface than 2.8 incision needles (with permission of Oertli Instrumente AG).

The Holding Force of Fragments in the C-MICS Tip is Lower

This is false. The holding force calculus is easily determined, and depends on the contact area with the material to be held. With special designs of tips the holding force is similar or better than that of a 2.8 mm phaco tip (106% vs. 100%) (Fig. 2).

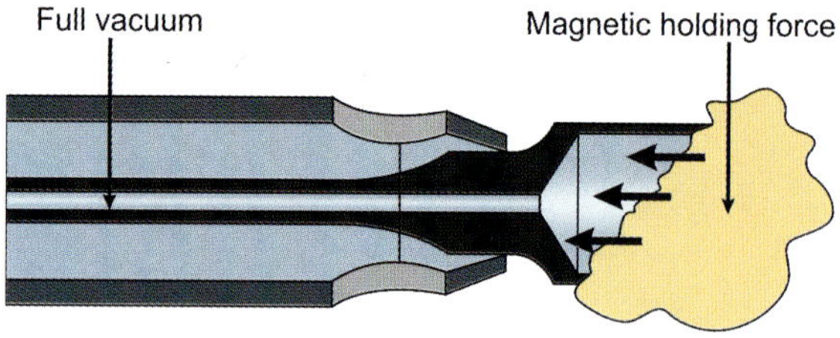

Fig. 2: The broader surface of contact of the tip along with fluidics augments the holding force.

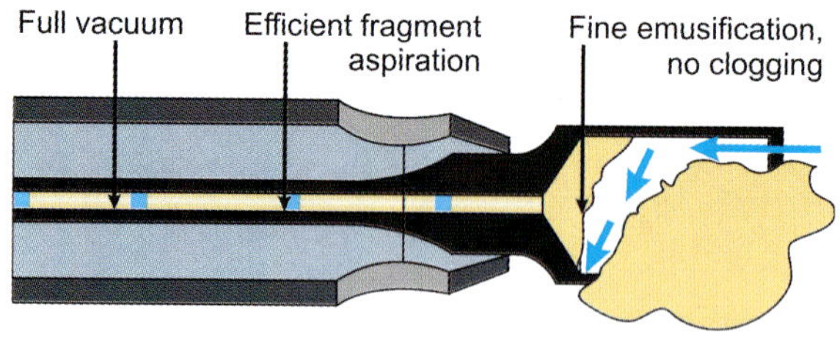

Fig. 3: Fine fragments are efficiently aspirated through the capillary inner tunnel of the phaco tip.

The Aspiration Power of a Microincision Tip is Low

This depends basically on the relation of size between the tip surface and the inner diameter of the aspiration needle and the vacuum settings. In the C-MICS the vacuum has to be set higher in order to have this effect (100–150 mm Hg above the normal vacuum settings, the surgeon is used to larger incision coaxial phaco technique) (Fig. 3).

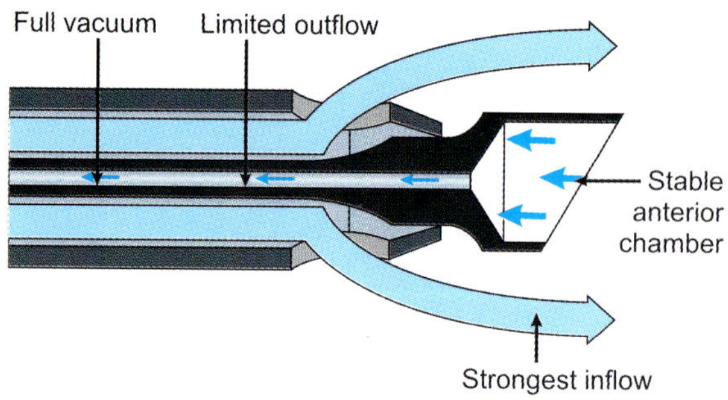

Fig. 4: No surge is produced at the tip of the Co-MICS needle because of fluidic pressure difference in the tip and inner tunnel is fully compensated by the needle design and the fluidic of the machine.

In C-MICS, Anterior Chamber Stability is Worse than with Wider Phaco Needles

Once again this depends in the design of the needle, the relationship with its diameter, surface of contact, the inflow higher than the outflow and the phaco machine. But it is basically a matter of proper fluidics management including that the inflow through the phaco sleeve does not flow to the tip of the needle (Fig. 4).

Fluidics and Regulation of Emulsification Energy

So all the misconceptions about microincision cataract surgery are wrong in particular regarding the coaxial technique especially since the modification of the phaco needles (CO-MICS 1.6 mm easyPhaco tip—Oertli Instrumente AG, Switzerland) and the Stellaris Microincision 1.8 mm tip (Baush & Lomb USA). Phaco systems, that allow better fluidics (Oertli Instrumente AG—Faros; CataRhex, OS3), allow safer coaxial or bimanual microincision surgery. Other machines that rely in sophisticated microprocessors, special tubing and softwares are also suitable for C-MICS (Bausch & Lomb—Stellaris; Millennium and Alcon Infiniti—Nanosleeve Microphaco needle), nonetheless the smaller surgeons can go is 1.8 mm incision size phaco. At this time the smaller C-MICS incision is 1.4–1.6 mm with the Oertli Faros Machine. It can be used with reusable or disposable tubing. There is no special software or hardware to add and the only thing to must modify is the increase in vacuum level 150 mm Hg above the normal values that surgeons use for large incision phaco.[10,12,15]

Regarding the optimization of ultrasound power, it works in four ways to disassemble the tissue in every phaco system.[5-7]

1. *Mechanic impact*: The mechanical force induced by the needle (Jackhammer effect) that cuts the tissue when knocking.
2. *Acoustic wave*: The propulsed water at +/- 1500 m/s depending of the phaco handpiece´s kHz features.
3. *Hydrowave*: The "liquid" force produced by the mechanic impact that tends to tissue displacement one over another.
4. *Cavitation*: The forming of bubbles because of cycles of implosion and expansion caused by the vibration of the phaco needle.

The newest research studies suggest that the Jackhammer effect initiates the tissue destruction by cutting it in big pieces that are the emulsified by the cavitation and hydrowaves effects. Authors should mention about the use of torsional phaco for no sleeve MICS since the cavitation process is present at the body of the phaco needle,[8-9] which causes inflammation and corneal edema and produces less self-

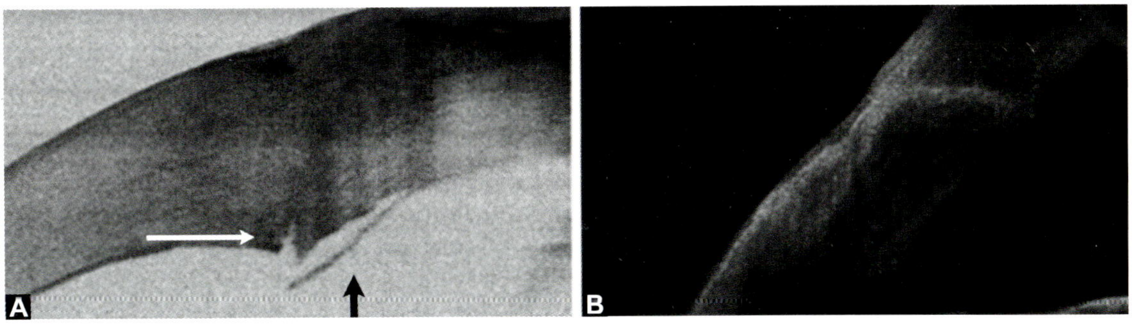

Figs 5A and B: (A) Inner lip incision open (fish mouth—green arrow/descemetocele—rose arrowhead) after torsional B-MICS. (B) Perfect wound apposition after C-MICS 1.6 mm

sealing incisions because of direct effect of the cavitation process against the corneal tissue (Figs 5A and B).

From authors' point of view, there are three main advantages of C-MICS compared to B-MICS:[6,7,12-14]

1. The incision is sealed by the silicone sleeve so less problems of oarlock in small incisions and no fluid loss around the instruments are faced in large incisions (Figs 6A and B).
2. The technique is similar to the standard larger phaco technique that the surgeon is currently using, so the learning curve is shorter.
3. No forced infusion is needed with outstanding chamber stability.

In conclusion, the C-MICS technique through 1.6 mm incision using specially designed phaco needles with peristaltic or venturi pumps allow us to obtain excellent surgical results with clearer corneas, less endothelial cell loss, less asymmetric induced astigmatism, more percentage of self-sealed incisions and probably less chances of postoperative infection complications.

References

1. Ernest PH, Lavery KT, Kiessling LA. Relative strength of scleral corneal and clear corneal incisions constructed in cadaver eyes. J Cataract Refract Surg. 1994;20:626-9.
2. Menapace R. Update on wound construction: indications, techniques, deformation resistance and corneal curvature changes. In: Vörösmarthy, et al. (Eds). 10. Kongress der DGII; Budapest. New York: Springer; 1996. pp. S27-40.
3. Rainer G, Menapace R, Vass C, et al. Surgically induced astigmatism following a 4.0 mm sclerocorneal valve incision. J Cataract Refract Surg. 1997;23:358-64.
4. Vass C, Menapace R. Computerized statistical analysis of corneal topography for the evaluation of changes in corneal shape after surgery. Am J Ophthalmol. 1994:118:177-84.
5. Rainer G, Menapace R, Vass C, et al. Corneal shape changes after temporal and superolateral 3.0 mm clear corneal incisions. J Cataract Refract Surg. 1999;25:1121-6.
6. Hayashi K, Yoshida M, Hayashi H. Postoperative corneal shape changes: microincision versus small-incision coaxial cataract surgery. J Cataract Refract Surg. 2009;35:233-9.
7. Radner W, Menapace R, Zehetmayer M, et al. Ultrastructure of clear corneal incisions. Part II: corneal trauma after lens implantation with the microstar injector system. J Cataract Refract Surg. 1998;24:493-7.

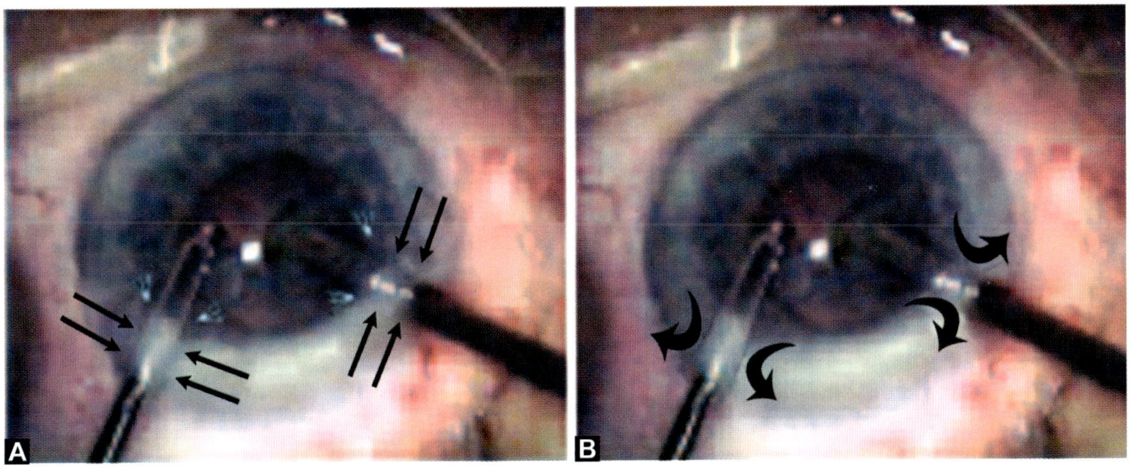

Figs 6A and B: (A) Tight wound with oarlock effect, and (B) large wound with loss of balanced salt solution around the instruments

8. Menapace R. Prevention of PCO. In: Kohnen T, Koch DD (Eds). Cataract and Refractive Surgery, Essentials in Ophthalmology. Berlin-Heidelberg New York: Springer. 2004. pp. 101-22.
9. Menapace R. Posterior capsulorhexis combined with optic buttonholing: an alternative to standard in-the-bag implantation of sharp-edged intraocular lenses? A critical analysis of 1000 consecutive cases. Graefes Arch Clin Exp Ophthalmol. 2008;246:787-801.
10. Vock L, Menapace R, Stifter E, et al. Posterior capsule opacification and neodymium: YAG laser capsulotomy rates with a round-edged silicone and a sharp-edged hydrophobic acrylic intraocular lens 10 years after surgery. J Cataract Refract Surg. 2009;35: 459-65.
11. Menapace R, Di Nardo S. How to better use fluidics with MICS. In: Aliò J, Fine H (Eds). Minimizing incisions and maximizing outcomes in cataract surgery. New York: Springer; 2009.
12. Berdahl JP, DeStafeno JJ, Kim T. Corneal wound architecture and integrity after phacoemulsification of coaxial, microincision coaxial, and microincision bimanual techniques. J Cataract Refract Surg. 2007;33:510-5.
13. Johar SR, Vasavada AR, Praveen MR, et al. Histomorphological and immunofluorescence evaluation of bimanual and coaxial phaco incisions in rabbits. J Cataract Refract Surg. 2008;34:670-6.
14. Werner L, Tetz M, Feldmann I, et al. Evaluating and defining the sharpness of intraocular lenses: microedge structure of commercially available square-edged hydrophilic intraocular lenses. J Cataract Refract Surg. 2009; 35:556-66.
15. Werner L, Müller M, Tetz M. Evaluating and defining the sharpness of intraocular lenses: micro-edge structure of commercially available square-edged hydrophobic lenses. J Cataract Refract Surg. 2008;34:310-7.

4

A Low Fluidics Strategy for Micro-Coaxial Torsional Phaco for Dense Cataracts

Khiun F Tjia (The Netherlands)

The nonrepulsive sideways shaving action of a phaco tip driven by torsional ultrasound technology, has dramatically changed the development of microincision cataract surgery and greatly accelerated the adoption of smaller incision phaco since 2005, when torsional ultrasound technology was first described.[1-3]

Torsional Versus Longitudinal Ultrasound

Thermal injury and/or corneal decompensation are much more common after phacoemulsification of dense lenses. Dense lenses also lengthen the surgical time needed to remove the lens material. Fluid usage increases with these cases since the longitudinal phaco procedures require higher fluidics settings to offset the resulting repulsion and loss of followability of the higher stroke length required with dense lens material. Dense nuclei require much greater longitudinal and torsional ultrasound power, i.e. stroke length for the emulsification process than do softer nuclei. However, the side to side shearing action of torsional ultrasound has proven to be more efficient and effective at emulsifying lens material. This increased efficiency and reduced repulsion have shown that higher fluidics parameters are not necessary to offset higher energy levels needed with dense lenses. The increase of the side motion of the phaco tip has not demonstrated a decreased followability or attractability of lens material with torsional ultrasound. In a previous study[4] of fluid volume required to remove the nucleus, longitudinal phaco was found to require 50% more balanced salt solution than torsional phaco. Consistent with this demonstration of efficiency with torsional ultrasound, a recent study[5] found a reduction in corneal endothelial cell loss with this technology.

Torsional Ultrasound and Microincision Cataract Surgery

The fluidics settings adaptation for micro-coaxial torsional phacoemulsification need to be addressed: a reduction of incision size implicates a reduced sleeve size and results in proportional decreased irrigation flow capacity. This requires a reduction in aspiration flow, which should directly correlate to the reduction in irrigation flow.

With torsional ultrasound, the efficiency of emulsification is still extremely efficient at low aspiration flow rates. The virtual lack of repulsion is responsible for the fact that routine phacoemulsification through microincisions is possible at very modest fluidics settings. Dissipated energy, fluid use, and procedure time are comparable between regular coaxial and 2.2 mm micro-coaxial phacoemulsification surgery.[6]

In the evolution towards even smaller incision micro-coaxial phaco surgery, studies of 1.8 mm incision phaco have already been described as very effective.[7,8]Smaller shaft phaco tips (700–800 μ) are desirable to guarantee sufficient irrigation flow.

Fluidics Settings with Torsional Ultrasound in Very Dense Cataract Cases

Cataract surgery has become safer and much more efficient with the advent of torsional phacoemulsification. However, this technology is even more valuable when applied to very dense nuclei and other complex surgical situations.

Phacoemulsification of a dense lens always presents a larger challenge to surgeons. Dense nucleus removal with the use of longitudinal ultrasound requires a higher amplitude of the vibrating metallic tip ("jackhammer effect") to emulsify and remove dense lens material. High fluidics settings are required to compensate for repulsion of longitudinal ultrasound. This results in increased turbulence and fluid use, and a higher incidence of corneal endothelial cell loss.

However, the side-to-side shearing action of torsional ultrasound has proven to be more efficient and very effective at emulsifying lens materially at moderate vacuum settings[9] and very low-flow aspiration flow settings.[10]In the longitudinal era, high vacuum settings were widely used to keep nuclear material close to the phaco tip in order to increase ultrasound efficiency and decrease the required ultrasonic energy.

Even today, when using torsional ultrasound, higher vacuum settings can draw softer lens material through the phaco tip and aspiration tubing without using significant ultrasonic energy levels. Dense lens material, however, needs to be completely emulsified prior to aspiration. Vacuum alone will not lead to any dense lens removal. The key to the superior efficiency, torsional ultrasound is the absence of any intrinsic repulsive effect of the side-to-side shaving motion of the phaco tip. Moderate vacuum is still largely sufficient to keep nuclear material at the phaco tip. After emulsification of whatever density of nuclear material, the milky substance of the emulsified lens matter poses very little resistance to aspiration, and therefore eliminates the need for high vacuum settings.

A very low aspiration flow (e.g. 15 mL/min; Fig. 1) will not aspirate a dispersive viscoelastic substance that protects the corneal endothelium.

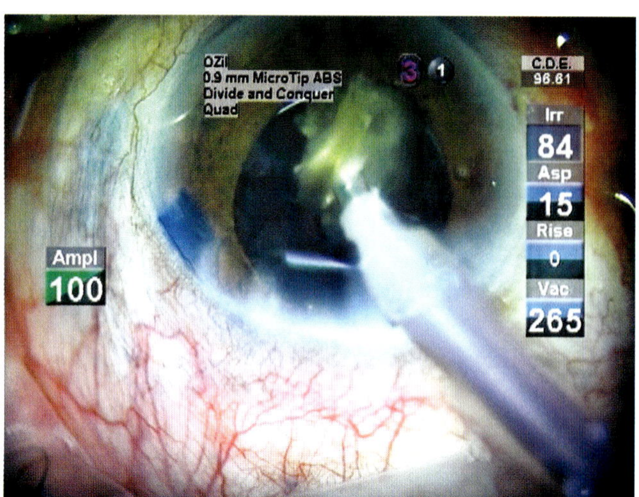

Fig. 1: 5+ nucleus with moderate vacuum setting of 300 mm Hg and 15 mL/min aspiration flow

The combination of a dispersive viscoelastic and very low-flow torsional phacoemulsification is my preferred strategy for very dense cataract surgery.[11]

Dispersive Viscoelastic Protection

Dispersive viscoelastic substances (e.g. Viscoat®, Alcon Laboratories, Inc.) are widely used to protect the corneal endothelium from the destructive effects of ultrasonic energy, fluid turbulence and/or direct impact of nuclear fragments.

The key of a low fluidics torsional phaco strategy is to leave the dispersive viscoelastic layer intact. A low aspiration flow setting is therefore mandatory to protect the fragile corneal endothelial cells.

Tip Choice for Torsional Ultrasound and Dense Nuclei

For very dense nuclei, 45 degree bevel tips[12] are more efficient compared to 30 degree bevel tips.

The 45 degree tips have a larger surface and make the nuclear pieces tumble around their axis whilst being emulsified. 30 degree tips drill more easily into the nucleus (lollipop) and emulsification halts when the sleeve obstructs further movement.

Our experience with traditional longitudinal ultrasound and very dense nuclei is that flared tip designs were prone to potential clogging of the tip. Clogging of a tip could lead to insufficient cooling of the tip and possible heating/burn of the corneal tunnel.

Because of the sideways ultrasonic movement of a tip with torsional ultrasound, the nucleus is emulsified in a different manner. The nuclear material at the tip and inside of a flared phaco tip is probably less emulsified compared to longitudinal ultrasound. There is also no significant repulsion and subsequent repositioning of the nucleus relative to the tip.

This could be an explanation for the higher incidence of clogging of flared tip designs with torsional ultrasound.

Flared Tip Design and Prolonged Occlusion

The oscillatory movement of the torsional tip is highly effective in shaving lens material. However, when a flared tip design is used, the mechanism does not cause aspirated material to be "jackhammered" into and through the tip as it is with traditional phacoemulsification. Therefore, it is important for the material to be broken up into relatively small pieces that can pass through the inner lumen of the tip without obstructing it. If torsional vibration is interrupted or larger fragments of dense lens material enter the lumen, tip obstruction may result.

These periods of prolonged tip occlusion halt the shaving process and decrease the tip efficiency.

The advantage of a bigger port opening is an increased holding surface and therefore holding power of the phacotip. With flared tips, the larger port opening narrows into a smaller size lumen shaft, which reduces the occlusion break surge. This type of flared phacotips were particularly advantageous when using longitudinal ultrasound technology, when high vacuum and aspiration flow settings were necessary to overcome the repelling effect of the longitudinal movement of the phacotip. With torsional ultrasound lower fluidics settings are more effective and safer.

A New Non Flared Tip Design for Micro-coaxial Phaco: 0.9 MiniTip

Especially for denser nuclei, flared tips repeatedly show brief periods of prolonged occlusion. This can sometimes even necessitate retraction of the Phaco handpiece to liberate the phacotip from nuclear material.

A new small non-flared tip has recently been introduced with an identical shaft lumen size as the MiniFlared tip of 570 microns. The outside diameter is even slightly smaller than MiniFlared tip, 800 versus 830 microns.

The slightly thinner wall is probably responsible for the lightly increased cutting edge tip displacement. During clinical evaluation, the 0.9 MiniTip performed very well, not showing any significant prolonged occlusion, enhancing the overall cutting efficiency, specifically for denser nuclei.

A comparison of the performance of several tip designs is shown in Table 1.

A comparison of dimensions is shown in Figure 2.

TABLE 1

Stroke	*Tapered Kelman*	*Mini-Flared OZil 12*	*Mini-Flared Kelman*	*0.9 Mini Tip Kelman*
At cutting edge	90 µm*	100 µm*	130 µm*	135 µm*

* Rounded to the nearest 10 µm.

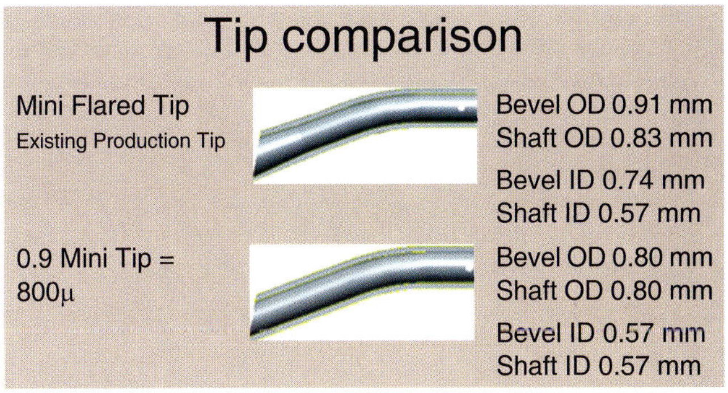

Fig. 2: Comparison of dimensions

Personal Settings Recommendations (Micro-tip/Tapered Tip and Ultrasleeve)

2.2–2.4 mm Incision for Very Dense Nuclei/Corneal Endothelium Dystrophy

Chop—for impaling and chopping the nucleus only

- Bottle height: 75–90 cm
- Aspiration flow: 20 mL/min fixed
- Vacuum: 450 mm Hg fixed
- Power: Burst mode, 20 ms, 50% fixed longitudinal ultrasound

Quadrant Removal—for emulsification of the nuclear pieces

- Bottle height: 75–90 cm
- Aspiration flow: 15 mL/min linear
- Vacuum: 300 mm Hg fixed
- Power: Continuous mode, minimum 50% linear to maximum 100% amplitude torsional ultrasound

References

1. Tjia K. Torsional lens removal technology. Presented at: XXIII Congress of the ESCRS. September, 2005; Lisbon, Portugal.
2. Tjia K. Total cataract removal procedure through a 2.0-2.2 mm incision using new torsional lens removal technology and new smaller sleeves. Presented at: XXIII Congress of the ESCRS. September, 2005; Lisbon, Portugal.
3. Tjia K. Trends in phacoemulsification. Ophthalmology Times Europe. 2005;1(1):32-4.
4. Tjia K. Efficiency of torsional versus longitudinal ultrasound. Cataract Refract Surg Today Europe. 2008;3(4):33-4.
5. Liu Y, Zeng M, Liu X, et al. Torsional mode versus conventional ultrasound mode phacoemulsification: randomized comparative clinical study. J Cataract Refract Surg. 2007;33(2):287-92.
6. Tjia K. Fluid use and ultrasound energy comparison between coaxial and micro-coaxial torsional ultrasound. Poster presented at: XXVI Congress of the ESCRS. September, 2008; Berlin, Germany.

7. Packard R. Microcoaxial phaco with 1.8 mm incisions using 2 phaco machines and IOL systems. Presented at: XXVI Congress of the ESCRS. September, 2008; Berlin, Germany.
8. Tjia K. Comparison between 1.8 and 2.2 mm microcoaxial torsional phaco. Presented at: XXVII Congress of the ESCRS; September, 2009; Barcelona, Spain.
9. Johansson C. Optimizing vacuum settings in torsional ultrasound phacoemulsification. Cataract Refract Surg Today Europe. 2008;3(4):24-7.
10. Tjia K. A low fluidics parameters strategy. Cataract Refract Surg Today Europe. 2007;2(2):52-3.
11. Tjia K. Iatrogenic zonular disaster. Cataract Refract Surg Today Europe. 2010;5(3):51-2,62.
12. Allen D. Comparison of efficiency of 30° and 45° Mini-Flared Kelman tips during torsional phacoemulsification. Presented at: XXV Congress of the ESCRS; September, 2007; Stockholm, Sweden.

5 Prechopping in Micro-coaxial Phaco

Alejandro Cruz-Hernández (Mexico)

Introduction

Cataract Surgery

An authentic search of excellence in which the main objective is to replace the cataractous lenses with an intraocular lens, implanted to correct the vision problems.

Other secondary objectives are to perform an ocular surgery with a minimum invasion, easy recovery and null or minimum complications, to obtain a clear vision, recover focus and, if it is possible, improve the far and near sight.

Today the above mentioned can be obtained. Thanks to technological advancements, the experience in optical surgical procedures, as well as the approximation on more precise intraocular lenses.[1]

Lens Hardness

The capsule molds the crystalline material which is a viscous, elastic, and flexible structure and allows the accommodation. The lens changes its hardness at least four times during its lifetime, leading to an increment of its viscosity and loss of elasticity. This process is known as nuclear sclerosis, an age-related change in the density of the lens nucleus which makes the accommodation impossible.

Today surgeons have the Lens Opacities Classification System III (LOCSIII), a system used for grading the lens hardness to decide the best surgical procedure to be practiced in a patient. Although, because of authors' experience they can assert that in practice this classification system couldn't provide this kind of information as the only way to certainly know the hardness of a material, in this special case the lens, is by touching it during the surgical procedure, with the advantage of using a manual device, reducing the use of ultrasonic waves.

Table 1 Classification of lens hardness according to Moh´s scale

Material	Hardness	Material that Could Damage It
10. Diamond	Very hard	Diamond
9. Corundum		
8. Topaz		
7. Quartz	Very hard to hard	Steel
6. Orthoclase		Titanium
5. Apatite	Hard to relatively hard	
4. Fluorite		
3. Calcite	Relatively hard to soft	Copper
2. Plaster	Soft to very soft	Fingernail
1. Talc	Very soft	

Source: http://www.allaboutgemstones.com/mohs_hardness_scale

There are different ratings to grade the hardness of materials that can be extrapolated in order to determine the best surgical procedure to be used.

Authors

We are taking into consideration the Mohs´s scale, which is an ordinal scale that characterizes the scratch resistance of various minerals through the ability of a harder material to scratch a softer. This scale is graded form 1 to 10, 10 being the hardest material (Table 1)

Steps to evaluate the hardness of lenses:

1. Touch the lens: Identify if it is harder or softer than the surgical material (the surgical material is generally made of steel or titanium).
2. Penetrate the lens: In its center or in line (it depends on how deep the surgical material can get).
3. Fracture: Apply lateral force to see how the central nuclei are separate from the lens.

Diagram of a Multiple Fracture

For an easiest comprehension-authors consider the lens as a circle, taking into account the following information:

1. The first fracture (FxA) is performed in the first half of the circle (if we consider this circle as a clock, the fracture must be performed from 6 o'clock to 12 o'clock) getting two semicircles, if it is possible two symmetric semicircles (Fig. 1A).
2. Next, another fracture is performed (FxB) aside to FxA, approximately at 2 mm from the right semicircle, repeating this same process in the left semicircle (FxC) getting four segments (Fig. 1B).
3. Following, the segments are to be rotated 90º jointly. Finally another fracture is performed at the center and vertical to the central segments (FxD) getting six segments (Fig. 1C).

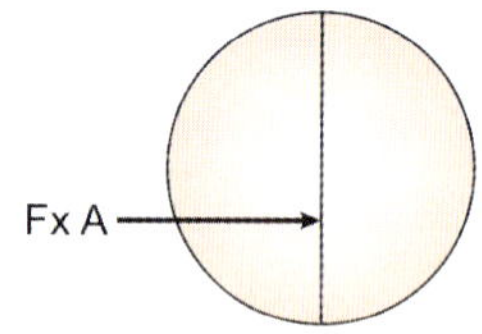

Fig. 1A: First fracture direction

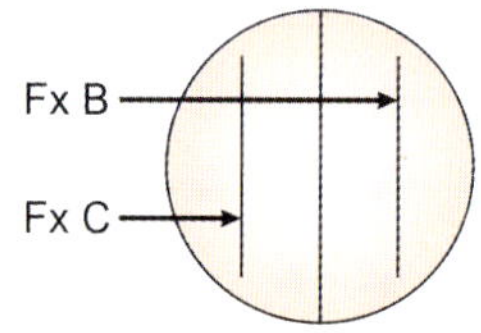

Fig. 1B: Second step includes two fractures

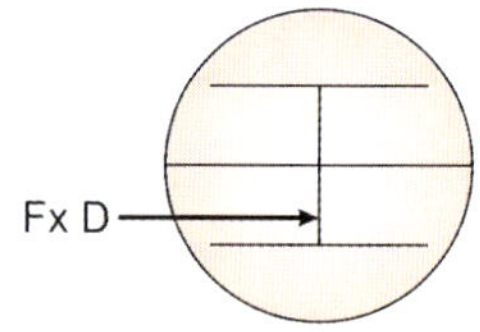

Fig. 1C: Third fracture at 90º

Surgical Procedure: Multiple Phacofracture[2]

Perform asepsis and antisepsis with iodine povidone 10% (periorbital) and 5% (superior conjunctival fornix). Minimal sedation and topical anesthesia (alcaine or tetracaine), surveillance with the anesthesiologist.

Technical Description

Incision

In this step authors describe a simple incision technique, generally using two hands, but this is optional as the surgeon must decide how to do it.

Eye incision at 110–130° at two levels, first using a crescent keratome to create a 2 mm tunnel which is used to penetrate a 2.2–3.2 mm keratome right into the cornea to get a squared and self-sealing incision, keeping the anterior chamber pressurized, in accordance to the experience of the author (Fig. 2A).

Next a viscous-elastic material is injected to regenerate the anterior chamber and protect the endothelium.

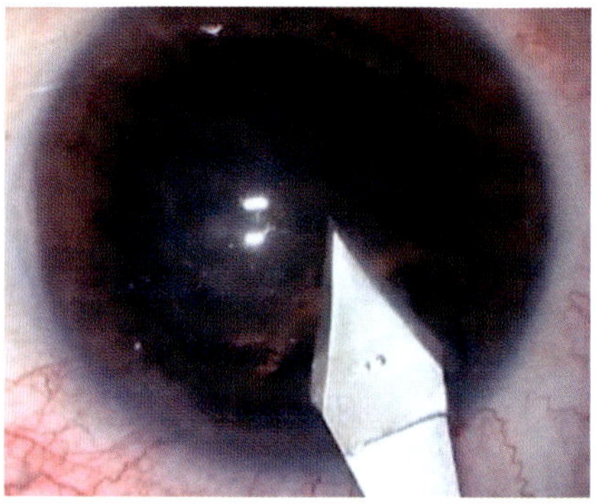

Fig. 2A: Incision

Capsulorhexis

Afterwards a 5–6 mm continuous curvilinear capsulorhexis is practiced. Using a small needle, the anterior chamber is incised in the center of the lens, displacing it to the right and elevating a segment of the chamber using a straight Utrata capsulorhexis clip, long lines, rounded handle, always pulling to the center to avoid radial damages. The incision of the capsule allows authors to work at first in the most complicated zone, making easier to work the rest of the chamber (Fig. 2B).

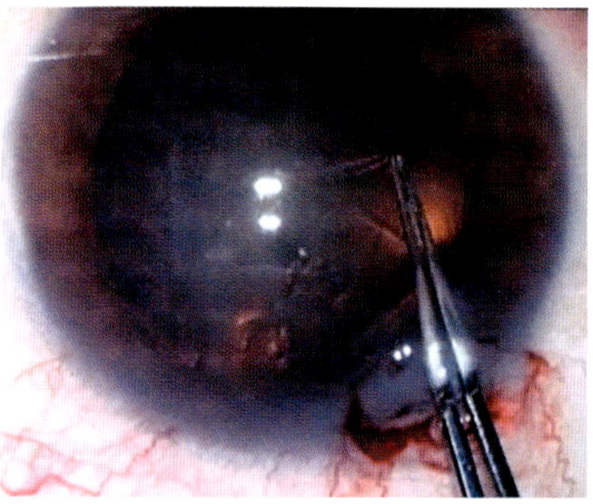

Fig. 2B: Capsulorhexis

Hydrodissection

Using a 0.22 cannula and a 3 cc syringe, hydrodissection is carefully made, guiding the cannula under the capsule where needed while verifying if the fluid wave could pass behind the lens, making the nucleus to rotate 180° to liberate the cortico-capsular attachments (Fig. 2C).

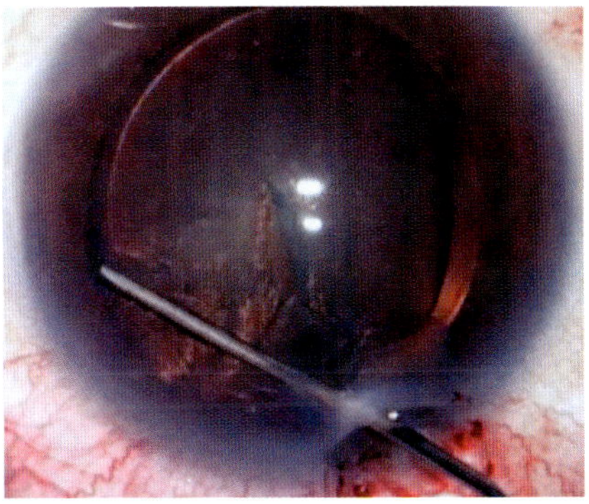

Fig. 2C: Hydrodissection

Lens Multiple Phacofracture

Next, using an Akahoshi´s Prechopper Combo, the mechanical fracture of the lens is effected. First authors start by touching the center of the lens to verify its hardness.

There are two ways to treat the lens:

1. *Soft lenses*

Directly penetrate the lens from the center through the central nucleus where the clips are to be opened to provoke the fracture of the nucleus.

2. *Hard lenses*

A groove is made over the surface of the lens, passing the clip two or three times (from back to front) just the same way you cut a crystal. The clip then is positioned in the middle of the groove lightly pressing the center of the nucleus. Then the lines of the clip are separated (Fig. 3A).

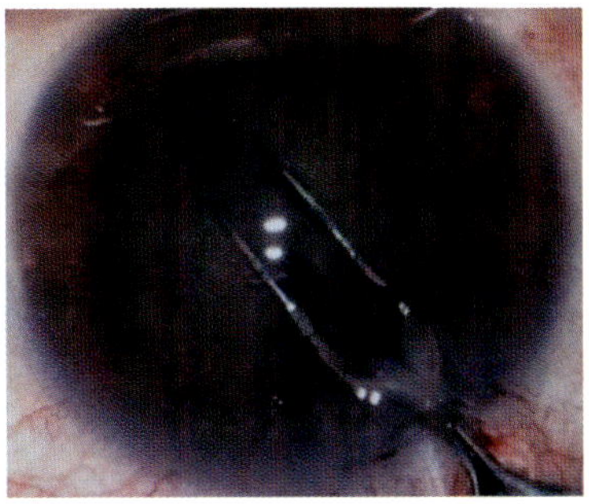

Fig. 3A: First fracture

In both cases, the next step is to position the clip at the end of capsulorhexis, aligned to the main fracture in order to make an incision in both sides of the area, making four lens segments (Fig. 3B).

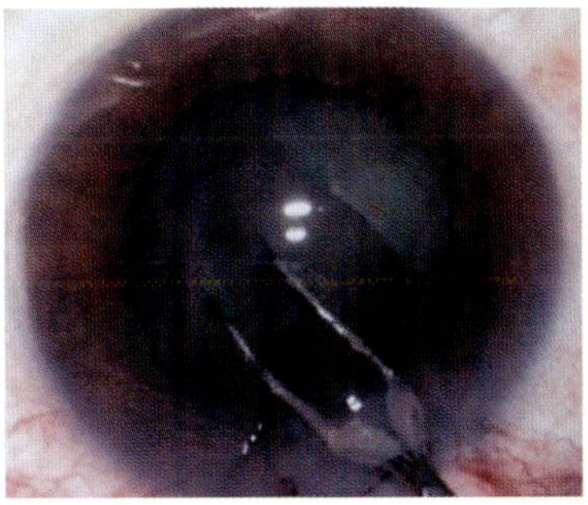

Fig. 3B: Creation of 4 nuclear fragments

Next the lens is rotated 90° to fracture both central segments using the following method:

1. The nearest segment is incised by its center in order to cause the fracture.
2. The way to handle the distal segment is by lining it from front to back, leaving the clip in the deepest side of this groove, opening and breaking the nucleus. This way you get a multiple fracture in six different segments making easier the phacoemulsification process (Fig. 3C).

This technique is daily used in an 80% or 90% of authors' patients.

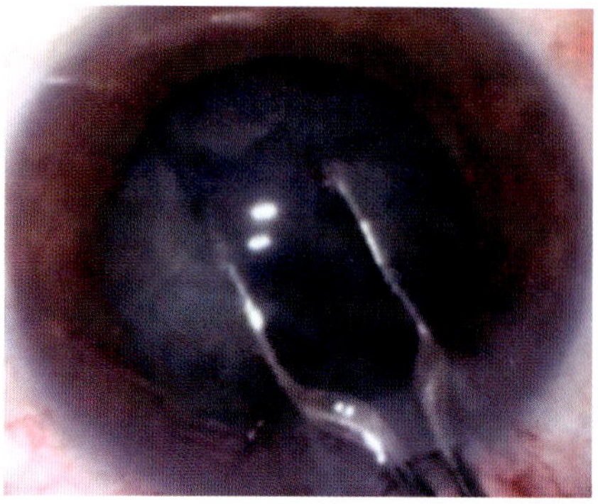

Fig. 3C: Fracture at 90°

Phacoemulsification of Segments

Using a titanium tip, if possible a 0.9–1.1 mm 45° flared Kelman, the farthest left central segment is removed by emulsifying and aspirating the area. The other central segments are removed clockwise, always by emulsifying the area (Fig. 3D).The lateral segments can be handled using the manual device making them to rotate lightly and bringing them to the special area to be removed, it is very important to check the back capsule.

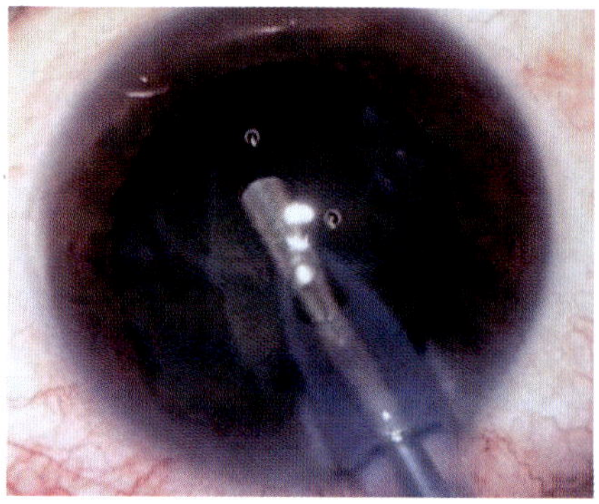

Fig. 3D: Phacoemulsification of nuclear pieces

How to Aspirate the Cortex?

Using a right or 45° irrigation-aspiration device the cortex is gently aspirated. The anterior chamber must always be pressurized, starting with the farthest area of the lens, moving clockwise and leaving the top cortical remnants that will be finally aspirated with a 90° irrigation-aspiration device (Fig. 3E).

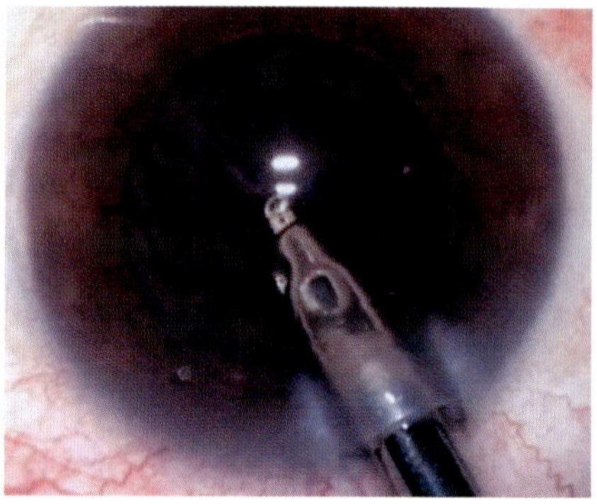

Fig. 3E: Coaxial cortical aspiration

TABLE 2 Parameters in phaco machine according to the surgical step

Surgical Stage	High (cm)	Vacuum (mm Hg)	Flux (cc/min)	Power
Segment removal	100–110	350–380 Lineal	40–45 Fijo	40–60% 30 ms Lineal Burst
Cortex irrigation-aspiration	95–100	400 Lineal	30–40 Fijo	—
Viscous-elastic material aspiration	90–100	400	40	—

Then, the capsule and the anterior chamber must be regenerated with a viscous-elastic cohesive getting prepared to implant the intraocular lens.

The anterior chamber could be gently washed with Cruz´s spatula (Fig. 3F).

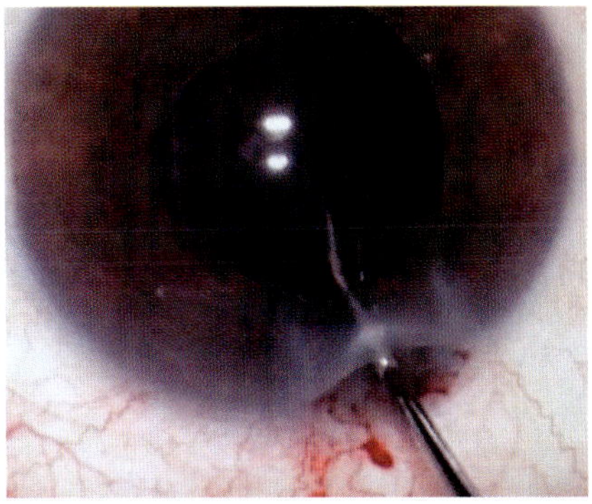

Fig. 3F: Use of the spatula

How to Implant the Intraocular Lens

The surgeon must select the intraocular lens depending on the characteristics of the patient, as well as the availability of an intraocular lens in the zone. If it is possible, it always has to be in the capsule and centered (Fig. 3G).

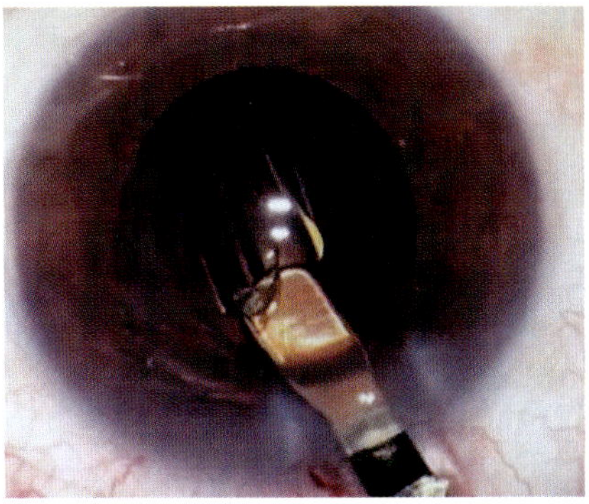

Fig. 3G: IOL implantation

Viscous-elastic material aspiration, anterior chamber regeneration and sewing up the opening with or without suture (Fig. 3H).

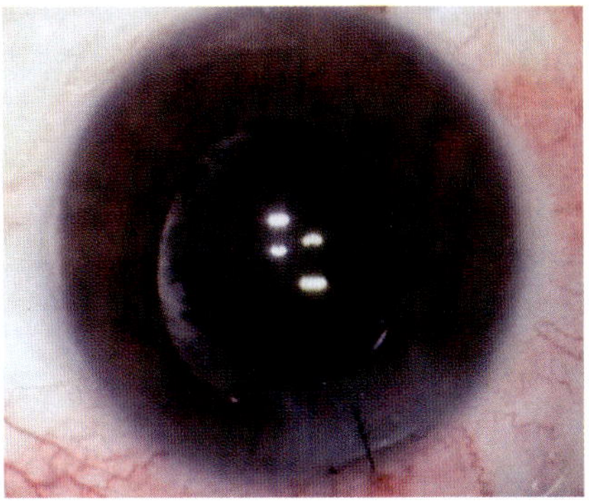

Fig. 3H: End of surgery

The multiple phacofracture is a technique accessible to all public if you recognize its perspectives, purposes, and that it involves technical components as well as skills and experience.[2]

A clinical and surgical review allows surgeons to personalize the therapeutic process to be used with each patient. This way surgeons can offer an excellent service and warranty the best visual results.

References

1. Paul S Koch. Converting to Phacoemulsification: Making the Transition In-The-Bag Phaco. New Jersey: Slack Inc.; 1992.
2. Barry S Seibel. Phacodynamics: Mastering the Tools and Techniques of Phacoemulsification Surgery. New Jersey: Slack Inc.; 1994.

6

Coaxial Microincision Cataract Surgery with Oertli Swiss Technology

Francisco Sanchez-Leon (Mexico)

Introduction

Stunning improvement of cataract surgery has been obsessed by the effort of decreasing surgical invasion to the eye, better technology used for cataract removal and intraocular lens (IOL) delivery in order to achieve early visual recovery as fast as possible. Since the concept of small incision cataract surgery created by Charlie Kelman (Fig. 1) in the early 70s, with the introduction of phacoemulsification, great efforts of modern cataract surgery has been guided technological development to the concept of microsurgery by decreasing the incision size.

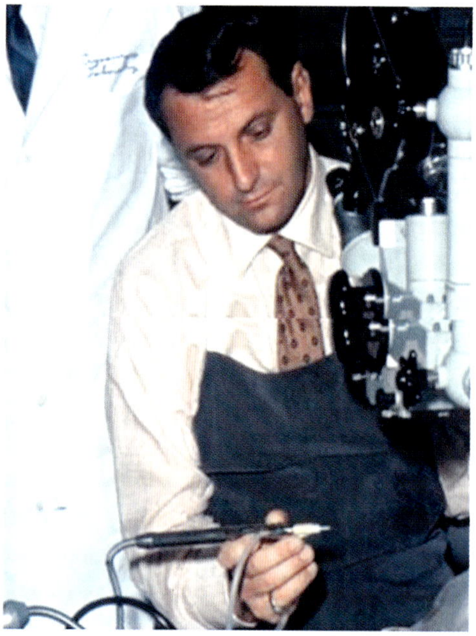

Fig. 1: Charlie Kelman patented phacoemulsification in 1967 (Greek word *"phako"* means lens, and *"emulsify"* means suspended fine particles in liquid)

The desire for small cataract surgery is driven to reduce trauma and astigmatism after phacoemulsification surgery and led to an evolution in phacoemulsification techniques.

Is there a Need for Further Downsizing of the Cataract Incision?

Cataract incisions must fulfill two requirements:

1. **Deformation resistance (wound stability):** To be safe, an incision must not open when manipulated in practice; a patient may rub the eye with a finger tip. Temporally located incisions are particularly exposed to such deformation and must be designed accordingly. Deformation resistance depends on the size and construction of the incision; it increases as it gets smaller and longer and when it incorporates a scleral portion.[1]
2. **Topographic neutrality (corneal stability):** Incisions must not induce corneal shape changes. Smaller incisions cause asymmetrical changes, which are properly picked up only with corneal topography. Topographical stability may be considered relevant within a pupillary zone of 5 mm.[2]

If temporally located sclerocorneal incisions (SCI) up to a size of 4 mm fulfill the requirements, then why should we struggle to further minimize the cataract incision? The answer is that the aforementioned is true only for sclerocorneal incisions. It has been demonstrated that 3 mm wide clear corneal incisions (CCI) are not safe enough and induce asymmetrical corneal flattening adjacent to the incision that encroaches on the 5 mm optical zone.[3,4] With temporal-superiorly or superiorly located incisions, this sectorial flattening effect increases significantly.[5]

While SCIs, due to conjunctival healing, allow for permanent sealing within one week, CCI take months to do so, thereby exposing the patient to a risk of endophthalmitis for an extended time. However, corneal incisions have become very popular since they are easy and fast to create, exclude intraoperative ballooning of the conjunctiva and are cosmetically appealing while avoiding patient disturbances due to conjunctival bleeding or foreign body sensations. However, to be safe and astigmatically neutral CCI must be further downsized.

How small must a safe CCI be? Deformation resistance of a CCI depends on the width and length of the incision. The smaller the incision, the shorter the incision can be while providing for the same amount of resistance against digital massage. Practically, a 2 mm x 1.5 mm incision should fulfill these requirements. Smaller incisions further optimize safety, as long as they are not overstressed during phaco and IOL insertion. Topographical impact on the central corneal zone has been shown to be negligible with a CCI size of 2.0 mm or smaller.[6]

What are the requirements for phaco and IOL technology? Phaco should provide maximum safety and efficiency. Safety means minimal incision trauma and maximum chamber stability. Efficiency means minimal phaco time and energy consumption. This should be achieved through the smallest incision possible. IOLs should provide easy and atraumatic insertion, auto-centration and stable fixation within the bag, circumferential barrier function against lens epithelial cell immigration and optimum optical performance. Implanting IOL's through smaller than appropriate incisions may cause permanent tissue trauma, and compromises the self-sealing properties.[7]

What incision sizes should be aimed for? Incision sizes are dictated by the IOLs to be inserted. Current IOLs may be divided into two subgroups: mini-incision IOLs, which fit through a 2.2–2.4 mm incision, and microincision IOLs, which fit through incisions smaller than 2 mm. In conjunction with appropriate phaco equipment, the latter allow for what has been termed 'sub 2 mm' or 'microincision' cataract surgery (MICS).

MICS through 2.2–2.4 mm incisions is achieved with current coaxial phaco and IOL technology. However, this is a trade-off. Simply reducing the size of a standard phaco needle, reduces holdability and energy output. Therefore, innovative phaco needle technology is mandatory (Fig. 2).

When reducing the shaft diameter, higher vacuum and flow settings may be used, at the same time suppressing postocclusion surge. By increasing the bevel angle of the needle, holdability (a function of the area of the opening) is augmented. The transition between the broad needle-head and the slim shaft increases the frontal projection area, which is proportional to the energy output. The slim-shaft allows for a sleeve that runs almost flush with the needle-head, which further reduces the incision size required, and avoids anteriorly directed infusion inflow, which tends to push particles away from the front opening of the needle. Together, this slim-shaft strong-bevel (SSSB) needle design fits into a concept that optimizes followability, holdability, energy transfer and surge suppression (Fig. 3).

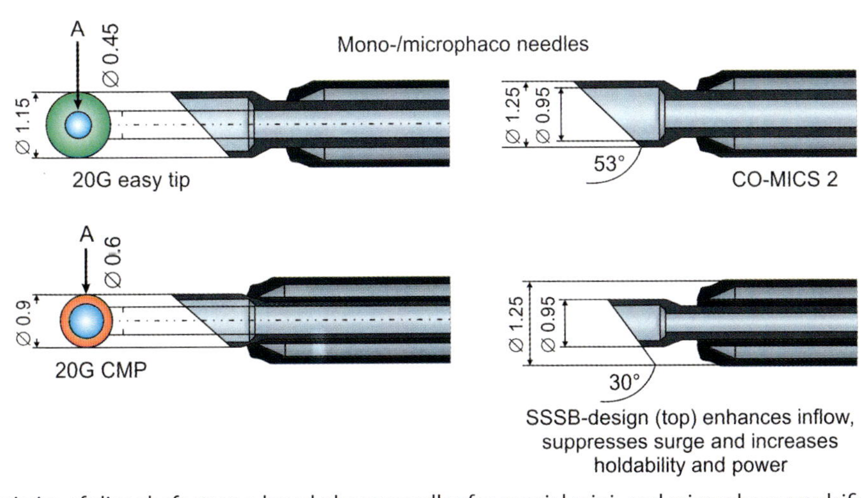

Fig. 2: Design characteristics of slim-shaft strong-bevel phaco needles for coaxial mini- and microphacoemulsification (*easy*Tip®2.2 mm, *easy*Tip®CO-MICS)

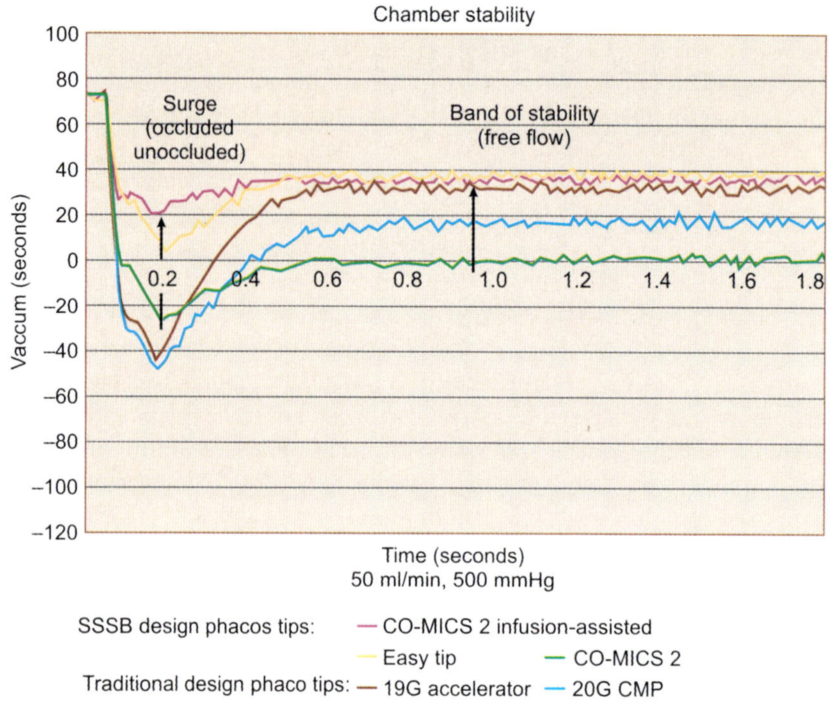

Fig. 3: Postocclusion surge and band of steady-state stability with different phaco tips including infusion assistance

Such a needle has recently been released by the Oertli® company—the *easy*Tip® 2.2 mm (Fig. 2, left). A significant decrease in phaco time and energy consumption in clinical tests has corroborated the theoretical advantage of this concept. Of the IOLs in market, several fit through a 2.2–2.4 mm incision. However, most of these (e.g. Alcon Acrysof® SN60WF, Zeiss-Acri.Tec AcriLyc 47LC) are one-piece acrylic IOLs with broad haptic-optic junctions with the injector tip docked to, and not inserted into, the incision. Broad junctions inherently interfere with capsular bending and, thus compromise the barrier function against immigrating lens epithelial cells, giving way to earlier and more pronounced after-cataract formation.[8,9] A singular exception is the Hoya AF-1 preloaded three-piece IOL, which has recently been fitted with an exquisitely sharp posterior optic edge and allows injection through a 2.4 mm incision, if properly designed.

Due to its slim junction design, the Hoya IOL may also be used in conjunction with posterior optic buttonholing for permanent eradication of any form of after-cataract formation.[10]

Traditional phacoemulsification involves an incision size approximately 3 mm. Bimanual sleeveless phacoemulsification reduces the incision size further by dividing the incision into two smaller incisions (Fig. 4). Additional advances in phacoemulsification systems allow surgeons to return to traditional coaxial phaco techniques or coaxial microincision cataract surgery (CO-MICS) defined by Alio as phacoemulsification surgery performed though incision

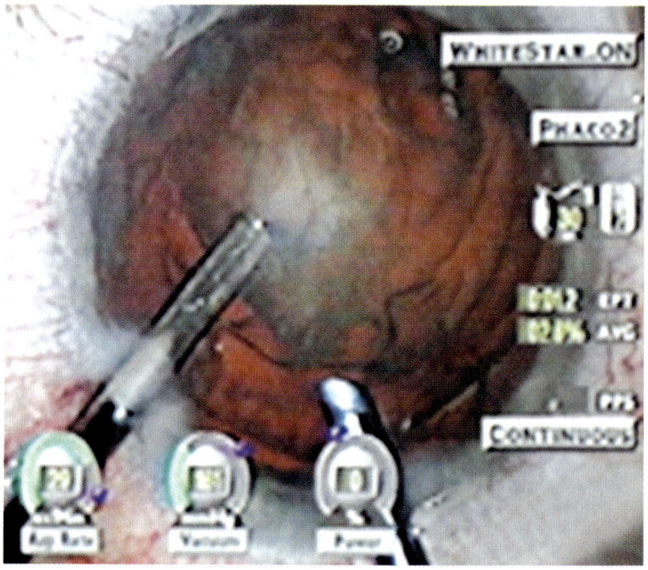

Fig. 4: Bimanual phacoemulsification divides the incision in two smaller incisions

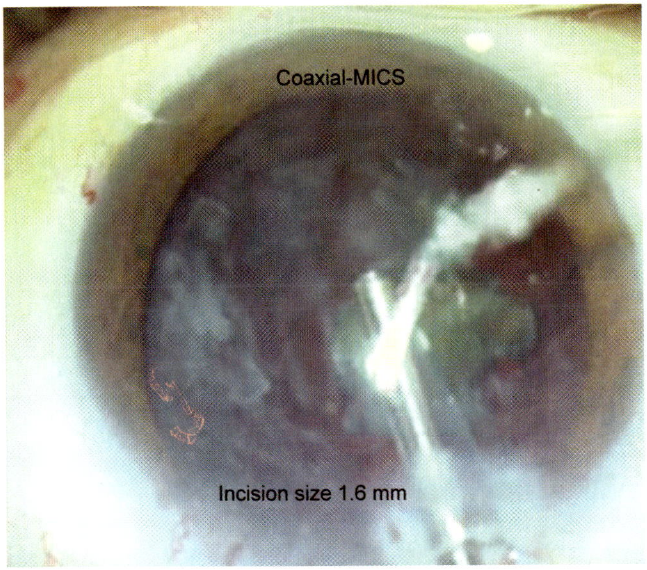

Fig. 5: Oertli phaco technology allows coaxial-microphacoemulsification through 1.6 mm

2 mm or less. Today, Oertli Instrumente offers options to perform the procedure through incisions as small as 1.6 mm (Fig. 5).

Coaxial Microincision Cataract Surgery Versus Bimanual

Coaxial Microincision Cataract Surgery

- Flexible silicone sleeve seals and protects the incision
- Superior inflow
- Less surge due to greater resistance of a smaller phaco tip
- Superb anterior chamber stability
- Rare leaking
- Useful in hard nuclear

Bimanual

- Excessive surgical trauma
- Wound leaking
- Flow-vacuum limitation
- Surge

Microincision Cataract Surgery through Sub 2 mm Incisions

Phaco Instrumentation

Microincision cataract surgery requires new technologies and surgical techniques if the efficacy and safety of phaco are to be preserved. For phaco, a microcoaxial or a biaxial approach can been chosen. For several years, the biaxial approach has been the only choice for real microincision phaco through incisions smaller than 2 mm. Recent improvements in phaco needle manufacturing technology have allowed implementation of the SSSB design into a coaxial micro-tip—*easy*Tip®CO-MICS by Oertli Instrumente (Fig. 2, right). This needle allows coaxial microphaco (MPE) through incisions as small as 1.4 mm when used with trumpet-shaped incisions. Clinical studies have demonstrated its efficacy and safety. However, inflow remains the limiting factor for high-fluidic settings. To compensate for this, infusion-assisted or hybrid phaco11 has been introduced and evaluated. In place of a phaco spatula, a special infusion spatula is inserted through the side port, which supplements the infusion inflow and allows for the manipulation of the cataractous lens during work-up and aspiration. The additional fluid supply allows the use of excessive vacuum and flow settings for maximum phaco efficiency while at the same time preserving a 'rock-solid' chamber. The safety limits were elaborated in an experimental setting. Vacuum limits of 600 mm Hg and flow rates of up to 50 mm Hg have been demonstrated to be safe. In a clinical study comparing the *easy*Tip®CO-MICS tip standard and hybrid techniques, less than half the phaco energy was required when infusion assistance was used. While allowing for phaco through incisions as small as those used with biaxial MPEs, coaxial MPE with SSSB tips offers the following advantages, especially when infusion-assisted: no incision leakage, which optimizes chamber stability; no tissue damage by the oscillating needle, which preserves the self-sealing ability of the incision; abundant infusion supply, allowing for work with excessive flow, which optimizes followability and needle occlusion; and usage of SSSB tip technology, which optimizes holdability and energy output while suppressing postocclusion surge. Thus, maximum efficiency and safety are provided while optimally preserving the tissue integrity and valve function of the incision[10-12] (Figs 6A to H).

Sleeve-Armed Coaxial or Sleeveless Biaxial Microphaco—Which Way to Go?

Proponents of sleeveless biaxial phaco argue that it requires a smaller incision and improves the flow characteristics in the anterior chamber. Although biaxial MPE is feasible, there are a number of downsides. In order to maintain a deep and stable chamber while using high fluidics, incision leak must be minimized. Sleeveless phaco needles tend to 'oarlock' a tight CCI or allow for continuous collateral

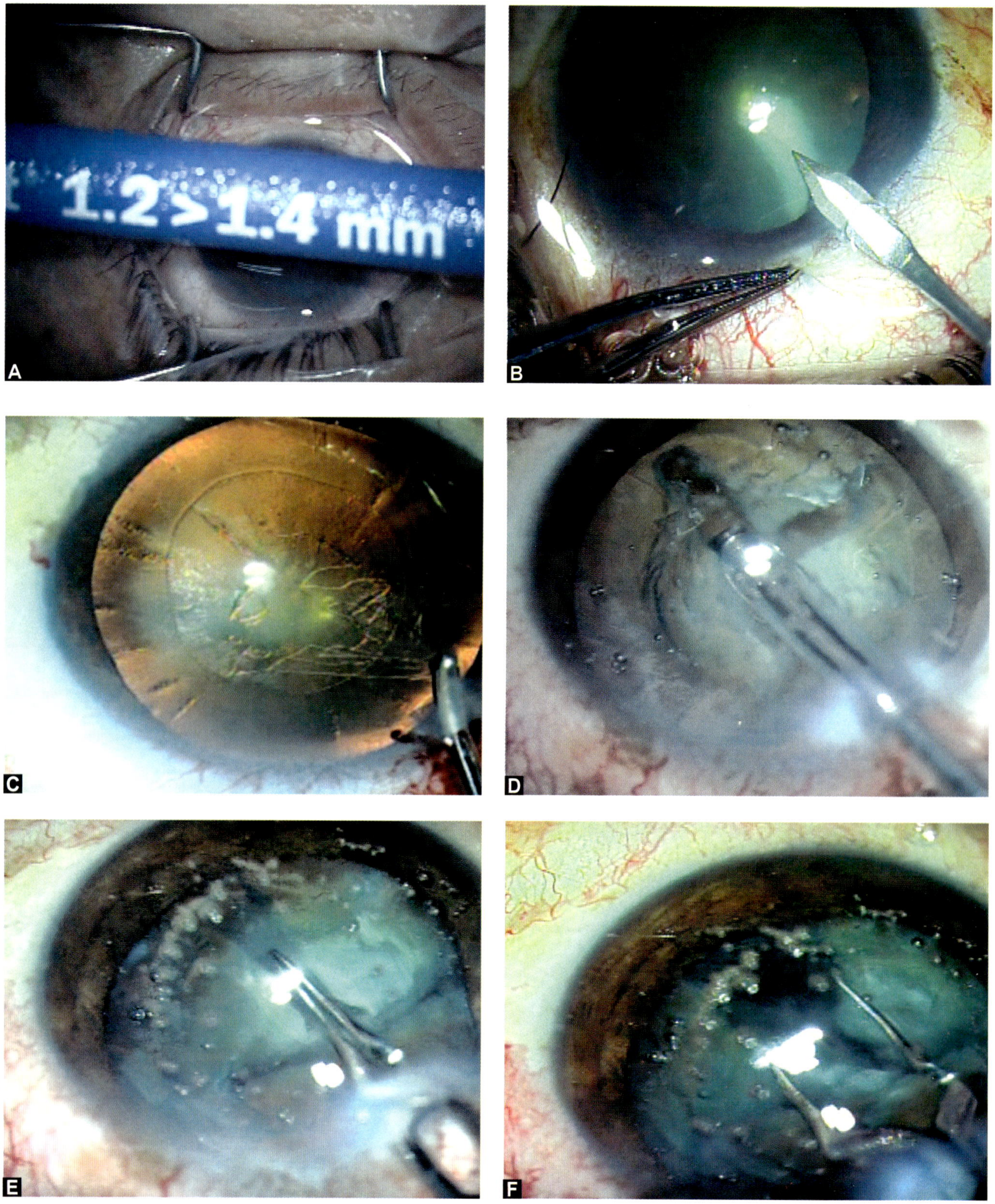
1.2>1.4 mm
A
B
C
D
E
F

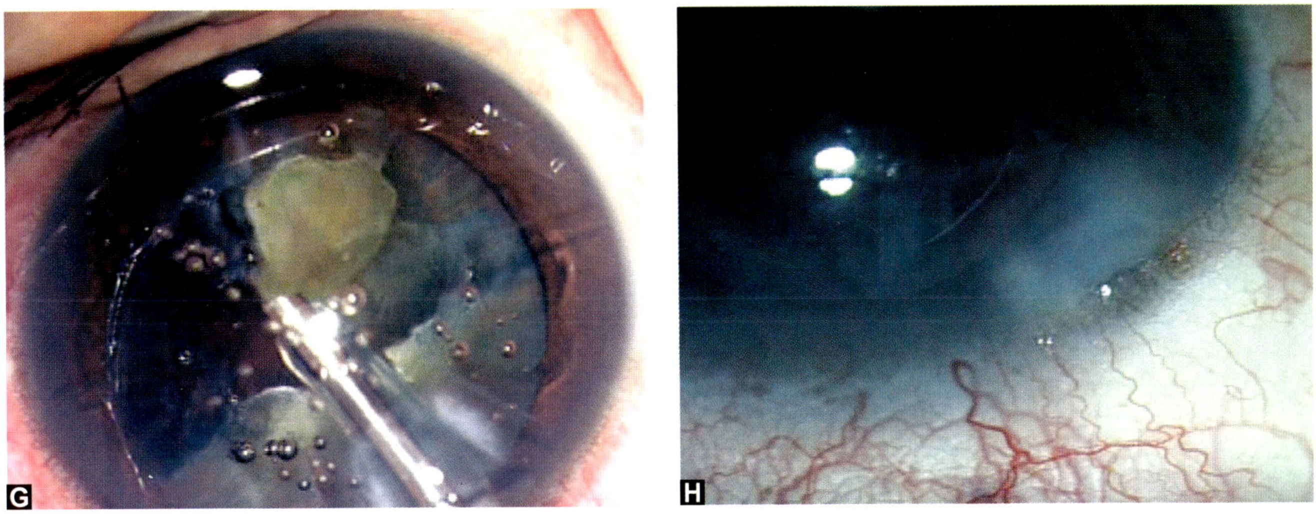

Figs 6A to H: Sequence of photos of coaxial microincision cataract surgery (CO-MICS) phaco through 1.4–1.6 mm incision. (A) MICS blade 1.4 mm; (B) clear cornea incision 1.4 mm; (C) Ikeda capsulorhexis forceps; (D) CO-MICS tip with silicone sleeve, through 1.4 mm, divide and conquer technique; (E) Inamura-Eagle prechopper; (F) Inamura-Eagle prechopper lens nucleus splitting; (G) CO-MICS tip with sleeve emulsifying nucleus fragments; (H) Corneal incision hydrated and sealed

wound leak with a wider CCI, which varies according to the changing angle of the instrument approach. There is no way of designing and sizing a CCI that seals the wound and spares tissue at the same time. Histological studies have demonstrated that both the stromal tunnel and the corneal valve are compromised in their morphology and function.[11,12] A soft-silicone sleeve snugly adapts to the slit incision and guarantees both atraumatic tight sealing and a greater infusion throughput. The new SSSB design optimizes phaco efficiency and safety by further increasing influx while running flush with the swollen needle head, which counteracts forward-directed flow. The infusion enters the chamber through the lateral openings of the sleeves and is re-attracted by the frontal opening of the phaco needle. The high fluidics allowed with this particular needle design and the incision tightness provided by the sleeve minimizes uncontrolled turbulences in the chamber by confining the fluid stream between the sleeve and needle openings to the tip of the handpiece. With infusion and aspiration separated, the fluid stream changes according to the relative positioning of the instrument openings and is superimposed by turbulences caused by the wound leak, which varies as the instruments manipulate the corneal wound. Also, the advantages of a slim-shaft needle cannot be fully exploited since the outer wall of a needle used with sleeveless phaco must run flush with the head for proper wound sealing. In order to be efficient, needles for sleeveless phaco must be thicker, or they will be less efficient if downsized in diameter for use in microincisions. Apart from the familiarity with the coaxial phaco techniques, these limitations are the main reason why sleeveless biaxial phaco has not gained widespread usage.

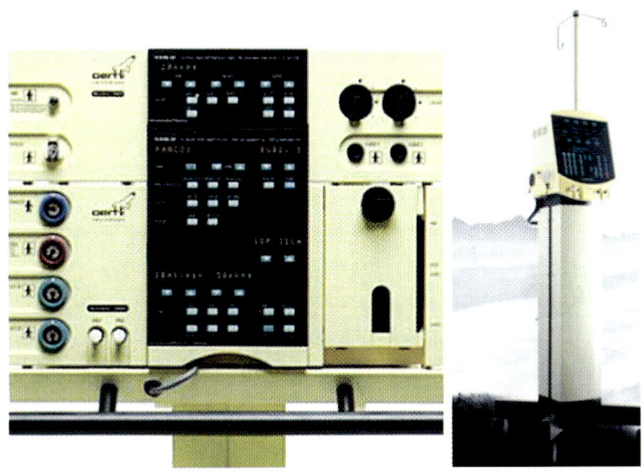

Fig. 7: Oertli® OS3, here with vitreoretinal extension and faros new phaco vitreoretinal platform

Oertli Instrumente AG offers three different models: Oertli® OS3, Oertli® Faros (Fig. 7) and Oertli CataRhex®SwissTech. All platforms support both coaxial and bimanual MICS. While (sleeveless) bimanual MICS requires adjustments of fluidics and "cool phaco" power settings, which are readily available on these platforms by

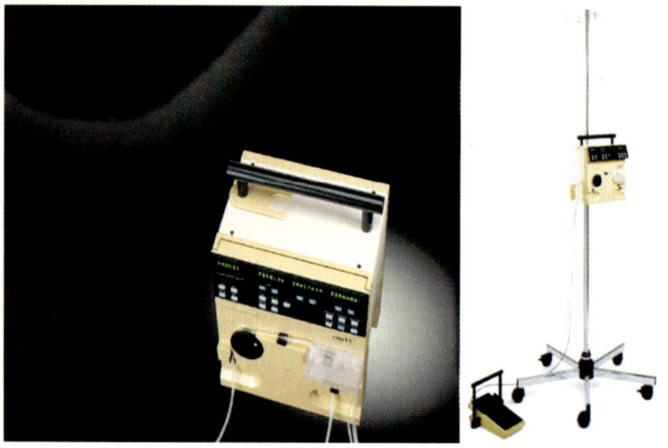

Fig. 8: CataRhex® SwissTech only weighs 5.6 kg and attaches to every infusion stand

simply pressing the cool micropulse (CMP) button, coaxial MICS with the Oertli CO-MICS tip needs an increase of vacuum.

When considering microsurgery procedure, why do we need to roll a 107 kg of weight (Alcon Infiniti®) into the operating theater to remove 200 mg of lens material, when we can take one big advantage of CataRhex® SwissTech portability, only weighs 5.6 kg and attaches to every infusion stand (Fig. 8).

CO-MICS Oertli Technology

From our personal experience CO-MICS has major advantages: (1) the sleeve seals the wound, thereby preventing fluid outflow. With sleeveless phaco tips, fluid loss is not only inevitable but also variable depending upon the relative orientation of the tip with regard to the wound. This leads to pressure fluctuations within the camber which may be difficult to counteract and carry the risk of chamber collapse in case of occlusion break (Figs 9A and B). (2) The sleeve protects the surrounding wound tissue from mechanical and thermal damage. With sleeve-less phaco tips, the wound slit must be kept as narrow as possible to provide a tight fit and thus avoid excessive fluid outflow. This may lead to tissue damage especially when instrument manipulation in a tight incision causes locking of the wound.

Equipments

No specific software or special tubing-systems or other modification is required to do CO-MICS with the OS3, Faros and CataRhex SwisTech platforms. All three equipments allow mounting to the Oertli Hexadisq phaco handpiece to perform phacoemulsification using three different incision sizes with three different of phaco tips and sleeve. Oertli technology permits 2.8–3.0 mm Excellerator, 2.2–2.4 mm Microcoaxial, 1.6–1.8 mm CO-MICS incision sizes with the use of same phaco handpiece (Fig. 10).

Today there are different phaco tips for each surgeon according to size and performance preference. No other technology allows wide range for choosing. We will describe some different phaco tips for each surgeon technique preference, from standard phacoemulsification 2.8–3.0 mm, following to MICS 2.2–2.4 mm and CO-MICS 1.6–1.8 mm (Figs 11A to D).

Oertli Instrumente produces special tips for bimanual sleeve-free cool phacoemulsification technique.

When appropriately adjusted, the front of the sleeve seals with the backside of the tip head, avoiding anteriorly

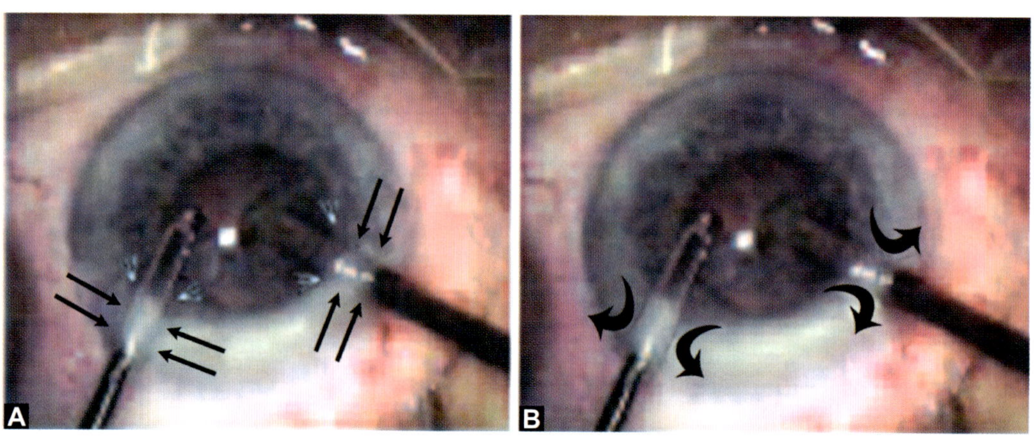

Figs 9A and B: The dilemma of sleeveless biaxial microphaco: tissue "oarlocking" versus wound leakage. (A) Tight wound fit, (B) Loose wound fit

	Excellerator	Microcoaxial	CO-MICS
	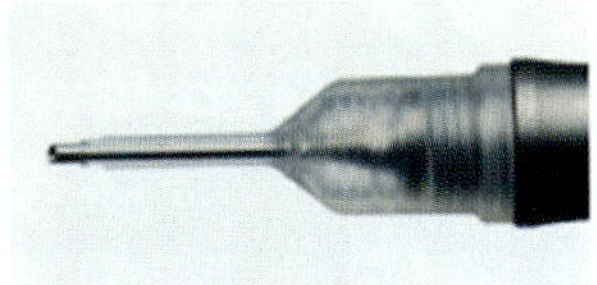	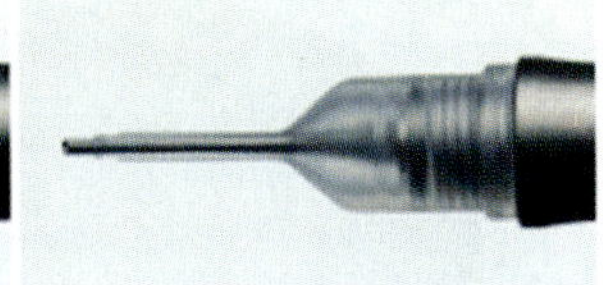	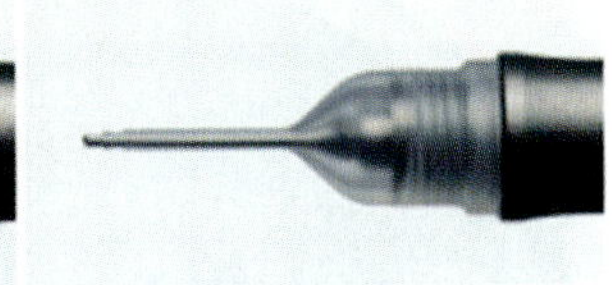
Incision size	2.8 - 3.0 mm	2.2 - 2.4 mm	1.6 - 1.8 mm
Phaco pack OS3	VV630011A	VV630011B	VV630011C
Phaco pack SwissTech	VV621011A	–	VV621011C
Reusable tip	VV800430	VV800730	VV800830
Reusable sleeve	VV603200	VV603220	VV603230
Aspiration tip 45°	VE655535	–	VE655515
Aspiration tip straight	VE655035	VE655035	VE655015
Bimanual I/A	VE65410x	VE65410x	VE65410x

Fig. 10: Examples of different Oertli phaco tips for each incision size are shown in image

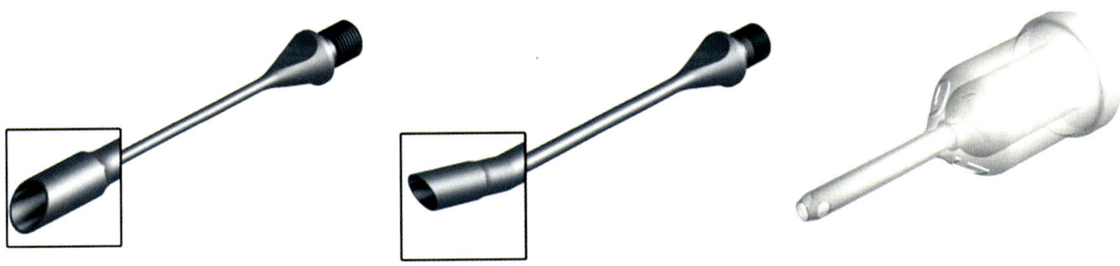

Fig. 11A: Titanium tip excellerator 2, 30° 2.8–3.0 mm (on left panel). Ergo Excellerator, for hard nuclei and narrow pupils, 30°(center). Irrigation sleeve silicone 19G Standard (on right panel)

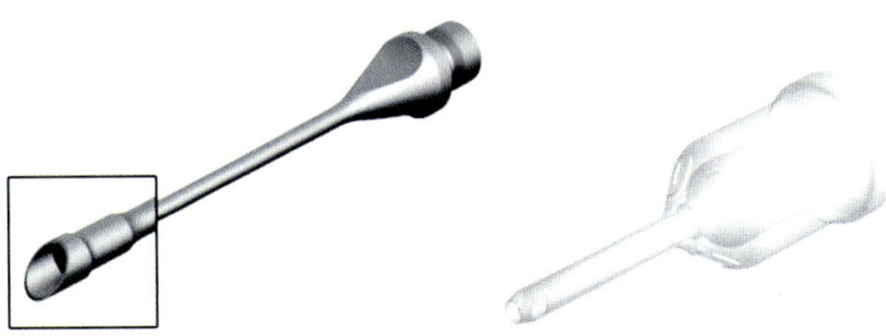

Fig. 11B: *Easy*Tip®2.2 mm for incisions of 2.2–2.4 mm, 40°. Irrigation Sleeve Silicone 20G for *easy*Tip®2.2 mm

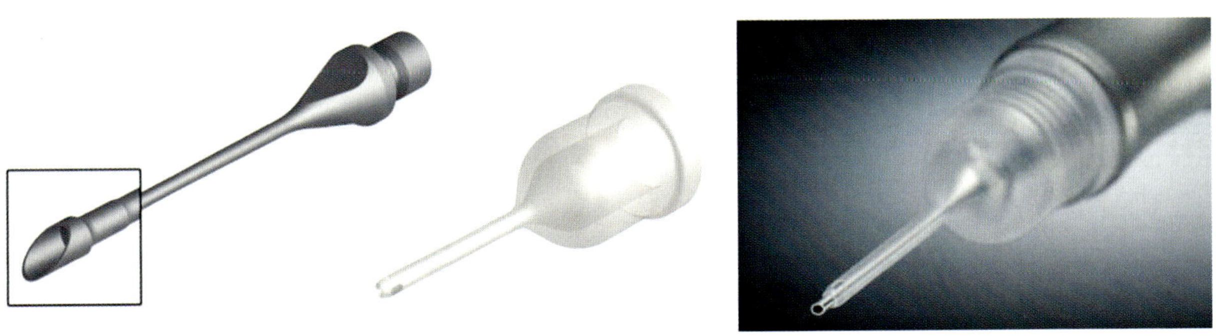

Fig. 11C: *Easy*Tip®CO-MICS for incisions of 1.6–1.8 mm, 53°. Irrigation Sleeve Silicone for *easy*Tip®CO-MICS

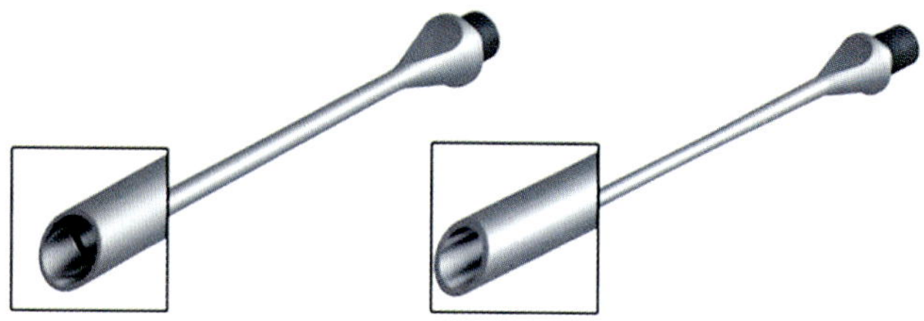

Fig. 11D: Special tips for sleeve-less phaco technique. 19G CMP titanium tip. 20G CMP titanium tip

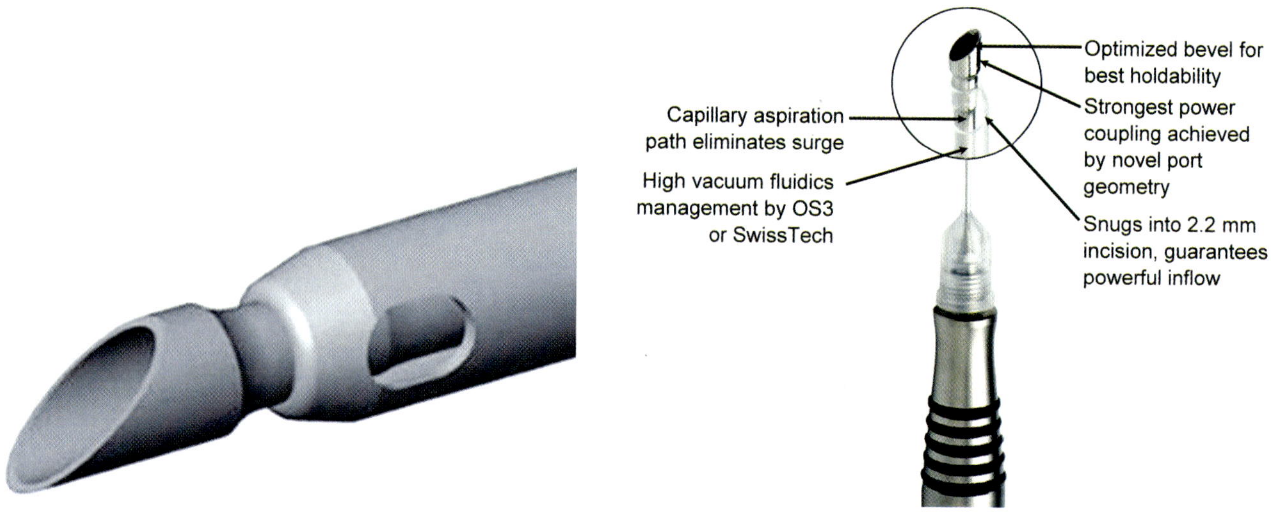

Fig. 12: Positioning of the sleeve in the Oertli CO-MICS2 instrumentation

directed inflow. With traditional tips, this coaxial inflow tends to push fragments away from the tip. With CO-MICS tip (2.2 mm incision) the irrigation fluid inflow is essentially confined to the side openings (Fig. 12)

Machine Settings

Excellerator, *easy*Tip®2.2 mm, *easy*Tip®CO-MICS works equally well either with venturi or peristaltic pumps of the Oertli OS3, faros and CataRhex SwissTech platforms. In the case of Oertli OS3 platform, both venturi and peristaltic pumps work ideally for any surgeon's preference.

Do not change flow settings (mL/min peristaltic) or venturi rise time (% venturi)

For grooving: Increase vacuum level by 50 mm Hg (peristaltic or venturi)

Fragment removal: Increase vacuum level by 150 mm Hg (peristaltic or venturi)

Phaco power and modulation needs no adjustment, keep preferred values and modulation mode. After first CO-MICS surgery, take into consideration, the possibility of further increasing the vacuum level and flow rate.

*Easy*Tip®2.2 mm, *easy*Tip® CO-MICS works excellent at high vacuum levels, provides excellent anterior chamber stability and suppresses surges. The phaco experience is different compared to standard 2.8 mm tip, is smoother and more "forgiving", and performance is superb.

*Easy*Tip®2.2 mm, *easy*Tip® CO-MICS tips provide astonishing phacoemulsification efficiency and chamber stability, inherent reduction of surge upon occlusion break and optimally preserves the integrity and self-sealing properties of the wound.

More Intelligent Technology

- Never before has so much intelligence, technology and capability been concentrated into such a small space
- Direct processor control instead of a fickle PC operating system
- Intelligent physical concepts instead of expensive sensor technology
- Reliable control elements instead of a complicated touch screen
- Varying intensities of ultrasound for every degree of hardness instead of unorthodox emulsification methods.

More Intelligent Design

- Rolling 107 kg of weight (Alcon Infiniti®) into the operating theater to remove 200 mg of lens material.

CataRhex® SwissTech is portable, only weighs 5.6 kg and attaches to every infusion stand

- Direct Access® responds to button actuation without the need for a multilevel user menu
- The stability of the I/A system does away with the need to change the bottle height
- A tubing set replaces the cassette
- Upgradeable to a posterior segment system.

More Intelligent Solution

- CataRhex® SwissTech will fit into the smallest operating theater
- Its simple operation hardly requires any training
- It requires less assistance thanks to a multifunction pedal
- The sensational pump system speed up operating times
- Purchase and maintenance are less costly
- Its portability enables it to be used at different operating venues
- The pressure sensor incorporated in the tubing set ensures total sterility.

Oertli utilize more sophisticated phaco control using CMP phaco, represents the leading-edge of technology. CataRhex®SwissTech is a match for any larger piece of equipment—both in terms of comfort, functions and safety as well as in respect of the operation result. But above all else—when efficiency is the benchmark.

CataRhex®SwissTech is a state-of-the-art phaco system with all of the functions necessary for modern anterior chamber surgery:

- Irrigation/aspiration
- Continuous irrigation
- Multi-mode phaco
- Occlusion-mode phaco
- CMP cool phaco
- Bipolar diathermy
- High-speed vitrectomy
- Bipolar capsulotomy
- Bipolar glaucoma surgery

CO-MICS with CataRhex®SwissTech

CataRhex®SwissTech is based on an innovative design concept, which offers particular advantages compared with conventional phaco systems:

- Genuine portability
- Unequalled lightness and compactness
- Fits into a pilot case
- Able to be mounted directly onto an infusion stand
- Simple tubing system with integral sensor
- Space-saving multifunction pedal, can be moved by foot

CataRhex®SwissTech has a particularly simple Direct Access®, control surface which ensures immediate access to every function:

- Fast and simple unit preparation
- Short change-over times between operations
- Simple to use, short learning phase
- Rapid programming and call-up of multimode programs
- Ergonomic control panel with bright displays and distinct push buttons
- Background programming with Para Programs
- Uncompromising Oertli® quality

CataRhex®SwissTech can be used in conjunction with all Oertli® surgical instruments including the particularly ergonomic TITANO range.

Direct Access® generates immediate vacuum. The SwissTech pump system is way ahead of the competition. It practically achieves the values of a modern venturi system. Only fractions of a second is needed to establish a vacuum. Perfect flow control for aspiration is achieved. Whether only very gentle or full power suction is required, the flow always remains under precise pedal control with the SwissTech. Even at the lowest flow rates, no noticeable rolling effect exists. It also provides contamination-free pressure measurement. The patented pressure measurement system rules out any contact with the sensor by the aspiration fluid, as long as anterior chamber is stable. The application of correct physical principles and the elimination of air from the fluidics system are the key elements underpinning the high chamber stability of the SwissTech. It allows you to employ the SwissTech's high vacuum and flow rate levels without a problem in modern surgical techniques.

The patented ultrasound technology for phaco emulsification has made decisive progress in recent years. Oertli® has played an important part in this development. That's why CataRhex®SwissTech offers you the very latest technology. Alternative methods like laser, Aqualase, Neosonix (Alcon Laboratories, Fort Worth, USA), sonic and even rotating systems offer neither medical nor economical advantages. Nothing comes close to the elegance of ultrasound, which can be used for all degrees of hardness. Even for a Clear Lens Exchange (CLE), the kind of case where the nucleus is soft, the low-energy system is highly effective. The latest developed methods of phacoemulsification, are trying to reduce the amount of energy delivered to the eye with the objectives to prevent the warming of the phaco tip, intensify the holding force to the nuclear pieces and make the infuson sleeve redundant (e.g. cool micropulse). These same concepts apply very easy to hard nucleus as well, as you should see in the Chapter 4 of this same textbook.

Occlusion Mode Phaco

In occlusion mode, the adjustment parameters of flow, phaco output and modulation method are vacuum dependent. Once a particular vacuum value is reached (occlusion), the desired parameters (e.g. pulse or reduced output) are immediately activated.

CO-MICS 1.6 mm

CataRhex®SwissTech is the ideal platform for coaxial MICS with 1.6 mm incisions. Just change the blade, not your technique. CO-MICS provides the same power as standard phaco. Holding force and chamber stability are even better than with larger incision sizes (Fig. 13). CataRhex®SwissTech offers four methods of output modulation.

1. Continuous Linear

- Standard method
- Very efficient
- Surgeon needs to set the output level himself
- Phaco intensity corresponds to the degree of pedal deflection

2. PULSE Modulation

- Reduces the emitted ultrasound energy
- Pulse frequency (up to 40 Hz) and cooling factors are freely selectable and not linked to the pedal position
- Pulse intensity corresponds to the pedal position

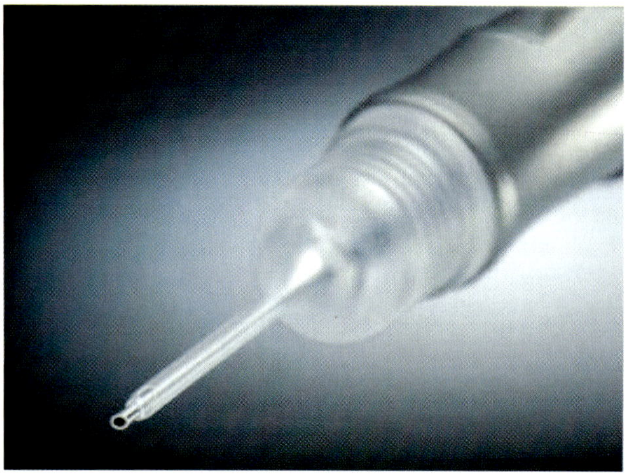

Fig. 13: CO-MICS 1.6 mm tip and sleeve

3. BURST Modulation

- Reduces the emitted ultrasound energy
- The duration and intensity of the bursts (packets of energy pulses) are freely selectable and not linked to the pedal position
- The pause between bursts is controlled by the pedal. The more the pedal is depressed, the shorter the pauses become

4. Cool Micropulse Phaco

- Genuinely cool phaco under all conditions—even at 100% phaco output
- The pulse frequency (up to 40 Hz) and cooling factors are freely selectable within the CMP phaco boundaries and remain unaffected by the pedal position
- The pulse intensity corresponds to the pedal position. Ideal for bimanual MICS
- In the CMP phaco setting, the phaco handpiece at its full output can be held by its bare tip with the fingers only. It is the most impressive proof of Cool Phaco.

Microincision Cataract Surgery

Irrigation/Aspiration: Safe and Fast Capsule Cleaning

Irrespective of whether you work bimanually or with a combined irrigation/aspiration (I/A) instrument, CataRhex SwissTech offers optimal suction and safety. Separate settings for cortex removal and capsule cleaning can be called up by pedal.

The new proportional override function enables you to suck up larger cortex particles accurately and quickly.

Proportional Override

A low vacuum near the capsule and high suction for larger cortex particles: seemingly a contradiction. Proportional override is the solution.

Surgeon should specify a safe vacuum value that is never exceeded in pedal setting 2 for every I/A program. If any cortex clogs the tip, then pedal setting 3 provides an increased vacuum of up to 600 mm Hg proportional to the pedal position at an unchanged aspiration flow rate.

Modern cataract surgery is striving for smaller and smaller incisions with the aim of making CCI that are as safe and topographically stable as possible. Recent innovations in both phacoemulsification and IOL technology have made MICS, defined as lesser than 2 mm incision, safe and effective. Biaxial sleeveless microphaco has recently been joined by sleeve-armed microcoaxial microphaco, which is made possible by the development of SSSB phaco needles, armed with micro-sleeves that run flush with an enlarged needle head. Such tip technology allows for a highly efficient and safe high-flow, high-vacuum phaco through incisions as small as 1.4 mm by providing high influx and suppressing surge while avoiding mechanical and thermal tissue damage. Two tips have so far been made available for mini-incision (2.2–2.4 mm) and microincision cataract surgery (1.4–1.6 mm, depending on the incision architecture used). With the micro-tip supplemented by additional flow through an infusion spatula ("infusion-assisted" or "hybrid" phaco), excessive flow and vacuum rates may be used, resulting in a two-fold efficiency as mirrored by the reduced phaco power required. IOL technology is lagging behind phaco technology. The challenge is to avoid trade-off with regard to implant stability and after cataract formation, as well as optical performance. Current MICS-IOLs are mostly hydrophilic acrylic one-piece constructions with insufficiently sharp posterior optic edges and broad haptic-optic junctions, both of which features compromise the optic-edge barrier effect. Recently, a hydrophobic three-piece IOL has been made available, which features a slim haptic junction and an exquisitely sharp optic edge and also allows for optional optic entrapment into a posterior capsulorhexis for lasting eradication of after-cataracts.

References

1. Ernest P, Lavery KT, Kiessling LA. Relative strength of scleral corneal and clear corneal incisions constructed in cadaver eyes. J Cataract Refract Surg. 1994;20:626-9.
2. Menapace R. Update on wound construction: indications, techniques, deformation resistance and corneal curvature changes. In: Vörösmarthy, et al. (Eds). 10. Kongress der DGII, Budapest. New York: Springer. 1996. pp S27-40.
3. Rainer G, Menapace R, Vass C, et al. Surgically induced astigmatism following a 4.0 mm sclerocorneal valve incision. J Cataract Refract Surg. 1997;23:358-64.
4. Vass C, Menapace R. Computerized statistical analysis of corneal topography for the evaluation of changes in corneal shape after surgery. Am J Ophthalmol. 1994:118:177-84.
5. Rainer G, Menapace R, Vass C, et al. Corneal shape changes after temporal and superolateral 3.0 mm clear corneal incisions. J Cataract Refract Surg. 1999;25:1121-6.
6. Hayashi K, Yoshida M, Hayashi H. Postoperative corneal shape changes: microincision versus small-incision coaxial cataract surgery. J Cataract Refract Surg. 2009;35:233-9.
7. Radner W, Menapace R, Zehetmayer M, et al. Ultrastructure of clear corneal incisions. Part II: corneal trauma after lens implantation with the Microstaar injector system. J Cataract Refract Surg. 1998;24:493-7.
8. Werner L, Tetz M, Feldmann I, et al. Evaluating and defining the sharpness of intraocular lenses: microedge structure of commercially available square-edged hydrophilic intraocular lenses. J Cataract Refract Surg. 2009;35:556-66.
9. Werner L, Müller M, Tetz M. Evaluating and defining the sharpness of intraocular lenses: micro-edge structure of commercially available square-edged hydrophobic lenses. J Cataract Refract Surg. 2008;34:310-7.
10. Menapace R, Di Nardo SH. How to better use fluidics with MICS. In: Aliò J, Fine H (Eds). Minimizing Incisions and Maximizing Outcomes in Cataract Surgery. New York: Springer; 2009.
11. Berdahl JP, DeStafeno JJ, Kim T. Corneal wound architecture and integrity after phaco evaluation of coaxial, microincision coaxial, and microincision bimanual techniques. J Cataract Refract Surg. 2007;33:510-5.
12. Johar SR, Vasavada AR, Praveen MR, et al. Histomorphological and immunofluorescence evaluation of bimanual and coaxial phaco incisions in rabbits. J Cataract Refract Surg. 2008;34:670-6.

Section 3

Biaxial Microincision Cataract Surgery

7 Biaxial Microincision Cataract Surgery

Mark Packer (USA)

The historical development of biaxial microincision cataract surgery (B-MICS) began in the 1970s when Girard attempted to separate infusion from ultrasound and aspiration, but abandoned the procedure because of thermal injury to the tissue.[1,2] Shearing and colleagues successfully performed ultrasound phaco through two 1.0 mm incisions using a modified anterior chamber maintainer and a phaco tip without the irrigation sleeve.[3] They reported a series of 53 cases and found that phaco time, overall surgical time, total fluid use and endothelial cell loss were comparable to those measured with their standard phaco techniques. Crozafon described the use of Teflon-coated phaco tips for bimanual high-frequency pulsed phaco and suggested that these tips would reduce friction and therefore allow surgery with a sleeveless needle.[4] Tsuneoka, Shiba and Takahashi determined the feasibility of using a 1.4 mm (19 gauge) incision and a 20 gauge sleeveless ultrasound tip to perform phaco.[5] They found that outflow around the tip through the incision provided adequate cooling, and performed this procedure in 637 cases with no incidence of wound burn.[6] Additionally, less surgically induced astigmatism developed in the eyes operated with the bimanual technique. Agarwal and colleagues developed a bimanual technique, "Phakonit," using an irrigating chopper and a bare phaco needle passed through a 0.9 clear corneal incision.[7] They achieved adequate temperature control through continuous infusion and use of "cooled balanced salt solution" poured over the phaco needle.

Soscia, Howard and Olson have shown in cadaver eye studies that phacoemulsification with the Sovereign WhiteStar system (Abbott Medical Optics Inc., USA), using a bare 19 gauge aspiration needle, does not produce a wound burn at the highest energy settings unless all infusion and aspiration are occluded due to the limited duration of energy pulses this technology delivers.[8,9]

There are many advantages of B-MICS. These include enhanced chamber stability—thanks to a more nearly perfectly closed system, better followability due to separation of infusion and aspiration and access to 360° of the anterior segment with either infusion or aspiration by switching instruments from one hand to the other. Furthermore, it permits using the flow of irrigation fluid as a tool to move material within the capsular bag or anterior chamber, prevention of iris billowing and prolapse in cases of intraoperative floppy iris syndrome (IFIS), and significantly decreased chance of vitreous prolapse in the case of a posterior capsular tear, zonular dialysis or subluxed cataracts—thanks to maintenance of a pressurized stream of irrigation from above.

Separation of irrigation from the aspirating phaco needle allows for improved followability by avoiding competing currents at the tip of the needle. In some instances, the irrigation flow from the second handpiece can be used as a gentle adjunctive surgical device—flushing nuclear pieces from the angle or loosening epinuclear or cortical material from the capsular bag while minimizing trauma to delicate intraocular structures. In refractive lens exchange (RLE) the lens material may be washed completely out of the bag and extracted with aspiration and vacuum only, so that no ultrasound is used and no instrument enters the endocapsular space, increasing the safety profile of this demanding procedure.[10]

A separate infusion stream is also beneficial when scrubbing troublesome plaques from the posterior capsule. Focusing the flow of fluid on the posterior capsule and putting the tissue on stretch facilitates capsule polishing with either a roughened or silicone-covered aspiration tip without entrapping the taut posterior capsule.

Perhaps the greatest advantage of the biaxial technique lies in its ability to remove subincisional cortex without difficulty. Brauweiler originally described switching infusion and aspiration handpieces between two microincisions as a means of reaching 360° of the capsular fornices and making cortical clean-up quick and safe.[11]

The ability to switch hands is also a significant advantage to instructors, who may find they must take over a case from a resident with opposite manual dominance.

Utilization of B-MICS offers an enormous advantage of maintaining a more stable intraocular environment during lens removal. This may be especially important in high myopes who are at a greater risk for retinal detachment following lens extraction. By maintaining a formed and pressurized anterior chamber throughout the procedure, there should be fewer tendencies for anterior movement of the vitreous body with a theoretical lower incidence of posterior vitreous detachment occurring from intraoperative manipulations, although future studies in this regard are warranted.

Finally, B-MICS is advantageous when IFIS occurs. Keeping the irrigator high in the anterior chamber tamponades the iris and keeps it from becoming floppy. As long as surgeons irrigate above the iris, it will not billow. Alternatively, surgeons can hydroexpress the cataract out of the capsular bag and carousel the endonucleus in the plane of the capsulorhexis. So that the epinucleus holds the iris back. In those IFIS cases where author cannot hydroexpress the lens, he dilates the pupil widely with Healon 5 (Abbott Medical Optics, Inc., USA), do their hydrosteps, and then perform one endolenticular chop. Next, author brings the nuclear material up to the irrigating chopper, which is kept above the iris, for disassembly and mobilization. The pupil can be redilated with Healon 5 in the case of constriction following epinucleus removal. By keeping the aspiration tip in occlusion, author goes circumferentially around the capsulorhexis, mobilizing cortex from the capsular fornices without bringing it out of the eye. Maintaining occlusion of the tip, immobilizes Healon 5, thus allowing the pupil to remain dilated. After the cortex has been removed from the fornix, author then removes it from the eye.

While the advantages described above relate principally to separation of irrigation from aspiration, some of the other major advantages of B-MICS relate to incision size. For example, there has been an improvement in control of most of the steps involved in endocapsular surgery due to increase chamber stability. Since viscoelastics do not leave the eye easily through these small incisions, the anterior chamber is more stable during capsulorhexis construction, and there is much less likelihood for an errant rhexis to develop. This added margin of safety is particularly noticeable in cases of zonular compromise such as pseudoexfoliation, traumatic zonular dialysis and after glaucoma filtering surgery, as well as in cases of intumescent cataract and nanophthalmos with a very shallow anterior chamber. The added chamber stability can also make a difference in control of the capsulorhexis in high myopia with an extremely deep anterior chamber and floppy capsule. Hydrodelineation and hydrodissection can also be performed more efficiently by virtue of a higher level of pressure building in the anterior chamber prior to eventual prolapse of viscoelastic through the microincisions.

In order to reap the benefit of these advantages, strict attention to detail is required. The first technique to master is construction of the incision. There is variability in incision size depending on the gauge of instrumentation used. Author prefers 20 gauge because he feels it offers greater control. Because the outer diameter of the 20 gauge tip is 0.9 mm, the circumference of the tip is 2.8 mm and the incision must measure 1.4 mm. An incision smaller than 1.4 mm stretches and tears causing loss of self-sealability. These microincisions are converted from a line to a circle upon introduction of the tip, and author wants them to resume the configuration of a line when the tip is withdrawn. Compromise the corneal collagen by stretching or tearing will reduce the likelihood that the incision will resume its virgin architecture at the end of the case. This can be minimized by using only trapezoidal-shaped incisions.

Capsulorhexis construction represents a significant hurdle in the biaxial learning curve. However, microincision capsulorhexis forceps permit a greater degree of precision and control, so much so that author advocates their use with any size of incision. The pinch type initiation of the capsulorhexis is particularly valuable in cases of zonular compromise since the forces acting on the capsule remain balanced. Even with a severely wrinkling capsule due to traumatic zonular dialysis, these extraordinarily delicate forceps permit moment-by-moment control of the capsulorhexis. This is important because capsulorhexis size is an important determinant of final lens position and therefore postoperative refractive status. Using microincisions enhances the precision of capsulorhexis construction not only because of the improvements in instrumentation, but also because there is not a tendency for the chamber to shallow as often occurs with a 2.5 mm incision due to return of viscoelastic.

As stated previously, the goal of cortical cleaving hydrodissection is to lyse the equatorial capsular-cortical connections, which will generally allow aspiration of the cortex, along with the mobilization of the epinucleus.

Hydrodelineation is performed to allow free mobility of the endonucleus within the epinuclear shell, allowing endocapsular nuclear disassembly within the safety cushion of the epinucleus. Hydrodissection and hydrodelineation may be performed just as described above for standard small incision surgery; the microincisions do allow egress of viscoelastic during this step so that there is not an increase risk of blowing out the posterior capsule due to over-pressurization. Of note, author found that the intraocular pressure during hydrodissection, as measured in the vitreous cavity of a cadaver eye, varies around means of 78–223 mm Hg regardless of whether a standard small incision or microincision are employed.[12] These were among the highest pressures that author recorded during the entire phacoemulsification and intraocular lens (IOL) implantation procedure. Clearly, if viscoelastic is prevented from exiting the eye, there is adequate pressure to rupture the capsule. This represents a special concern to users of high zero-shear-viscosity ophthalmic viscosurgical devices, who should ensure that a path for egress is prepared with a track of balanced salt solution from the cannula tip to the incision.

The surprising fact about horizontal and vertical chopping techniques with biaxial phaco is how little they differ in terms of hand movement from standard small incision coaxial phaco. Seeing the bulkier irrigating chopper in the eye and getting used to the heavier feel in one's hand represent the major differences; the actual chopping techniques are the same. The stream of irrigation fluid from the chopper or manipulator can function as an efficient tool within the eye and is one of the most significant advantages of biaxial phaco, a key reason to abandon coaxial. In particular, washing subincisional endo- or epinuclear material into range of the phaco tip permits enhanced safety and control. An example is RLE with an accommodative IOL in high myopia, probably the situation in which author is most concerned about maintaining the integrity of the capsule. Not only would compromising the capsule increase the risk of posterior segment complications but it may also result in an inability to implant the IOL of choice for the procedure. With biaxial RLE, no instrument other than a cannula and a stream of fluid ever need to enter the endolenticular or endocapsular space; author can hydroexpress the soft lens material into the anterior chamber with the stream of irrigation fluid and carousel it safely from the eye with fluidics alone. Cortical cleaving hydrodissection achieves a clean capsule without ever placing an aspiration tip below the level of the capsulorhexis and the absence of ultrasound energy allows for the safest, most minimally invasive procedure possible, both exemplifying the enhanced margin of safety with this approach.

If there is a breach of the posterior capsule, however residual lens material can generally be removed while maintaining irrigation in the anterior chamber and disallowing vitreous prolapse. With biaxial phaco it is possible to switch from a phaco tip to an aspirator to a vitrector if necessary without ever compromising chamber stability. The approach, once a tear is recognized, consists of continuous irrigation in the anterior chamber while lens material is removed from the bag. Once the bag is clean, a dispersive viscoelastic is injected at the level of the posterior capsule while irrigation is still maintained; only once the viscoelastic has fully tamponaded the break and filled the chamber, the irrigator is removed. The IOL can then be inserted into the ciliary sulcus or the capsule through a standard temporal clear corneal incision. In the case of sulcus placement the optic is pushed posteriorly through the capsulorhexis prior to final clean up. Once viscoelastic is removed, the triamcinolone staining technique described by Burk is utilized to ensure a completely vitreous-free environment in the anterior segment.[13]

Author has found this technique to be simple, efficacious and safe since most of the lens extraction is occurring in the plane of the iris, away from the posterior capsule and the corneal endothelium. Nevertheless, details are very important with this technique as it is not very forgiving. Consider these concepts in beginning to apply B-MICS:

- Balancing inflow and outflow is critical. Most initial difficulties relate to chamber stability and fluid dynamics
- Conversations with an experienced B-MICS surgeon are extremely helpful—both for preparation before and for troubleshooting after the initial cases
- Surgical equipment representatives are a very good resource for technical information
- Have a phaco machine surgical representative, especially one with B-MICS experience, present in the operating room for the first few cases to adjust the machine settings during surgery as needed. This leaves the nurses/technicians free to concentrate on the new procedure steps and equipment
- Decrease aspiration flow rates for initial B-MICS cases because, due to the smaller caliber of the irrigator, effective aspiration flow rates are higher with B-MICS than in coaxial phaco. This results in faster movement of material within the eye at a given aspiration setting

- Decrease the vacuum setting for initial B-MICS cases to help prevent chamber fluctuations due to postocclusion surge. Once the flow parameters are worked out and the chamber is stable, vacuum can be gradually increased again.
- The phaco tip is used without a sleeve, but it is useful to place a cutoff sleeve on the phaco handpiece to prevent spraying of balanced salt solution during ultrasound. The sleeve must be cut off very close to the hub—if the stump of the sleeve is longer than about 1 mm, it can limit the phaco tip's excursion into the eye.
- Initially, B-MICS makes nuclear disassembly easier in some aspects and more difficult in others. It is made easier by improved chamber stability and followability, and it is made more difficult by the bulkier irrigating choppers and smaller, more restrictive incisions. Once adjusted to the instruments and smaller incisions, however B-MICS is a superior technique for nuclear disassembly.

Examining each step in a model case enhances understanding. Following hydrodissection and hydrodelineation, the phaco needle is first embedded proximally with high vacuum and 40% power. In the left hand is a vertical chopper which will be used to split the nucleus in two. As vacuum builds to occlusion a rapid rise time enables the phaco needle to quickly grasp the endonucleus. At the point occlusion is reached the aspiration flow rate drops to zero. Author then moves into foot position two so that high vacuum is maintained and the power goes to zero. The blade of the irrigating vertical chopper is brought down just distal to the phaco tip as author lifts up slightly with the phaco needle. As a full thickness cleavage plane develops, dividing the nucleus in two, author separates his hands to ensure a complete chop.

The lens can then be rotated with the irrigating chopper so that the first heminucleus can be chopped and consumed. If there is a disparity in size, the larger half is moved distally and a quadrant size piece is chopped off and consumed. The remaining quadrant of the first heminucleus is then impaled with the phaco tip and aspirated. Total effective phaco time (EPT), or the amount of time that ultrasound would have been turned on had it been running on 100% continuous power, is a useful parameter to follow and to this point was less than half a second. That means author used about half a second of the maximum ultrasound power that the machine can produce to remove half of the nucleus thereby minimizing thermal injury and maximizing safety.

The second half of the nucleus is next addressed by rotating it with the irrigating chopper so that it is in the distal capsule. The phaco needle is embedded in the smaller heminucleus which is then subdivided with the irrigating chopper, again using high vacuum and low levels of power. As the final quadrant is grasped and pulled centrally for aspiration, the sharp blade of the irrigating chopper is turned sideways as a safety precaution.

When addressing the epinucleus, author reduces his settings, turns down the vacuum and flow rate and trims the rim of the epinucleus, preventing the epinucleus from flipping into the phaco needle with the stream of irrigation fluid or the irrigating chopper itself. The advantage of the trimming procedure lies in the aspiration of cortical material from behind the epinuclear shell. In most cases this step eliminates the need for irrigation/aspiration prior to IOL insertion. Once three quadrants of the epinuclear shell have been rotated and trimmed the final quadrant is used to flip the epinuclear bowl into the phaco needle. Following aspiration of the epinucleus, the capsule is entirely clean of cortex.

In conclusion, B-MICS with a vertical chop technique allows efficient lens extraction with rapid visual rehabilitation. This procedure demonstrates some of the tangible benefits of separating inflow from outflow, use of irrigation fluid as an instrument to mobilize material and reduced effective phaco time.

References

1. Girard LJ. Ultrasonic fragmentation for cataract extraction and cataract complications. Adv Ophthalmol. 1978;37:127-35.
2. Girard LJ. Pars plana lensectomy by ultrasonic fragmentation: 1984--Part II: Operative and postoperative complications--avoidance or management. Ophthalmic Surg. 1984;15:217-20.
3. Shearing SP, Relyea RL, Loaiza A, et al. Routine phacoemulsification through a one-millimeter non-sutured incision. Cataract. 1985;2:6-11.
4. Crozafon P. The use of minimal stress and the Teflon-coated tip for bimanual high frequency pulsed phacoemulsification, presented at the 14th Meeting of the Japanese Society of Cataract and Refractive Surgery, Kyoto, Japan, July 1999.
5. Tsuneoka H, Shiba T, Takahashi Y. Feasibility of ultrasound cataract surgery with a 1.4 mm incision. J Cataract Refract Surg. 2001;27:934-40.

6. Tsuneoka H, Shiba T, Takahashi Y. Ultrasonic phacoemulsification using a 1.4 mm incision: clinical results. J Cataract Refract Surg. 2002;28:81-6.
7. Agarwal A, Agarwal A, Agarwal S, et al. Phakonit: phacoemulsification through a 0.9 mm corneal incision. J Cataract Refract Surg. 2001;27:1548-52.
8. Soscia W, Howard JG, Olson RJ. Bimanual phacoemulsification through 2 stab incision. A wound-temperature study. J Cataract Refract Surg. 2002;28:1039-49.
9. Soscia W, Howard JG, Olson RJ. Microphacoemulsification with WhiteStar. A wound-temperature study. J Cataract Refract Surg. 2002;28:1044-6.
10. Fine IH, Hoffman RS, Packer M. Optimizing refractive lens exchange with bimanual microincision phaco-emulsification. J Cataract Refract Surg. 2004;30:550-4.
11. Brauweiler P. Bimanual irrigation/aspiration. J Cataract Refract Surg. 1996;22(8):1013-6.
12. Khng C, Packer M, Fine IH, et al. Intraocular pressure during phacoemulsification. J Cataract Refract Surg. 2006;32(2):301-8.
13. Burk SE, Da Mata AP, Snyder ME, et al. Visualizing vitreous using Kenalog suspension. J Cataract Refract Surg 2003;29(4):645-51.

8

MICS (Minimally Invasive Cataract Surgery): How to Perform the Transition? Which Instruments should I Use? How to Use the Phaco Machine?

Jorge L Alio (Spain)

The Continuous Transition of Cataract Surgery

Cataract surgery is one of the most frequently performed surgeries and millions of the eyes are operated each year in the entire world. The first modern cataract surgery was done by Sir Harold Ridley in 1949 with the implantation of the first polymethylmethacrylate (PMMA) intraocular lens (IOL). The incision was longer than 10 mm, the IOL was not perfect, and the surgery was complicated.

The spectacular progress of the cataract surgery technique in the 1980 and 1990 of the twentieth century leads to diminish the surgical trauma and percentage of the complications connected to the maneuvers and energy delivered into the eye. The technical progresses made possible to think about diminish the incision size. The idea to make the cataract surgery bimanually without phaco tip sleeve was started in the end of the 1980. This method was described by Shearing in 1985. But the idea of diversification of the liquid was the main step to develop new surgical techniques, new surgical tools and new surgical possibilities.

Better visual outcome, aggressiveness surgery, separated infusion, minimal phaco power, new surgical tools and fluidics management evoke new idea of surgery—microincision cataract surgery (MICS).

In 2001 Jorge Alio registered the concept of MICS as the surgery performed through incisions of 1.8 mm or less. Understanding this global concept implies that it is not only about achieving a smaller incision size but also about making a global transformation of the surgical procedure towards minimal aggressiveness.

Separated fluidics, high volume of the liquids and high vacuum also become in the new tool. Especially in the case of the soft cataracts lens opacities classification system I or II (LOCS I or II) the use of the ultrasound can be diminished or practically eliminated. The high vacuum and infusion chopper use permits the mass breaking and aspiration without ultrasound power. The phacoemulsification of the harder grade of the cataract needs to be supported by minimal doses of the ultrasound energy. Nowadays the small doses of the ultrasound power and MICS concept can eliminate the phaco tip overheating and the thermal injury of the cornea. These ideas diminish surgical trauma and improve cataract surgery refractive result.

The complications with MICS can occur during learning curve. Transition to MICS needs to understand the principles of MICS ideas and technique. In the first time of transition, the problems with fluidics, anterior chamber stability and wound integrity can occur.[1,2]

The Transition to Microincision Cataract Surgery

Incision

Diminishing of incision is the most interesting and important parameter of the modern surgery. Following the minimization idea smaller incision means lower wound dimension, less eye traumatism and faster healing.

Small wound construction satisfies the principles of the self-sealing incision. The wound closing is more efficient and the leakage is not observed in short period of postoperative time. The watertight construction of the wound diminishes the iris prolapses complications. Faster wound healing reduces possibility of the bacterial infection. The reduction of the surgically induced astigmatism (SIA) by the small incision becomes more important advantage in the field of cataract and refractive lens surgery.[3]

Reduction of the cataract surgery incision leads to:

- Corneal tissue damage reduction
- Faster recovery of the wound
- Higher stability of the eye during surgery
- Easier capsulorhexis, hydrodissection performance
- Diminishing of the postoperative complications
  - (a) Wound leakage
  - (b) Risk of endophthalmitis
  - (c) Surgically induced astigmatism
- Improves optical quality of the cornea

The idea of the small incision leads to progress in the instruments adaptation, machine construction, software programming. The small incision demands new technology of the foldable lenses. In the future probably it will make the incision smaller.[2-4]

Fluidics

The fluid management is essential in MICS. The proper setup of machine with the balanced values protects the eye and helps the surgeon to pass through the all stages of the surgery without complications.

The fluid inflow should be balanced by outflow, but the balance should be corrected based on the sufficient eye ball tension. The pressure of the infusion should make the infusion larger than the outflow of the liquid. This difference between inflow and outflow keeps the proper anatomy of the anterior segment of the eye and becomes the powerful tool in the breaking of the cataract masses. During the occlusion high under pressure in the phaco aspiration tip can break the masses without using of ultrasound power. At this moment fluidics become powerful tool in the process of the surgery. MICS fluidics is more efficient than in the micro coaxial surgery. The gas forced infusion (GFI) support is obligatory in the MICS surgery. The continuous flow of the infusion liquid is supported by the gas which is delivered with

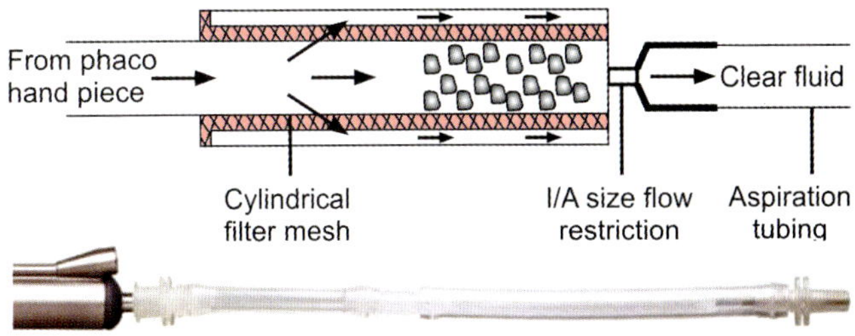

Fig. 1: Cruise Control™ System (STAAR Surgical Company, Monrovia, CA, USA) and Stable Chamber™ System (Bausch & Lomb Inc. Rochester, NY, USA)

the pressure to the infusion bottle. The GFI helps to stabilize and maintain the inflow of the liquid on the high level. This keeps the anterior chamber constant and permits to cool the tip. It equilibrates the intraocular pressure (IOP) during the whole surgery. It is very important to keep IOP stable in the case of severe retinal degenerations, proliferative vitreoretinopathy (PVR), neovascularizations and vascular diseases. Deregulation of the pressure can lead to anterior chamber collapse and intrasurgical hypotony of the eye like in the standard coaxial phacoemulsification.

Some of the platforms such as the Accurus or Millennium are supported by internal pump. The Infinity platform needs to be supported by external air pump connected with the air filter.

Other fluid problem is the postocclusion time and problems connected to the high vacuum and insufficient inflow. This dangerous circumstance can happen when occluded mass is aspirated suddenly by the tip and the pressure of the anterior chamber suddenly decreases. Some phaco machines have software to prevent the surge. The Abbott Medical Optics (AMO) Sovereign has virtual model of anterior chamber and in the moment of occlusion the pump decreases the vacuum. The use of the Flow Restrictors can also solve the problem. The restrictor can be connected to the aspiration tube. Small filters restrict the flow, and surge does not exceed the limit values. The possibility of the anterior chamber collapse and rupture of the posterior capsule is practically eliminated[5] (Fig. 1).

Power Modulation

Varying the power modulation during phacoemulsification can be safe and efficient method to improve the efficacy of cataract surgery. Pulsing ultrasound can dramatically diminish energy delivered into the eye. Changing on, off-times and shortening the time of pulse surgeon can achieve better result in cataract mass emulsification and corneal wound and endothelial cell protection. It is very important that very short power modulation like hyper pulse and ultra pulse can dramatically decrease possibility of wound burn during MICS surgery. During the on-time cycle the cornea is heating but during the off-time cycle phaco tip and cornea are cooling. Also short pulse energy seems to be more effective because it produces more cavitational energy than continuous power. The use of torsional phaco can additionally diminish the delivered energy. With use of torsional phaco, practically surgeon can eliminate the longitudinal ultrasound power or use it only in minimal way with the hard cataract. The active use of power modulation seems to change MICS to more efficient surgery.[5,6]

Microincision Cataract Surgery Instruments

MICS is bimanual procedure. Two incisions with the same diameter allow using the same instruments by the both wounds. This advantage is very helpful to clean the anterior and posterior capsule, remove cortical and nuclear fragments. The access to all regions of the anterior segment is ideal. The construction of the instrument permits to perfect maneuvers and liquid steam direction protects the posterior capsule integrity and endothelium stability.

MICS 18G

To perform MICS surgery, surgeons can use two types of the instruments depending on the incision size preferred by them. Surgeons can use tools for standard MICS (18 G instruments) and micro-MICS (22 G instruments).

To perform standard MICS 18 G surgery, surgeon needs instruments specially designed for 1.5 mm incision. To make incision the calibrated knife is necessary. The Alio MICS Knife (Katena Products, Inc. Denville, NJ, USA) has trapezoid shape 1.25 mm/1.4 mm/2.0 mm, which is necessary to make incision of the desired shape and dimensions. The other opportunity is the diamond knife with the same proportions. (Figs 2 and 3).

The shape and dimension of the knives permit to make incision which is perfectly adapted to the MICS phaco tip of 0.9 mm. The incision is watertight, keeps the anterior chamber stable and permits perfectly the maneuvering in the anterior chamber. The borders of the incision are perfectly adapted to close without suturing. The small amount of the fluid during hydration ascertain in incision closing.

Continuous curvilinear capsulorhexis (CCC) is essential in the each type of the phaco surgery. To make the capsulorhexis through the 1.25 mm incision, the micro forceps is obligatory. The Alio MICS Capsulorhexis Forceps (Katena Products, Inc. Denville, NJ, USA) is 23G tool. This instrument is perfectly perpetrated to do tearing of the anterior capsule by the pointed catch which is situated at the end of the forceps. The CCC is easy with this thin and delicate forceps (Fig. 4).

During each capsulorhexis, the maintaining of the stable anterior chamber is essential. The disproportion between incision and tool can make conduct to the ophthalmic viscosurgical devices (OVD) leakage during the CCC and tear the capsule outside. With the 1.25 mm incision and 23G instrument practically it does not happen.

Hydrodissection and hydrodelineation are the next stage of the surgery which permit to separate the lens from the capsule and divide the lens layers. This maneuver can be done by each type of the cannula preferred by surgeon but the washout of the OVD from the anterior chamber before is essential. The small incision and high density of the OVD can block the incision and lead to the increase the pressure in the anterior chamber and be dangerous for the stability of the posterior capsule.

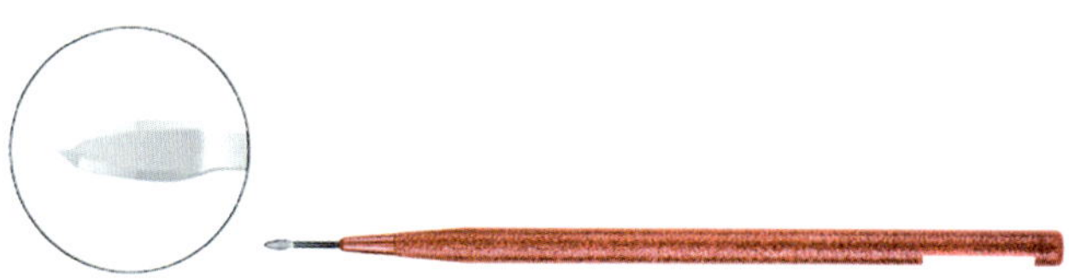

Fig. 2: Alio MICS metal knife (Katena Products, Inc. Denville, NJ, USA)

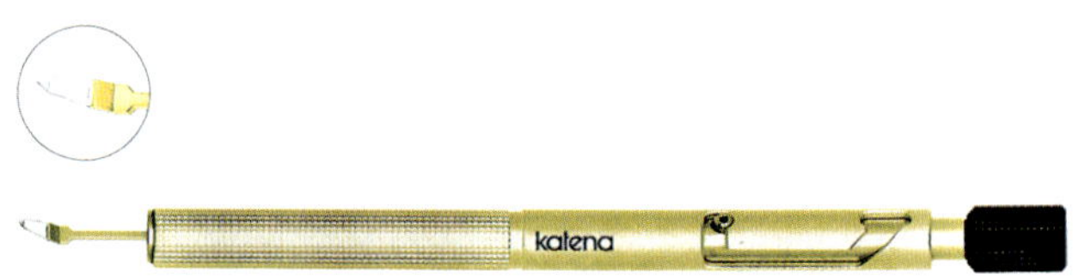

Fig. 3: Alio MICS diamond knife (Katena Products, Inc. Denville, NJ, USA)

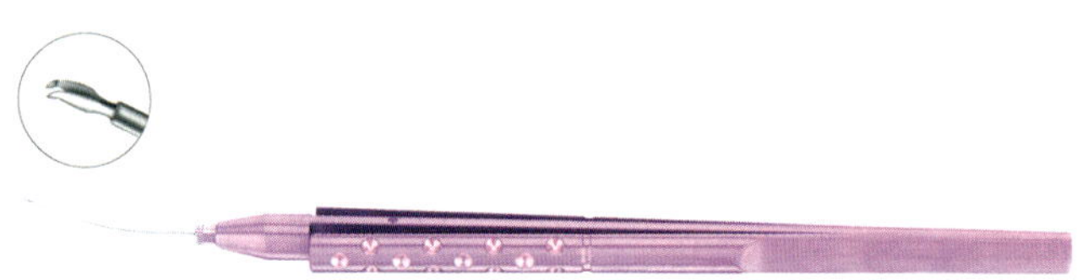

Fig. 4: Alio MICS Capsulorhexis forceps (Ketana Products, Inc. Denville, NJ, USA)

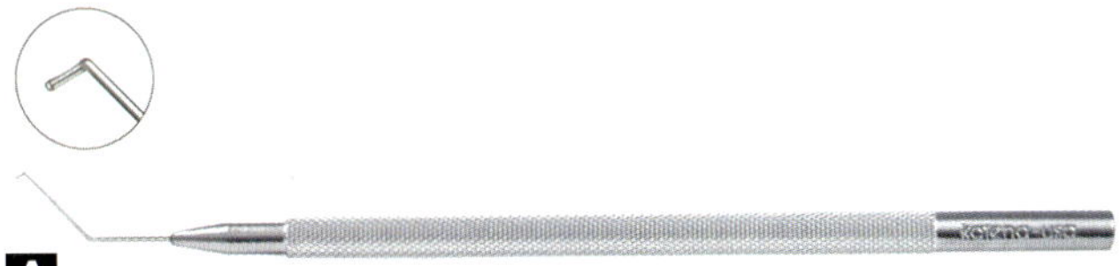

A

B

Figs 5A and B: (A) Alio-Rosen MICS Phaco Prechopper, and (B) Alio Scimitar Prechopper microincision cataract surgery (Katena Products, Inc. Denville, NJ, USA)

Prechopping can facilitate the surgery. This stage of the surgery is based on the mechanical division of the lens by the two prechoppers. This simple maneuver can be done by Alio-Rosen MICS Phaco Prechopper (Katena Products, Inc. Denville, NJ, USA) or by Alio Scimitar MICS Prechoppers (Katena Products, Inc. Denville, NJ, USA) (Figs 5A and B).

The shape of Scimitar prechopper is designed to perform and facilitate the 700 μ surgery. The Scimitar prechopper has a curved tip with a blunt end and a sharp inferior edge. The choppers are crossed by situating symmetrically opposite oneself. Now, cutting movements are being made by gently crossing prechoppers. The cut will be made from the perimeter to the center of the nuclei. Internal edge has a sharp edge that facilitates the incisions of the lens masses. When the cut is made, two dividing hemispheres are made. The nucleus is then rotated about 90º and then for the second time prechopping is repeated as described.

Next stage of the surgery is phacoemulsification of the cataract lens. MICS permits to do surgery bimanually. One port is for the irrigating chopper and the second is for the aspiration phaco tip without the silicon sleeve. MICS gives opportunity to perform phacoemulsification from both sides, by right and left hand any time at all stages of surgery. It depends on corneal astigmatism, surgeon preferences, intraoperative conditions.

For the standard MICS surgery, surgeons use two types of the irrigating choppers: Alio original Fingernail MICS Irrigating Hydromanipulator, and Alio MICS Irrigating Stinger (Katena Products, Inc. Denville, NJ, USA) (Figs 6 and 7).

First irrigating hydromanipulator fingernail helps to remove rather soft cataracts. There is irrigation hole on the bottom lower side of the tool. The hole's diameter is 1 mm. It has also very thin walls to increase internal diameter of instrument. This irrigation cannula is assuring infusion in borders 72 cc/min. A large infusion directed to the bottom assures the excellent flow of liquids and also a fast and effective chilling phacoemulsification tip. An outstanding stability of the anterior chamber is assured through the function infusion and directs the liquid to the lens masses at the bag back, independently from high vacuum sets of phacoemulsification machine. The strength of the stream permits the bag to be held in a safe distance from the phacoemulsification tip and at the same time enables convenient manipulations of tools and lens masses. Additionally, this stream can clean the back bag from remaining cortical cells. A very fertile directed stream to the back bag is provided with the preservation of cells endothelium corneas before mechanical and thermal damage. The irrigation hole can be found situated on the side of the irrigating probe or on top and this can result in the turbulences in the anterior chamber. This effect can damage the endothelium cells and stabilities of the anterior chamber.

The tool which allows the removal of harder cataracts is Alio MICS Irrigating Stinger. This tool has a 19G diameter, and it is equipped with a tip at the end which is angled downwards. This tool is useful to chop off segments or dividing masses of the nucleus in the phacoemulsification tip.

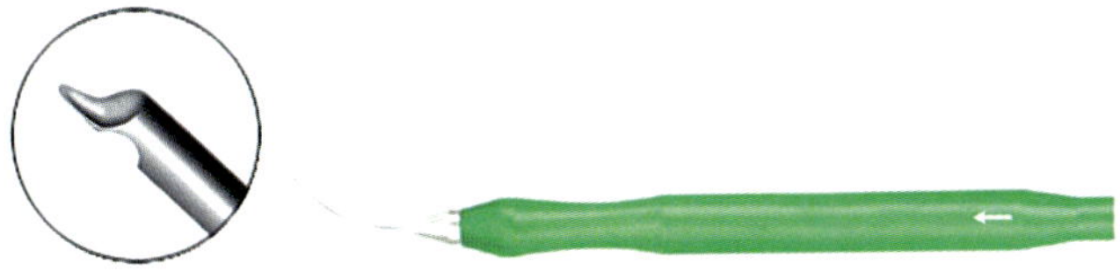

Fig. 6: Alio original Fingernail MICS Irrigating Hydromanipulator (Katena Products, Inc. Denville, NJ, USA). Not in use now

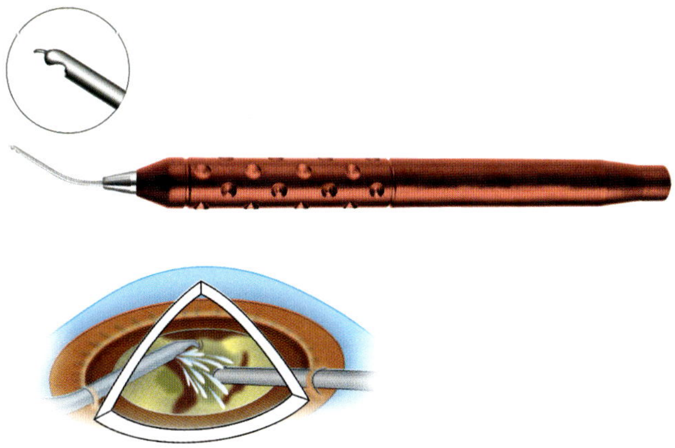

Fig. 7: Alio MICS Irrigating Stinger (Katena Products, Inc. Denville, NJ, USA)

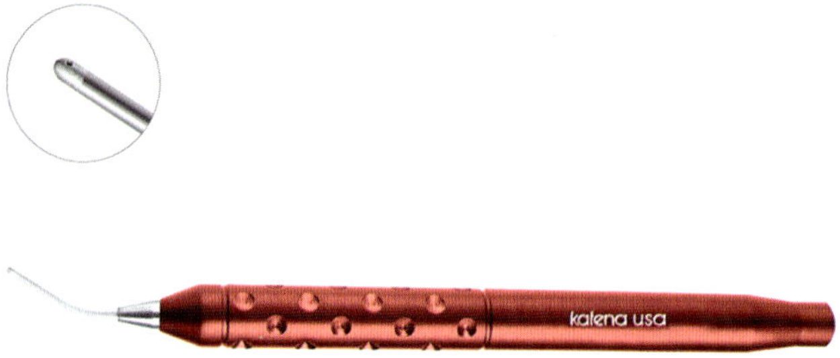

Fig. 8: Alio MICS Aspiration Handpiece (Katena Products, Inc. Denville, NJ, USA)

For removing remains of cortical masses is serving Alio MICS Aspiration Handpiece (Katena Products, Inc. Denville, NJ, the USA) (Fig. 8).

There is a tool especially designed for delicate and safe manipulations within the anterior chamber. It has a diameter of 18G. The cylindrical shape allows this tool to gently manipulate within the surgical wound. At the same time the port diameter of 0.3 mm assures the stability of the hydrodynamic of liquid within the anterior chamber. This handpiece allows to remove remained masses from the bag and the full comfort of polishing the bag back.[7]

MICS 22G

The Alio Stinger irrigating chopper Duet System (Redmond, Washington, USA) is the 22G inferior opening instrument. It has one hole on the inferior side of the cannula and provides the infusion stream directly backward, forcing cataract fragments to levitate towards the phaco tip pointed to masses and posterior capsule. This also allows maintaining anterior chamber deep and holding the capsule far from the phaco-tip. The fluid infusion with GFI is sufficient for 0.7 mm MICS demand. The end of the stinger is equipped with a pointed tip which is angled downwards. It enables to break masses with ease and provide them to aspiration hole[7] (Fig. 9).

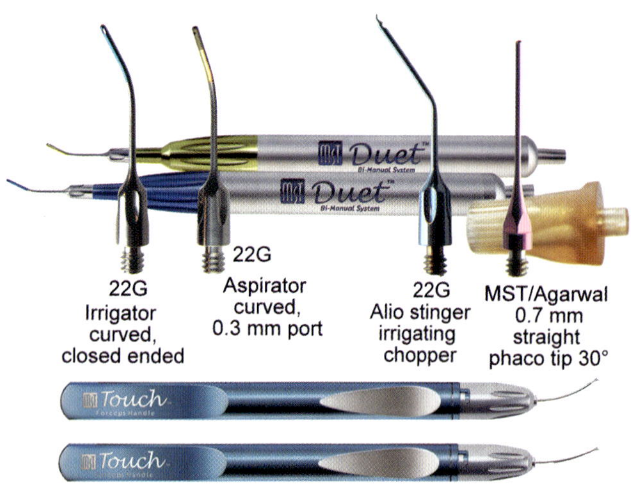

Fig. 9: The 0.7 mm (22 G) Duet® System Alio Stinger Irrigating Chopper

Microincision Cataract Surgery Phacoemulsification Platforms

Microincision cataract surgery can be made with the help of practically each type of the phaco platforms supported by venturi pump. This type of the pump is very powerful and effective in the vacuum construction. The surgery on venturi pump machine is the high vacuum and constant vacuum surgery. The vacuum about 550 mm Hg is very easy to achieve in few milliseconds in all of these types of machines. Other types of the pumps like peristaltic are not such effective.

In the case of soft cataracts having placed under pressure of 500–550 mm Hg, surgeons can only use Alio MICS hydromanipulator irrigating fingernail. This makes it possible to divide and aspirate fragment masses of the lens without using ultrasound or using ultrasound in the minimum way. The torsional phacoemulsification with the oscillatory, mechanically moving tip can be helpful. Ultrasound energy can be eliminated. The Kelman Tip and Infinity System (Alcon Laboratories, Inc.) equipped with OZil energy are preferred. In the case of hard cataracts, when total occlusion tip is not causing aspiration of masses, stinger Alio MICS irrigating chopper would be more useful. This headpiece has a narrow edge at the end which divides the masses and allows easy aspiration of the phacoemulsification tip. The fragmented elements of the hard cataracts are now easily aspirated using the high under pressure and in rare moments using of the ultrasound energy. Usually, MICS is performed with up to 4% ultrasound power and fewer than 10 seconds of real phacoemulsification time.

Alcon Accurus 600

This device functions very well in MICS. Accurus device has the exerted inflow, high rate of the under pressure, advanced steering pump and fast efficiently in reacting. This system is very useful for the MICS surgery. In the table, author offers settings for cataract grade 3 (LOCS III) (Table 1).

TABLE 1 Accurus 600 Alcon settings for 19G MICS

Quad	Phacoemulsification power	20%
	Vacuum	300 mm Hg
	Irrigation	90
	Mode burst	30 ms

TABLE 2 Infinity Alcon settings for 19G MICS

Chop	Phacoemulsification power	0
	Dynamic rise	0
	Vacuum	150
	Irrigation	110
	Torsional amplitude	Limit 40 On: 20 Off: 40
	Aspiration rate	15
Quad	Phacoemulsification power	0
	Dynamic rise	2
	Vacuum	500
	Irrigation	110
	Torsional amplitude	Limit 80 On: 20 Off: 40
	Aspiration rate	30
Epi	Phacoemulsification power	0
	Vacuum	28
	Irrigation	110
	Torsional amplitude	Limit 30 On: 20 Off: 40
	Aspiration rate	28

Note: For 21G MICS forced air infusion with air pump is necessary

Alcon Infinity

This is a device with a highly efficient pump and good software which is effective in practice. The torsional phaco is the system which perfectly complements need to diminish the surgical trauma during cataract surgery. This lateral movement system of the phacoemulsification tip practically eliminates the ultrasound energy. For infinity most useful settings are shown in Table 2.

Bausch & Lomb Millennium

The Millennium is also adapted to lead the operation in the MICS mode. This highly efficient device has the software which reduces the power of ultrasound used for a surgery. It has modes: pulse, singles burst, fixed burst and multiple burst. The Millennium updated by the mode pulsed, pulse lets for creating the model of cycle 250 milliseconds "on-time". It is a cut which considerably reduces the energy. In Table 3, standard settings for MICS are shown.

TABLE 3 Millennium Bausch & Lomb settings for 19G MICS

Sculpture	Bottle height	100 cm
	Maximum bottle infusion	40 mm Hg
	Fixed vacuum	200 mm Hg
	Fixed ultrasound	10%
	Duration	20 ms
	Duty cycle	60%
Quadrant	Bottle height	100 cm
	Maximum bottle infusion	40 mm Hg
	Fixed vacuum	470 mm Hg
	Fixed ultrasound	10%
	Duration	20 ms
	Duty cycle	60%
I/A	Bottle height	80 cm
	Maximum bottle infusion	40 mm Hg
	Maximum vacuum	550 mm Hg

Note: For 21G MICS forced air infusion with air pump is necessary

AMO Sovereign WhiteStar

The WhiteStar device is working well in mode of ultra pulse around 6 milliseconds on and 12 milliseconds off. For this device a height of the bottle is 90 cm, aspiration flow rate 26 mL/min, vacuum for nuclear emulsification 400 mm Hg, and for epinucleus 200 mm Hg.

MICS Intraocular Lenses

MICS cataract surgery develops postoperative astigmatism in the minimal way. In up to 80% of MICS patients the corneal astigmatism is less then 0.5 D. Only the 25% of coaxial cataract surgery patients have astigmatism less than 0.5 D. MICS is the useful method to do a cataract surgery with refractive surgery. MICS caused the foldable lenses evolution and now they can be implanted through 1.5 mm incision or less (Table 4). The lenses should fulfill the high technology. Most of them are made of hydrophilic acrylic biomaterial. But only some of them can be used to MICS incision. Compression during injecting can damage the lens. The lens ruptures can occur. Decompression can also be a matter of damage of the lens. For MICS IOL, it should fulfill the following requirements. The IOL should be implantable through a sub 2.0 mm incision.

Table 4 Microincision intraocular lenses

No.	Name of the Lens	Company
1	Zeiss-Acri.Tec MICS IOLs Family	Zeiss-Acri.Tec, Berlin, Germany
2	Akreos AO Microincision MI60	Bausch & Lomb, Rochester, New York, USA
3	IOLtech MICS lens	IOLtech, La Rochelle, France and Carl Zeiss Meditec, Stuttgart, Germany
4	TetraFlex KH-3500 and ZR-1000	Lenstec, St. Petersburg, Florida, USA
5	MicroSlim, SlimFlex IOL	PhysIOL, Liège, Belgium
6	CareFlex IOL	W20 Medizintechnik AG, Bruchsal, Germany
7	AcriFlex MICS 46CSE IOL	Acrimed GmbH, Berlin, Germany
8	Hoya Y-60H	Hoya Corporation, Tokyo, Japan
9	Miniflex IOL	Mediphacos Ltda., Minas Gerais, Brasil

After unfolding, the IOL shouldn't have any structural, mechanical changes or optical alteration or deformation. Haptics of the lens should defend from decantation. The structure of the lens should protect from posterior capsule opacification (PCO). Some of the lenses can have a problem with PCO but precise cleaning of the capsule can prevent the epithelium proliferation.[8] Lenses shouldn't induce halos, glare, night-vision phenomenon, aberrations or scattering. Microincision IOLs are the following:

Acri.Tec MICS's Lenses

Surgeon can use Acri.LISA for multifocals implantation. (Fig. 10). For toric implants and cases with more than 3.00 D of astigmatism, surgeon can use the toric Acri.Tec IOL, marking the axis of the implantation at the slit-lamp prior to surgery. Acri.Smart 48S and Acri.Smart 46S are the lenses with the optical diameter 5.5 mm and 6 mm. It is biconvex, equiconvex, nonangled lenses with hydrophobic surface. They can be implanted on both sides. Acri.Smart 48S IOLs have water content of 25% in its fully hydrated state. Acri. Smart lenses are designed with square truncated edges. The edge thickness corresponds to standard designed IOLs and is in the range 0.25–0.27 mm. The lens is made from acrylic material, a copolymer of hydroxyethylmethacrylate and ethoxymethacrylate with an ultraviolet absorber. The optic power of this lens ranges from 0.00 D to 32.00 D. Acri. Smart glide system with Acri.Glide cartridge is used to implant lens. Acri.Smart 48S are the lenses can be injected through 1.5 mm incision or smaller. They are very easy to apply. After injection the lens unfolds very quickly and with the control. It has no tendency to decentration or to tilt. The adhesion between posterior capsule and lens is perfect.[9] Wehner et al. investigation seems to confirm the stability of the Acri.Smart 46S lens. There was no decentration and rotation of this lens during 19 months observation after MICS surgery. No unwanted complications occurred.[10]

Clinical Results

Forty-five eyes with cataract grade 2, 3, 4 (LOCS III) were operated by MICS. The incision size was 1.46 mm (1.4–1.9 mm). Six months after operation 98.9% of the patients had best-corrected distance visual acuity (BCDVA) 20/25 (0.7 decimal value) or better and 71.3% of the patients had distance uncorrected distance visual acuity (UCDVA) 20/32 (0.6 decimal value) or better. The safety index for distance vision of the procedure was 2.5 and the efficacy index of the procedure was 1.8.

Ninety percent of the patients had a near best-corrected near visual acuity (BCNVA) of 20/25 (0.8 decimal value). 60% of the patients had a near uncorrected near visual acuity (UCNVA) of 20/32 (0.6 decimal value) or better. The mean add for near was +1.5 D or less in 70% of cases

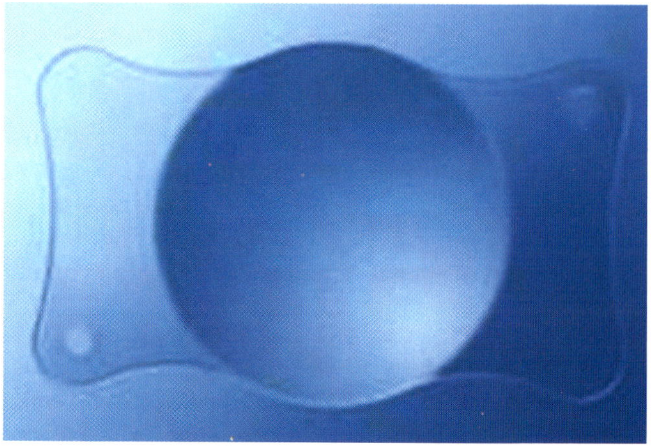

Fig. 10: Acri.LISA 366D multifocal intraocular lens (Zeiss-Acri.Tec, Berlin, Germany)

and was +2.0 D in 26% of cases. The safety index for near vision of the procedure was 1.4 and the efficacy index of the procedure was 0.9. It can indicate that Acri.Smart has a pseudoaccommodative ability. In this study none of the lenses shoved any change in position, decentration, tilt and posterior capsular opacification (PCO).[11]

Akreos AO MI60 Microincision is a hydrophilic acrylic with 26% hydration rate. Optic measures 6 mm and has a 360° posterior ridge-barrier to prevent PCO. Haptics geometry consists of 4-point support system, haptics angled at about 10°. Akreos has an aspherical optic. Akreos MI60 is an aspheric lens, reduces the aberrations and improves contrast sensitivity.

Akreos AO MI60 can be implanted with a 1.8 Viscoglide cartridge and Viscoject lens injection system (Medicel AG, Wolfhalden, Switzerland). This type of lenses has no tendency to decentration or PCO (Fig. 11).

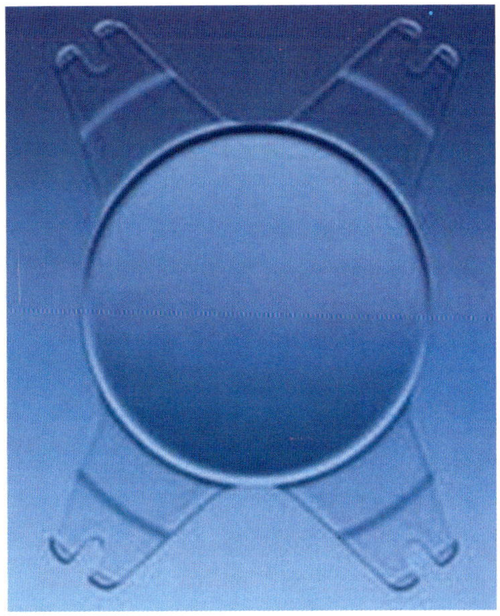

Fig. 11: Akreos AO MI60 microincision (Bausch & Lomb, Rochester, New York, USA)

IOLtech MICS lens (IOLtech, La Rochelle, France, and Carl Zeiss Meditec, Stuttgart, Germany) is biconvex. The total diameter is 12.0 mm and the optic diameter is 5.5 mm. The angulation is 13° between haptics and optics. This is the hydrophilic acrylic and monobloc lens. This lens has a square edge. The diopters range from +10.5 D to +25.5 D. The lens can be implanted with disposable injector and microincision cartridge. This lens shows pseudoaccommodative effect (Fig. 12)

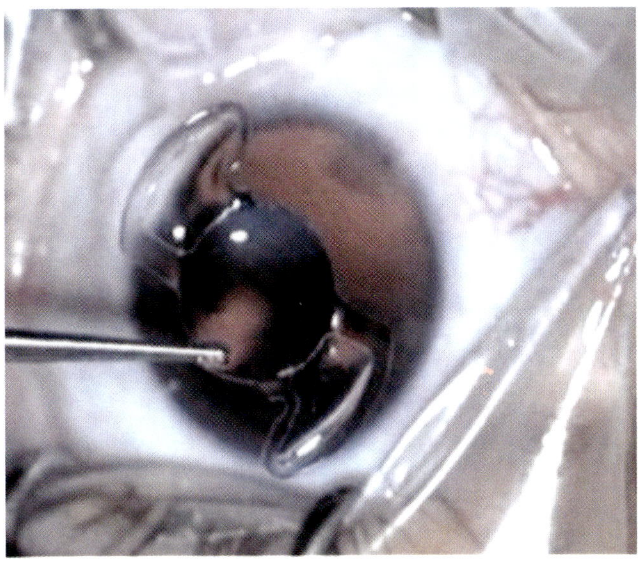

Fig. 12: IOLtech MICS lens

Verges et al. [European Society of Cataract and Refractive Surgeons (ESCRS) congress, Portugal 2005, and London 2006] showed data of 48 patients who underwent MICS surgery and implantation of IOLtech MICS lens through 1.8 mm incision. After 1 year follow-up 92% of the patients reported UCDVA 20/25 and 96% BCDVA more than 20/25. 65% of the patients achieved near visual acuity J3 with distant correction and 98% of the patients J5. Only two patients needed Nd:YAG capsulotomy.

TetraFlex KH-3500 and ZR-1000 (Lenstec, Inc. St. Petersburg, Florida, USA) is the accommodating MICS IOL. It is made from hydroxyethylmethacrylate, consists of 26% water and a material is highly flexible. The lens is 11.5 mm of total length and 5.75 mm optic length with square edges. It is one-piece lens. The lens is available in powers from +5 D to +36 D. The TetraFlex KH-3500 uses injector with 1.8 mm cartridge (Fig. 13).

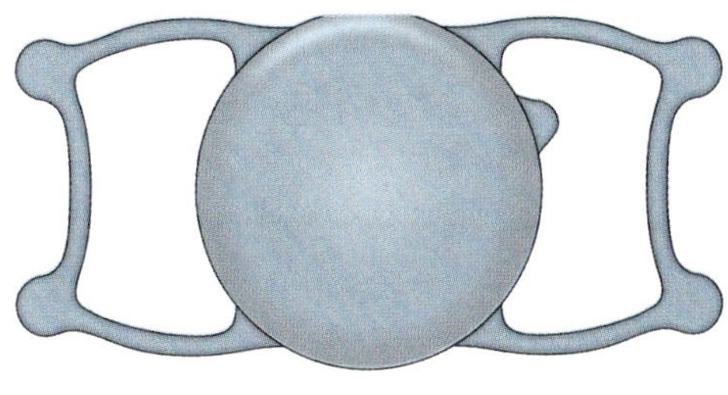

Fig. 13: TetraFlex KH-3500

Chitkara at the ESCRS Winter Refractive Surgery Meeting 2004 reported the mean accommodation achieved binocularly was 3.42 D. Moreover, 89% of the patients achieved J3 or better unaided binocular near vision at 6 months, and 100% achieved J5 or better.

ZR-1000 is the new one-piece lens from Lenstec. The length of this lens is 11.0 mm. The diameter of the optic is 5.5 mm and is made in square edge technology. The optic type is equiconvex and the haptic is plate. The angulation is 0°. This lens is made of 26% water content acrylic. The diopters of lens range from +10.0 D to +30.0 D. No clinical data is available for this lens (Fig. 14).

MicroSlim and SlimFlex MICS IOLs (PhysIOL, Liège, Belgium) is a hydrophilic acrylic lens with biconvex optics. Optic diameter is 6.15 mm, and overall diameter is 10.75 mm. The angulation is 5°. The power of the lens range is from +10.0 D to +30.0 D. This lens can be injected using Viscoject™ Injector and 1.8 Viscoglide cartridge (Medicel AG, Wolfhalden, Switzerland). No clinical data is available for this lens (Fig. 15).

Vryghem et al. presented on Congress of the ESCRS 2006 his experience in SlimFlex IOL implantation through 1.5 mm incision. The group of 50 patients underwent bilateral MICS with lens implantation. After 6 weeks, mean best-corrected visual acuity (BCVA) was 1.04. Less than 1% of the patients complained about halos or glare, and 3% of lenses resulted in small damage of the optic or haptics. No clinical data is available for this lens.

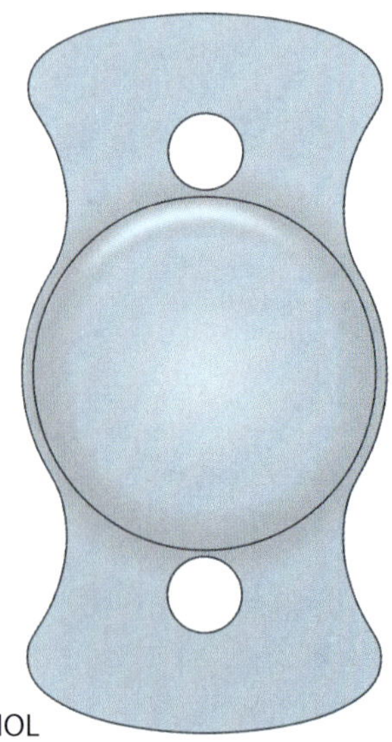

Fig. 14: ZR-1000 IOL

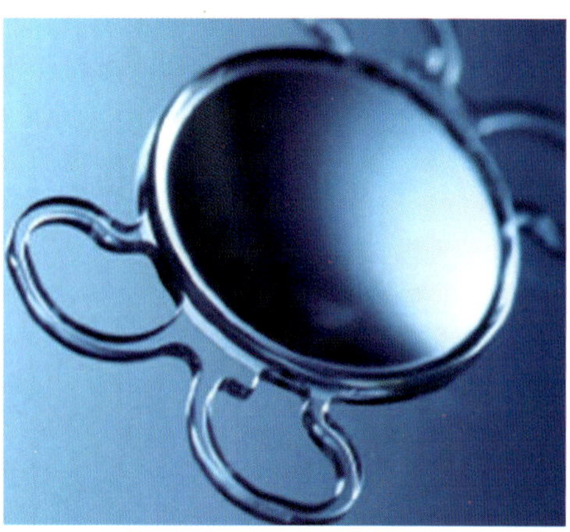

Fig. 15: MicroSlim IOL

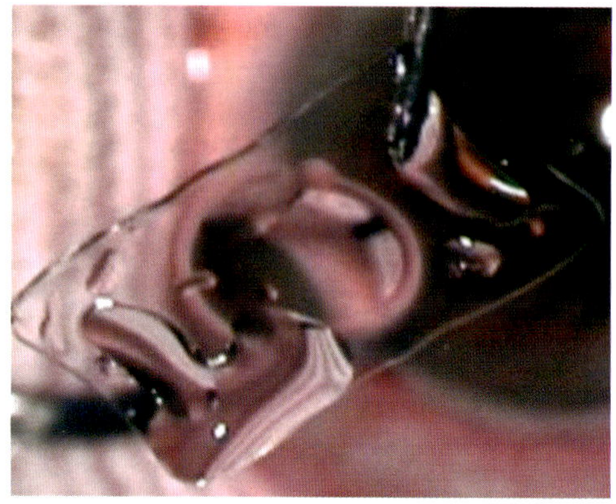

Fig. 16: AcriFlex MICS 46CSE IOL

CareFlex IOL (W20 Medizintechnik AG, Bruchsal, Germany) is a 26% hydrophilic acrylate, one-piece lens. Optic size is 5.8 mm, overall length is 10.5 mm and the haptic angulation is 0°. The optic design is a biconvex. The recommended anterior chamber depth is 5.1 mm. The lens is available from +10.0 D to +30.0 D. No clinical data is available for this lens.

AcriFlex MICS 46CSE IOL (Acrimed GmbH, Berlin, Germany) is made of 25% acrylic hydrophilic. The superficial is hydrophobic. The lens diameter is 11.0 mm and optic diameter is 6.0 mm. This is a monobloque type lens with perforated haptics. The angulation is 0°. The optic is biconvex with sharp edges. The lens is available from +15 D to +27 D. The clinical data is not available for this lens (Fig. 16).

Hoya Y-60H (*Hoya Corporation,* Tokyo, Japan) *is* a quite new lens for micro surgery. This is hydrophobic foldable lens. The clinical data is not available, but Tsuneoka described possibility of implantation of this lens through 1.7 mm incision. He used Hoya F-1 cartridge to inject the lens[12] (Fig. 17).

Miniflex IOL (Mediphacos Ltda., Minas Gerais, Brasil) is also new MICS surgery lens can be implanted through 1.8 mm incision. The material is Flexacryl® Hybrid Acrylic which brings together hydrophobic and hydrophilic monomers. The optics is aberration neutral. The lens can be implanted through 1.8 mm incision using a docking technique. The lens was presented on ESCRS 2008 in Berlin by Carlos Verges (Fig. 18).

Fig. 17: Hoya Y-60H MICS IOL

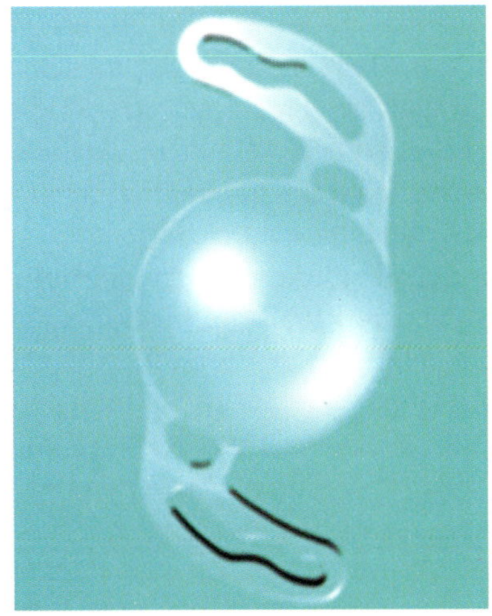

Fig. 18: Miniflex IOL

Finally, authors concluded that MICS IOL is not only the normal classic IOL which is adapted to MICS incision, these lenses are the other type of intraocular IOL. New technique and new idea of the construction lead to create thin and stable MICS IOL with the optical quality as good as standard intraocular IOLs.[8,13]

MICS IOL characterizes:

- Thin optic and haptic
- Perfect characteristic of compression
- Very good optical quality
- Long-term stability after implantation

MICS Outcomes

Astigmatism Control with MICS

Among the major advantages of MICS, the diminution of surgical trauma is resulting in reduction of SIA, aberrations and improvement of the optical quality of the cornea after surgery.

Degraded optical quality of the cornea after incisional cataract surgery would limit the performance of the pseudophakic eye. Thus, it is important not to increase or to induce astigmatism and/or corneal aberrations after cataract surgery. Even with MICS, surgeon could achieve reduction of the astigmatism and higher-order corneal aberrations.

The optical quality of the cornea plays an important role in recovery of visual function after cataract surgery, and this is determined by combination of corneal and internal aberrations generated by the IOL and those induced by the surgery. These corneal refractive changes are attributed to the location and size of the corneal incision. The smaller incision, lower aberrations mean better optical quality.

Authors have described the improved control on corneal SIA with MICS when compared to conventional 3 mm phacoemulsification. A great advantage of MICS is the reduction of SIA and that the microincisions do not produce an increase in astigmatism (Fig. 19).

The shorter the incision, the less the corneal astigmatism, as it was estimated that the magnitude of the SIA studied by vector analysis is around 0.44–0.88 D, rising as the size of the incision increases. This is considered important because cataract surgery today is considered more and more a refractive procedure.

Also, small-incision surgery (3.5 mm incision without suture) does not systematically degrade the optical quality of the anterior corneal surface. However, it introduces changes in some aberrations, especially not in rotationally symmetric terms such as astigmatism, coma and trefoil.

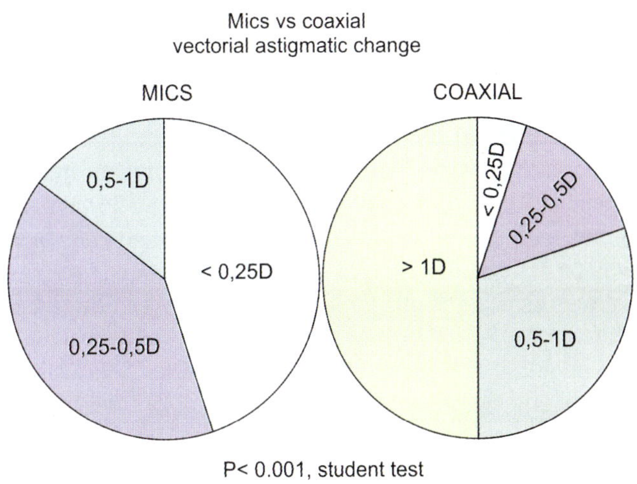

Fig. 19: Comparison of MICS and coaxial vectoral astigmatic change

Therefore, one has to expect better results and lesser changes with sub 2 mm incision (MICS). This is supported by the finding that the corneal incision of less than 2 mm had no impact on corneal curvature. Going hand in hand with the modern concept of making cataract surgery a refractive procedure by controlling and even decreasing astigmatism and higher-order astigmatism (HOA) by using MICS, which is the state of the art.[14] Authors can say that MICS sub 2 mm incision effectively decreases the induction or changes in corneal aberrations (higher-order astigmatism) during cataract surgery.

Corneal Aberration with MICS

Nowadays cataract surgery is not only a removal of a opaque lens but also it is a part of refractive surgery. Surgeons can obtain precise IOL power calculation, they can reduce residual astigmatism and do surgery without SIA and finally improve the corneal optical quality after cataract surgery. The final visual function is determined by the aberrations produced by the implanted IOL and corneal aberrations changed by the postsurgical incisions. The smaller incision means lower aberrations and the better optical quality.[15,16]

Authors Elkady and Alio in prospective cumulative interventional nonrandomized, noncomparative study of 25 eyes of 25 patients show that after the MICS incision smaller than 1.8 mm, there was no statistical difference in corneal power, corneal astigmatism before and 3 months of follow-up after surgery.[17] The RMS value of the total corneal aberrations decreased slightly after MICS (mean 2.15 ±2.51 μm preoperatively, 1.87 ±1.87 μm at 1 month, and 1.96 ±2.01 μm at 3 months); there was no statistically significant difference between the two follow-up visits (both P = 1.00, Bonferroni). Analysis of individual Zernike terms showed a mean astigmatism of 0.85 ±0.74 μm preoperatively, 0.65 ±0.44 μm at 1 month, and 0.69 ± 0.46 μm at 3 months and a mean spherical aberration of -0.11 ±0.25 μm, -0.09 ±0.25 μm and -0.19 ±0.13 μm respectively. Coma decreased (mean 0.45 ±0.40 μm preoperatively, 0.39 ±0.36 μm at 1 month and 0.42 ±0.44 μm at 3 months respectively); there was no statistically significant difference between the two follow-up visits (both P = 1.00, Bonferroni). The mean HOA was 0.47 ±0.26 μm preoperatively, 0.59 ±0.32 μm at 1 month and 0.54 ±0.25 μm at 3 months; there was no statistically significant difference between the two follow-up visits (both P > 0.47, Bonferroni) (Fig. 20).

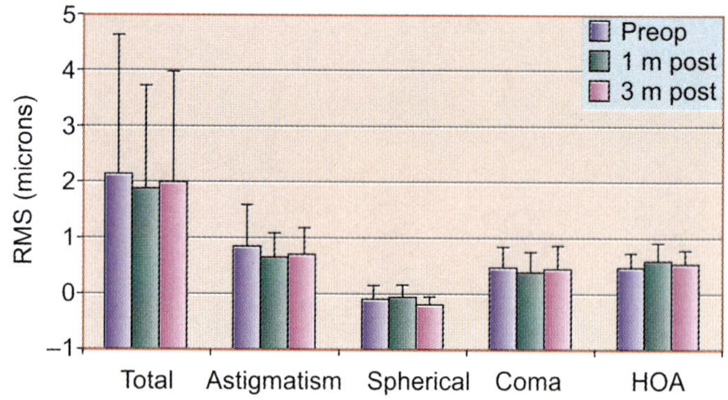

Fig. 20: Corneal aberrations (Seidel coefficients) with a 6.0 mm aperture diameter over time
Abbreviations: Preop = Preoperative; m = Month; HOA = Higher-order astigmatism

All aberration values except HOA decreased slightly, with no statistically significant differences between the follow-up visits. All aberration values were stable for 3 months after surgery, indicating that successful MICS depends on preventing induction of HOAs as well as a surgically neutral and stable procedure. Successful MICS gives visual quality equal to that in persons of the same age without pathology and leads to good patient satisfaction.[16,17]

Clinical Efficacy of MICS

Advantages of MICS in the field of the refractive result as astigmatism control and aberration neutrality are supported by many papers of the various authors as described above. But surgeons should evaluate the other area of the MICS surgical technique. For each cataract surgeon, it is very important to compare available surgical techniques in the field of surgical technology and clinical efficacy. Seven years of MICS was an opportunity to evaluate this technique by many authors.

Relatively fast method to compare is evaluation of the surgical machine parameters settings. Alio et al. comparing study of the MICS and coaxial phacoemulsification shows large difference between amounts of energy delivered into the eye. The effective phaco time (EPT) of the MICS surgery was more than four times lower than in the coaxial group and the astigmatism was almost three times lower than in the coaxial group. This means that intraocular injury connected with the phacoemulsification should be lower in the MICS group.[14] Also, Kurz et al. indicate in publication important decrease of phacoemulsification time in MICS group comparing to coaxial surgery.[18] The Kahraman study shows decrease of phacoemulsification time in the MICS group comparing to coaxial group (P = 0.001).[19] Also, Tanaka study shows lower ultrasonic output in the bimanual group than in the coaxial group. Tanaka correlates it with better efficiency of nuclear treatment, including nuclear compliance, crushing and flexor hinge in the case of bimanual procedure.[20] The other studies did not show difference in the total surgery time between MICS and coaxial phaco.[14,21] The other study described by Crema et al. shows the total ultrasound time was lower in the coaxial phacoemulsification group than in the MICS group; the means were 0.50 minutes ±0.33 (standard deviation) and 0.82 ±0.39 minutes respectively. The mean ultrasound power was similar between groups (mean 10.1% ±3.76% and 10.0% ±4.0% respectively).[22] Nowadays surgeon can also compare MICS and micro-coaxial phaco. Cavallini study of MICS shows shorter total surgery time (P = 0.04) and lower balanced salt solution consumption (P = 0.004) of the MICS group.[23]

The phacoemulsification process always affects the corneal endothelial cells. Wilczynski et al. comparison study of the endothelial cell density shows that there is no difference in the MICS group and micro-coaxial group in the loss of the endothelium.[24] Also, Kahraman et al. study evaluates the endothelial cell loss in the MICS and coaxial group but the results show the minimal difference between both groups. There were no statistically significant differences between preoperative and postoperative anterior chamber flare or endothelial cell loss.[19] No significant differences in corneal endothelial cell loss or endothelial morphology were found between MICS and standard incision techniques in Mencucci et al study.[21] Morphology of the cells was not different in the MICS and coaxial group in the study of Mencucci or Kahraman.[19,21] The comparative study of Crema et al. indicates lower cell loss in the coaxial group. The mean central corneal endothelial cell loss at 3 months was 4.66% ±6.10% in the coaxial phacoemulsification group and 4.45% ±5.06% in the MICS group and at 1 year, 6.00% ±6.72% and 8.82% ±7.39% respectively. Postoperative inflammation in the anterior chamber evaluated by laser flare photometry was the same in MICS and coaxial groups in various studies.[14,18,19] Also, Wylegala et al. in the article about corneal thickness after coaxial phacoemulsification or MICS indicate the difference in the postsurgery corneal edema. MICS reduces risk of corneal edema when comparing to standard coaxial phacoemulsification.[25]

The wound integrity and the self selling properties of the MICS and coaxial incisions are currently one of the most important agents in the endophthalmitis prophylaxis.

Irreversible changes may affect the cornea. Every incision of the cornea evokes the change of corneal curvature. The study of Kaufmann et al. confirms that MICS incision offers astigmatic neutrality in the cataract surgery, it supports the idea of MICS as the refractive procedure.[26] In a study by the authors (Jorge L Alio, P Klonowski) of this chapter, they proved that MICS and microphaco provided similarly good incision quality and optically neutral incisions. The MICS incision respected corneal prolateness more, with less corneal edema in the short term and less induced corneal aberrations in the long term.[27] In the other studies, Tong et al. support the perfect MICS optical result. Cataract surgery related changes in corneal wavefront aberrations were dependent on incision size. The MICS technique had advantages over the small incision cataract surgery technique in minimizing the destructive effect of the large incision size on the optical quality of the cornea.[15] Denoyer et al. compared MICS with conventional coaxial surgery. This study shows that MICS could improve the optical performances of the pseudophakic eye reducing in 3 months surgically induced corneal higher-order aberrations. The postoperative root mean square of 3rd to 6th was lower in MICS group 0.705 ±0.285 μm versus 0.956 ±0.236 μm in coaxial group, and it was significantly different (P < 0.001), and the root mean square for the 3rd to 6th order ocular aberration was lower in MICS 0.308 ±0.122 μm versus coaxial group 0.488 ±0.172 μm with significant difference (P = 0.002).[28] The latest publication of Saeed et al. show the smooth but significant difference between MICS and standard coaxial phacoemulsification in terms of uncorrected visual acuity recorded 1 hour and 2 weeks postoperatively. Nine eyes (18%) and one eye (2%) achieved an uncorrected visual acuity (UCVA) of C6/12 at 1 hour following MICS and coaxial phacoemulsification respectively, and this difference was statistically significant (P = 0.02). The authors conclude that mean UCVA at 1 hour and at 2 weeks following cataract surgery was not significantly different between eyes undergoing MICS and coaxial phacoemulsification. However, a greater proportion of patients achieved a UCVA of C6/12 following MICS when compared with coaxial phacoemulsification.[29] These results support other MICS investigations, smaller corneal complications, better incision leads to faster recovery and superior refractive result.[29] Astigmatic neutrality in biaxial microincision cataract surgery confirm Kaufmann et al. article. His investigation comparing keratometry of the surgical and nonsurgical eye shows the astigmatic neutrality of the sub 2 mm cataract surgery. The difference between groups was not statistically significant.[30] Wilczynski et al. article also confirm these results.[31]

Combining MICS and limbal relaxing incisions (LRI) cataract surgery can achieve superior refractive result. Ouchi et al. compares results of MICS and LRI-MICS groups. Statistically significant difference between both groups in UCVA is not surprising, but conclusion is very important. Limbal relaxing incision with bimanual MICS is an easy-to-follow combined surgery to correct pre-existing astigmatism with predictable accuracy. It confirms that MICS is SIA-neutral procedure.[32]

Quality of vision also depends on the quality of the lens implanted in the eye. Greater compression of the lens in the cartridge was a challenge for the MICS lens. But the results of comparative studies of standard lenses and MICS lenses were exceptionally good for MICS lens. There is no single method of assessing the surgical safety. Surgeon can only take into account data from the publication but also important is the opinion of surgeons. Most of them are very satisfying because of stable intraocular environment during lens removal especially in patients with high myopia, who are at greater risk of retinal detachment after lens extraction.[33] Practically MICS surgery can be performed under the stable anatomical conditions with the permanent use of the irrigating chopper.[34] Authors can conclude as Muller et al. in the article about MICS, the advantages of MICS are less corneal astigmatism and fewer corneal surface irregularities, with favorable implications for visual quality and early rehabilitation. In the effort toward smaller incisions, special interest should be given to wound integrity, especially regarding the risk of endophthalmitis but tissue laceration can occur and smaller incisions are superior only if they cause less trauma.[35,36] However bimanual MICS seems to be superior over the other surgical techniques because of the better refractive result, better fluidics, greater manual control and lower surgical time.[37] Authors have found this technique to be simple and safe.

Conclusion

MICS is a well established surgical technique for cataract removal. MICS offers distinctive advantages in terms of eliminating SIA and reducing the changes in the aberration pattern of the cornea to the minimum. MICS is the technique that best matches the concept of premium IOLs, as the control and correction of astigmatism and corneal aberrations seems to be mandatory at this moment in modern cataract surgery. Proven evidence exists to state that MICS is the best surgical option today for cataract removal, both biaxial and coaxial sub 2 mm incision. Micro-MICS (sub 1 mm surgery) is a feasible surgery, with the same standards and advantages of MICS, but IOL technology should be further developed in order to use these sub 1 mm incisions for IOL implantation, something not feasible today. Future evolution on IOL technology and new surgical tools will make MICS the gold standard of cataract surgery, as biaxial technique, separating irrigation and aspiration functions, once new energies allow the nucleus to be softened and the cataract to be aspirated injecting a lens refilling substance. Biaxiality and sub 1 mm, even punctual surgery, are pending further development in the coming years.

References

1. Alió JL, Klonowski P, Rodriguez-Prats JL, et al. Microincisional cataract surgery (MICS). In: Garg A, Alio JL, Fine IH. et al. (Eds). Mastering the Techniques of Advanced Phaco Surgery. New Delhi: Jaypee Brothers Medical Publishers (P) Ltd.; 2008. pp. 121-36.
2. Alió JL, Klonowski P, El Kady B. Microincisional lens surgery. In: Kohnen T, Koch DD, (Eds). Essentials in Ophthalmology. Cataract and Refractive Surgery. Berlin, Heidelberg: Springer; 2009. pp. 11-24.
3. Alio JL, Rodriguez-Prats JL, Galal A. Micro-incision cataract surgery. Highlights of Ophthalmology International, Miami, 2004.
4. Alio JL, Agarwal A, Klonowski P. 0.7 mm microincision cataract surgery. In: Alio JL, Fine IH, (Eds). Minimizing Incisions and Maximizing Outcomes in Cataract Surgery. Berlin, Heidelberg: Springer; 2010. pp. 13-25.
5. Alió JL, Klonowski P, Rodriguez-Prats JL, et al. Microincision cataract surgery (MICS). In: Cavallini GM, Perez Arteaga A, Malyugin B, et al. (Eds). Instant Clinical Diagnosis in Ophthalmology: Lens Diseases. New Delhi: Jaypee Brothers Medical Publishers (P) Ltd.; 2008. pp. 155-85.
6. Alió JL, Rodriguez-Prats JL, Klonowski P, et al. MICS: Cirugia de la catarata por microincision. In: Lorente R, Mendicute J. (Eds) Cirugia Del Cristalino. Tomo I. Sociedad de Española. Macline S.L. 2008. pp. 539-44.
7. Alio JL, Klonowski P, Rodriguez-Prats JL. MICS instrumentation. In: Alio JL, Fine IH. (Eds). Minimizing Incisions and Maximizing Outcomes in Cataract Surgery. Berlin, Heidelberg: Springer; 2010. pp. 25-37.
8. Cleary G, Spalton DJ, Hancox J, et al. Randomized intraindividual comparison of posterior capsule opacification between a microincision intraocular lens and a conventional intraocular lens. J Cataract Refract Surg. 2009;35:265-72.
9. Alió JL, El Kady B, Klonowski P. Acri.Lisa with MICS. In: Goes FJ (Ed). Multifocal IOLs. New Delhi: Jaypee Brothers Medical Publishers (P) Ltd.; 2009. pp. 201-10.
10. Wehner W. Microincision intraocular lens with plate haptic design. Evaluation of rotational stability and centering of a microincision intraocular lens with plate haptic design in 12-19 months of follow-up. Ophthalmologe. 2007;104:396-8.

11. Alió JL, Rodriguez-Prats JL, Vianello A, et al. Visual outcome of microincision cataract surgery with implantation of an Acri.Smart lens. J Cataract Refract Surg. 2005;31:1549-56.
12. Tsuneoka H. Implantation of a new Hoya-IOL, Y-60H, through a 1.7 mm corneal incision. In: Ashok Garg, Howard Fine, Jorge L. Alio, (Eds). Mastering the Techniques of Advanced Phaco Surgery New Delhi: Jaypee Brothers Medical Publishers (P) Ltd; 2008. pp. 209-13.
13. Alio JL, Klonowski P. MICS intraocular lenses. In: Alio JL, Fine IH (Eds). Minimizing Incisions and Maximizing Outcomes in Cataract Surgery. Berlin, Heidelberg: Springer; 2010. pp. 209-20.
14. Alió JL, Rodriguez-Prats JL, Galal A, et al. Outcomes of microincision cataract surgery versus coaxial phacoemulsification. Ophthalmology. 2005;112:1997-2003.
15. Tong N, He JC, Lu F, et al. Changes in corneal wavefront aberrations in microincision and small-incision cataract surgery. J Cataract Refract Surg. 2008;34:2085-90.
16. Nochez Y, Favard A, Majzoub S, et al. Measurement of corneal aberrations for customisation of intraocular lens asphericity: impact on quality of vision after micro-incision cataract surgery. Br J Ophthalmol. 2010;94(4):440-4. Epub 2009 Oct 14. 2009.
17. Elkady B, Alió JL, Ortiz D, et al. Corneal aberrations after microincision cataract surgery. J Cataract Refract Surg. 2008;34:40-5.
18. Kurz S, Krummenauer F, Gabriel P, et al. Biaxial microincision versus coaxial small-incision clear cornea cataract surgery. Ophthalmology. 2006;113:1818-26.
19. Kahraman G, Amon M, Franz C, et al. Intraindividual comparison of surgical trauma after bimanual microincision and conventional small-incision coaxial phacoemulsification. J Cataract Refract Surg. 2007;33:618-22.
20. Tanaka T, Koshika S, Usui M. Cataract surgery using the bimanual phacoemulsification technique with an Accurus system and Mackool microphaco tip. J Cataract Refract Surg. 2007;33:1770-4.
21. Mencucci R, Ponchietti C, Virgili G, et al. Corneal endothelial damage after cataract surgery: Microincision versus standard technique. J Cataract Refract Surg. 2006;32:1351-4.
22. Crema AS, Walsh A, Yamane Y, et al. Comparative study of coaxial phacoemulsification and microincision cataract surgery. One-year follow-up. J Cataract Refract Surg. 2007;33:1014-8.
23. Cavallini GM, Campi L, Masini C, et al. Bimanual Microphacoemulsification versus coaxial miniphaco-emulsification: prospective study. J Cataract Refract Surg. 2007;33:387-92.
24. Wilczynski M, Supady E, Loba P, et al. Comparison of early corneal endothelial cell loss after coaxial phacoemulsification through 1.8 mm microincision and bimanual phacoemulsification through 1.7 mm microincision. J Cataract Refract Surg. 2009;35:1570-4.
25. Wylegała E, Rebkowska-Juraszek M, Dobrowolski D, et al. Influence of 3.0 mm incision coaxial phacoemulsification and microincision cataract surgery (MICS) on corneal thickness. Klin Oczna. 2009;111:207-11.
26. Kaufmann C, Krishnan A, Landers J, et al. Astigmatic neutrality in biaxial microincision cataract surgery. J Cataract Refract Surg. 2009;35:1555-62.
27. Elkady B, Piñero D, Alió JL. Corneal incision quality: microincision cataract surgery versus microcoaxial phacoemulsification. J Cataract Refract Surg. 2009;35:466-74.
28. Denoyer A, Denoyer L, Marotte D, et al. Intraindividual comparative study of corneal and ocular wavefront aberrations after biaxial microincision versus coaxial small-incision cataract surgery. Br J Ophthalmol. 2008;92:1679-84.
29. Saeed A, O'Connor J, Cunnife G, et al. Uncorrected visual acuity in the immediate postoperative period following uncomplicated cataract surgery: bimanual microincision cataract surgery versus standard coaxial phacoemulsification. Int Ophthalmol. 2009;29:393-400.
30. Kaufmann C, Krishnan A, Landers J, et al. Astigmatic neutrality in biaxial microincision cataract surgery. J Cataract Refract Surg. 2009;35:1555-62.
31. Wilczynski M, Supady E, Loba P, et al. Comparison of surgically induced astigmatism after coaxial phacoemulsification through 1.8 mm microincision and bimanual phacoemulsification through 1.7 mm microincision. J Cataract Refract Surg. 2009;35:1563-9.
32. Ouchi M, Kinoshita S. Prospective randomized trial of limbal relaxing incisions combined with microincision cataract surgery. J Refract Surg. 2009;26:1-6.
33. Fine IH, Hoffman RS, Packer M. Optimizing refractive lens exchange with bimanual microincision phacoemulsification. J Cataract Refract Surg. 2004;30:550-4.
34. Sallet G. Viscoless microincision cataract surgery. Clin Ophthalmol. 2008;2:717-21.
35. Müller M, Kohnen T. Incisions for biaxial and coaxial microincision cataract surgery. Ophthalmologe. 2010;107:108-15.
36. Weikert MP. Update on bimanual microincisional cataract surgery. Current Opinion in Ophthalmology. 2006, 17: 62-7.
37. Paul T, Braga-Mele R. Bimanual microincisional phacoemulsification: the future of cataract surgery?. Curr Opin Ophthalmol. 2005;16:2-7.

9 Safety: MICS versus Coaxial Phaco

George HH Beiko (Canada)

Core Messages

1. Microincisional cataract surgery (MICS) is a recent innovation upon standard coaxial cataract phacoemulsification.
2. MICS meets the safety benchmark of coaxial phacoemulsification and surpasses it in some aspects.
3. Visual rehabilitation and outcomes with MICS meet or surpass that of coaxial phacoemulsification.

Introduction

The separation of irrigation and aspiration in cataract surgery, termed "biaxial technique", was first described in the early 1970s.[1,2] In 1985, Shearing advocated the use of the biaxial technique for cataract extraction; however, his technique required the enlargement of the incision to 7 mm in order to insert the intraocular lens (IOLs).[3] It was not until the advent of the ability to modulate power in phacoemulsification that sleeveless phaco tips could be inserted safely through small incisions and microincision surgery was born.

Microincision cataract surgery (MICS) was first coined by Prof J Alio in 2001 to describe cataract surgery through sub 2.0 mm incisions.[4] The term "MICS" was patented by J Alio in 2003 (personal communication, J Alio).

The benefits of the biaxial approach in MICS are described in other chapters of this book, but briefly can be listed as (from Brooks L and Ciprés MC 1.8 mm Biaxial White Paper. A review of the literature; Bausch & Lomb internal document):

- Better control of rhexis
- Improved surgical efficiency by decreased effective phaco time
- Better fluidic control
- Enhanced chamber stability
- Better followability through fluid dynamics by separation of irrigation and aspiration so as to minimize opposition between the two
- Access to entire anterior chamber with either irrigation or aspiration by inserting the instruments through either incision
- Ease of removal of subincisional cortex; lower posterior capsular opacification rates
- Increased ability to handle complications; including the ability to avoid areas of zonular weakness
- Ability to use the irrigating fluid as a tool to manipulate material within the capsular bag or anterior chamber
- Reduction of vitreous prolapse in cases of posterior capsular tear or rupture
- Increased suitability for complicated cases
- The purpose of this chapter is to investigate the safety of MICS by looking at visual outcome, incision damage, corneal changes and complications.

Visual Outcomes

The true test of a new technique or instrument in cataract surgery is visual outcome. Whenever a new lens is introduced, the point of comparison is the visual outcome compared to the current standard lens. Similarly, at the very least, MICS should be able to attain vision comparable to standard coaxial phacoemulsification; otherwise, any perceived benefit would be compromised.

Howard Fine and colleagues compared visual outcomes with bimanual phaco with standard phaco in a number of phaco systems and found that vision was improved similarly, irrespective of the technique[5] (Fig. 1).

In studying the visual rehabilitation following cataract surgery, it has been reported that MICS patients gain vision faster than coaxial patients. Kurz et al.[6] studied 70 patients prospectively, equally divided between MICS and coaxial;

Machine	Coaxial results	Bimanual results
Series 20000 Legacy with Neosonix	96%	93%
Millennium with phaco burst	100%	95%
Staar Sonic Wave*	74%	100%
Sovereign phaco system with Whitestar technology	94%	95%
		*P < .01

Fig. 1: Percentage of eyes with uncorrected visual acuity of 20/40 or better, 2 to 24 hours postoperatively, comparison of coaxial and bimanual phaco[5]

Post operative BVCA in Biaxial MICS compared with Coaxial Small Incision Clear Cornea Cataract Surgery[15]			
	Biaxial MICS	Coaxial MICS	P value
Pre-op	20/40	20/40	0.970
3 hour post-op	20/40	20/63	
	(20/400-20/25)	(20/400-20/15)	
1 day post-op	20/25	20/30	0.018
	(20/50-20/15)	(20/400-20/15)	
3 days post-op	20/25	20/30	0.002
	(20/30-20/15)	(20/400-20/15)	
7 days post-op	20/25 (20/40-20/15)	20/25 (20/200-20/15)	0.605
8 days post-op	20/20	20/25	0.015
Note: MICS 35 eyes, final incision size 1.5 - 1.7 mm; 35 eyes, final incision size 2.75 mm			

Fig. 2: Visual rehabilitation following cataract surgery; Comparison of MICS and coaxial techniques[6]

their findings are reproduced in Figure 2 and demonstrate a smaller interquartile range in MICS.

MICS has been reported to have a significantly decreased mean total phaco time and mean effective phaco time[6,7] (Fig. 3). As phaco time is believed to be directly related to corneal damage; less phaco time should translate into less corneal trauma and quicker visual recovery.

In point of fact, it has been reported that MICS brings about more rapid visual rehabilitation due to reduced postoperative inflammation as a result of decreased chamber turbulence.[8-10] Similarly, it has been reported that postoperative inflammation using flare readings were decreased significantly in MICS eyes compared to coaxial phaco eyes at one week (Krootila K, Matilla J. Effect of fluidics on postoperative outcomes in bimanual phaco using the Whitestar micro-pulse technology. Presented at ESCRS annual meeting, 2006). Thus, decreased inflammation should also mean faster visual recovery.

EPT for biaxial mics versus coaxial phaco[11]			
	MICS	Coaxial phaco	P value
Mean phacoemulsification time (s)	0.38 ± 0.41	0.41 ± 0.44	0.259
Mean total phacoemulsification (%)	5.28 ± 3.91	19.2 ± 10.98	0.001
Mean effective phacoemulsification	2.19 ± 2.77	9.2 ± 12.38	0.001

Fig. 3: Comparison of effective phaco time; MICS versus coaxial.[7] ("Mean effective phacoemulsification" was defined as the mean effective phaco time in seconds in this study as it "represented the estimated phacoemulsification time if 100% phacoemulsification power in continuous mode had been used"[7])

In terms of visual rehabilitation, MICS has certainly been demonstrated to be similar to coaxial phaco, and in some authors' hands, to be superior since visual recovery occurs sooner.

Incision Damage

Examination of the incision should reveal the extent of trauma or injury at the incision sites. Ideally, the incision should allow access to the eye without compromising the ability of the incision to seal postoperatively and to minimize the amount of permanent change such as induced astigmatism.

In a scanning electron microscope comparison study of incision damage in cadaver eyes[11] (Fig. 4), it has been suggested that incision leakage occurred in all MICS eyes under test conditions when the Intraocular pressure was raised to 125 mm Hg for 30 seconds and in none of microincisional coaxial eyes under similar conditions. It was also reported that whitening of the incision occurred in four or five MICS eyes, suggesting that incision burn would occur. However, the criticism of this study has been made that the investigators were inexperienced with MICS and that incision construction was inaccurate (personal communication, J. Alio).

In a similar cadaver study, the changes in incision architecture were also studied by the authors who compared MICS with microincisional coaxial incisions (Weikert M, Koch D. Corneal wound architecture in bimanual and coaxial microincisional cataract surgery; ESCRS Annual Meeting, London, 2006). It was found that both types of incisions were slightly larger postoperatively compared to the incision made; however, Descemet's tear extensions were greater at the MICS phaco site than the microincisional coaxial phaco site while tears were similar at the irrigation

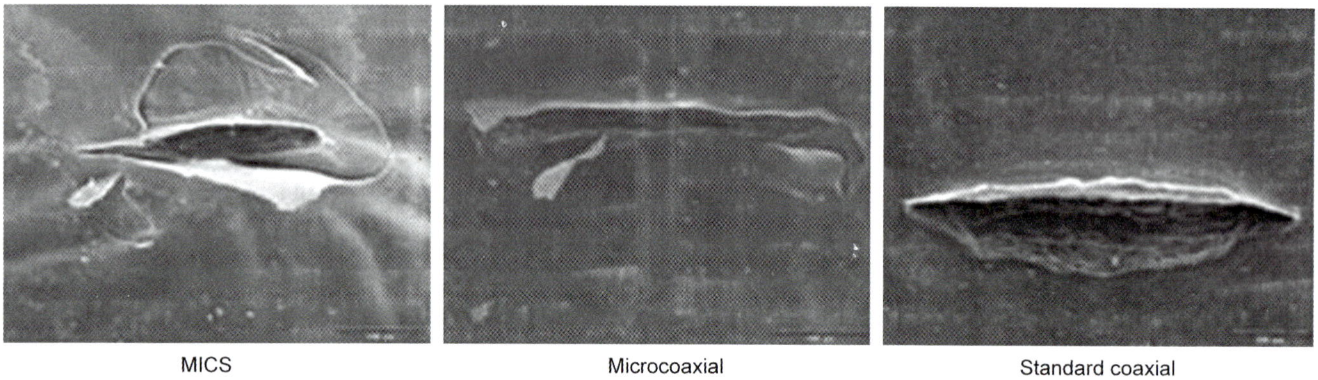

Fig. 4: Scanning electron microscope images of endothelial surface of clear corneal incisions after phacoemulsification in cadaver eyes[11]

sites in both. Also, endothelial cell loss (ECL) was similar in both, although there was greater loss near the phaco site of microincisional coaxial than MICS and no difference at the irrigation site in both. This study would suggest that although minimal differences exist between MICS and microcoaxial incisions, there is likely no significant impact on corneal endothelial function, incision leak or induced astigmatism when the two are compared.

Corneal Incision Burn

Corneal incision burns (Fig. 5) can result in significant distortion of the incision, resulting in the necessity of incision closure with sutures and significant induced astigmatism. Incision burns occur as a result of thermal damage to corneal collagen, and this occurs when tissue temperatures exceed 60°C.[12,13] It is for this reason, that irrigating sleeves on the phaco tip were introduced in traditional coaxial phaco. When considering conversion to sleeveless phaco for MICS, this is of paramount concern as there is a perception that the loss of the irrigating sleeve will allow friction of the phaco tip with the cornea tissue, causing incision temperatures to rise and incision burns to occur.

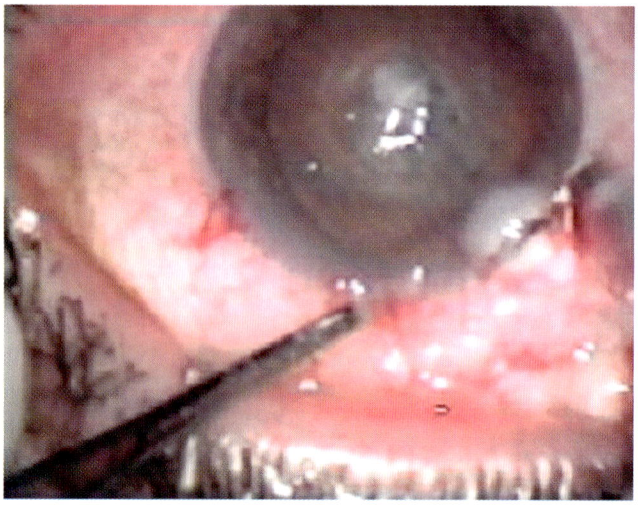

Fig. 5: Corneal incision burn

In MICS, it is almost a necessity for the phaco tip to make contact with the corneal tissue when microincisions are employed. Power modulations of phaco energies through variation of burst and pulse modes have allowed the safe use of sleeveless phaco tips in direct contact with corneal tissue without the creation of corneal incision burns. The proof of this is as follows.

Steinert and Schafer (Steinert RF and Schafer ME. Thermal energy and turbulence with WhiteStar and conventional phacoemulsification. Presented at annual meeting of ASCRS 2003) used a thermal camera in a laboratory setup to investigate the rise in temperature, comparing continuous ultrasound with Whitestar micropulse technology (Abbott Medical Optics, Santa Ana, USA). Their findings were that continuous ultrasound resulted in a phaco tip temperature of 61°C, while the Whitestar micropulse phaco tip temperature never rose above 35°C. Thus, clinically, continuous ultrasound would induce incision burn while the Whitestar settings would prevent this due to the decrease of at least 20°C in incision temperature, and well below the 60°C which would cause incision burn.

In a cadaver eye study, using sleeveless phaco, it was found that the incision temperature never rose above 41.8°C and that the incision remained clear.[9]

Clinically, using a thermocouple attachment in cataract patients, it has been shown that a sleeveless phaco tip with Whitestar modulations results in temperature rises in the 24–34°C range; far short of the temperature for incision burn.[14]

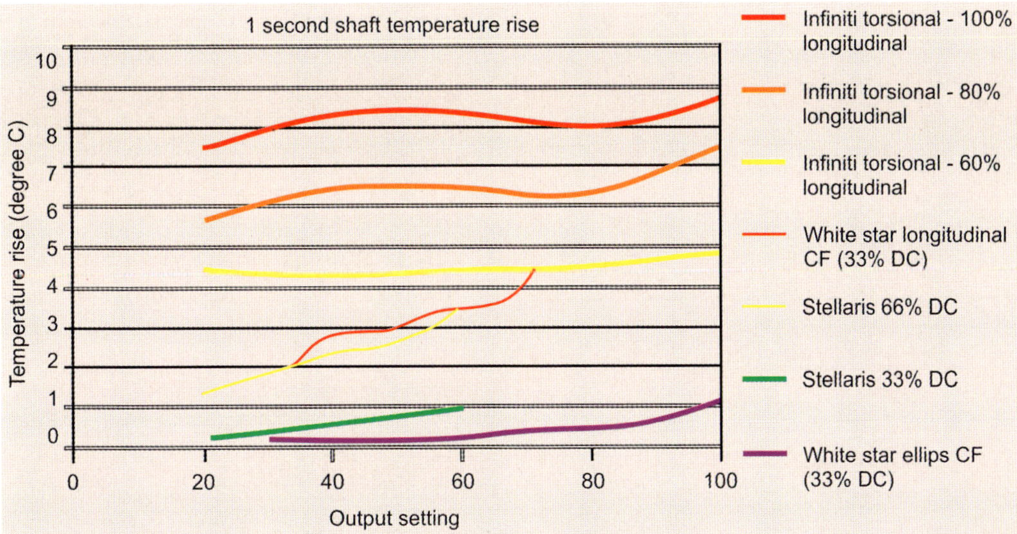

Fig. 6: Temperature rise in shaft of phaco tip after 1 second. (Schafer ME. Thermal characterization of phacoemulsification tips. Presented at ESCRS Annual Meeting. Berlin, 2008)

Similarly, other clinical studies have also determined that the wound temperature with MICS does not rise above 40°C under normal clinical conditions[15] (Fabian E. Bimanual phaco and temperature using new phaco-software (WhiteStar). Presented at ESCRS 2002, Nice, France). In a series of 637 patients who underwent MICS, there was no report of corneal incision burn.[16]

As corneal incision burn is dependent on the temperature, the impact of ultrasonic phaco handpieces, tip geometries and operating modes is significant. In a laboratory setting, it has been shown that there are differences between the various phaco systems currently available. Using high speed thermal imaging of phaco tips, it was found that the greatest temperature rise was with the Alcon Infinity system with torsional handpieces; Bausch & Lomb Stellaris and AMO Signature with Ellips had the least temperature rise, as demonstrated in Figure 6. (Schafer ME. Thermal characterization of phacoemulsification tips. Presented at ESCRS Annual Meeting. Berlin, 2008).

Thus, not only is there considerable laboratory and clinical evidence to support the use of sleeveless phaco tips in MICS but also some indication that the AMO Signature Ellips system may be the least likely to cause incision burn.

Corneal Changes

Clarity

Clarity of the cornea following cataract surgery is an indication of the trauma incurred during surgery. In a study comparing MICS and standard coaxial phaco, no difference was found between the techniques[3] as Figure 7 illustrates.

Thus, MICS and standard coaxial phaco, at the very least, induce comparable minimal trauma to the eye.

Induced Corneal Aberrations

As cataract surgery has evolved over the past two decades, so have corneal incisions decreased from greater than 10 mm with intracapsular cataract extraction (ICCE), 8–10 mm with extracapsular cataract extraction (ECCE), 6.0–7.0 mm with phaco and polymethylmethacrylate (PMMA) lenses, and less than 3.5 mm with phaco and foldable IOLs. With each incremental decrease in incision size, there has been a decrease in induced corneal

Machine	Coaxial Results	Bimanual Results
Series 20000 Legacy with Neosonix (Alcon Laboratories, Inc., Fort Worth TX)	98%	100%
Millennium with Phaco Burst (Bausch & Lomb, Rochester, NY)	100%	100%
Staar Sonic wave (Staar surgical company, Monrovia CA	95%	100%
Sovereign phaco system with Whit-estar Technology (Advanced Medical Optics, Inc, Santa Ana, CA	100%	97%
*P < .05 for all comparisons		

Fig. 7: Percentage of eyes with clear corneas, 2–24 hours postoperatively[5]

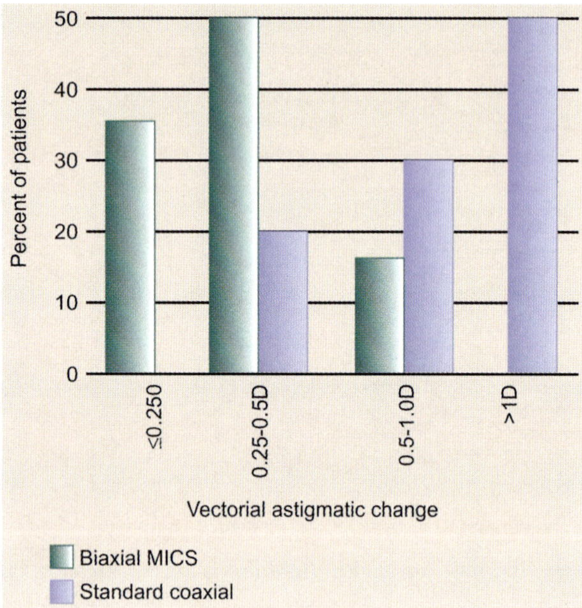

Fig. 8: Vectoral astigmatic analysis of surgically induced astigmatism in biaxial MICS compared with coaxial cataract surgery (from Alio et al.)[7]

Comparative results on corneal astigmatism for Microincision Cataract Surgery versus Small Incision Cataract Surgery			
	MICS	SICS	P value
Preoperative Δ Sim K (D)	0.7 ± 0.34	0.66 ± 0.38	0.669
Postoperative Δ Sim K (D)	0.78 ± 0.38	1.29 ± 0.68	0.001
Note. Δ Sim K represents the difference in power between the steep and flat meridians MICS: 30 eyes, 1.7 ± 0.1 mm; SICS: 30 eyes, 3.2 mm			

Fig. 9: Changes in the simulated keratometry values; comparison of MICS and coaxial cataract surgery[19]

Comparative results on corneal astigmatism for Microincision Incision Cataract Surgery versus Small Incision Cataract Surgery[10]			
Spatial Frequency (cpd)	MICS	SICS	P value
0.5 MTF	3.13 ± 0.30	2.75 ± 0.63	0.004
0.1 MTF	9.37 ± 3.72	7.24 ± 3.43	0.134
Note. MIcs: 30 eyes, 1.7 ± 0.1 mm; SICS: 30 eyes, 3.2 mm MTF (modulation transfer function) are the metrics to indicate retinal image quality from an incoming object			

Fig. 10: Comparison of MTF with MICS and coaxial phaco

astigmatism. Scleral incisions have been associated with less induced astigmatism than corneal incisions.[17]

In a prospective, randomized study of 100 patients, comparing MICS and standard coaxial phaco, Alio et al.[7] analyzed the surgically induced astigmatism using vectoral analysis. The MICS group had a mean incision size of 1.71 ±0.21 mm compared to the coaxial group of 3.1 ±0.25 mm. They reported a mean change of 0.36 ±0.232 D in the MICS group compared to a significantly greater increase of 1.2 ±0.74 D in the standard coaxial phaco group. An interesting finding was that more than 50% of the coaxial group had more than 1 D of induced astigmatism while none of the coaxial group had this (Fig. 8).

Similar reports of decreased induced corneal astigmatism have been reported by other authors.[16,18,19] Koch reported an induced astigmatism of less than 0.25 D at 4 weeks postoperatively with 2.0 mm incision; this decreased to less than 0.075 D by 6 months postoperatively (Koch D. Cataract surgery through a 2.0 mm incision: Results of bimanual phaco-chop technique and acrylic IOL implantation. ASCRS Meeting 2003, San Francisco, USA). Ke Yao et al.[19] found that the change in the simulated keratometry value was greater in the coaxial group (3.2 mm incision) versus the MICS group (1.7 mm incision) (Fig. 9). Thus, corneal induced astigmatism following MICS is significantly less than standard coaxial and approaches almost zero change.[20]

Not only can lower order aberrations of astigmatism be affected by cataract surgery, but also higher order aberrations. A 3.2 mm superior clear corneal incision "induced consistent and significant changes in several corneal Zernike terms (vertical astigmatism, trefoil and tetrafoil) resulting in a significantly increased overall corneal (root-mean-square) RMS wavefront error".[21] However, the 3.2 mm incision did not induce significant changes in spherical aberration or coma terms. The amount and orientation of the aberrations induced depended on the surgical meridian and incision location.

In contrast to the 3.2 mm incision, MICS does not induce any change in total RMS value.[20]

When optical quality is evaluated, it has been found that implantation of microincision IOLs with MICS results in at least similar modulation transfer function (MTF) values as standard IOLs in coaxial cataract surgery.[22] In fact, Ke Yao et al. reported a significantly better MTF values at a spatial frequency of 0.5 MTF with MICS in their study of MICS versus coaxial surgery[19] (Fig. 10). Thus, MICS provides similar or better quality of vision than coaxial.

If the corneal higher order aberrations are measured preoperatively and postoperatively, and a comparison is made of MICS versus 3.2 mm coaxial cataract surgery, an increase in induced coma has been reported in the latter group (Bellucci R, Morselli S. Aberration control in cataract surgery with the Akreos MI60 microincision IOL.

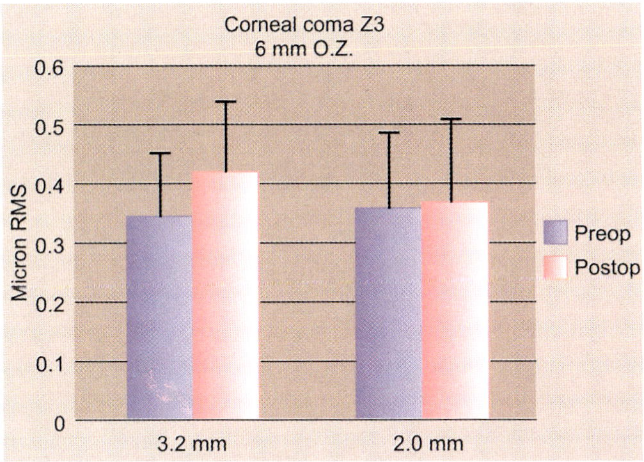

Fig. 11: Comparison of total corneal coma; MICS versus coaxial cataract surgery (from Bellucci R, Morselli S. Aberration control in cataract surgery with the Akreos MI60 microincision IOL. ASCRS Presentation. Chicago, 2008)

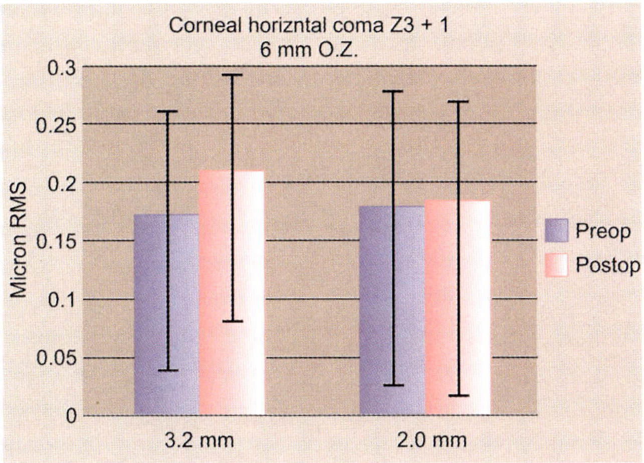

Fig. 12: Comparison of horizontal corneal coma; MICS versus coaxial cataract surgery (from Bellucci R, Morselli S. Aberration control in cataract surgery with the Akreos MI60 microincision IOL. ASCRS Presentation, Chicago,2008)

ASCRS Presentation. Chicago, 2008). This increased coma would result in degradation of the quality of vision (Figs 11 to 13).

All studies support the conclusion that smaller incisions with MICS result in less induced corneal aberrations, whether of lower order (astigmatism) or higher order (coma). Lower aberrations result in better vision.

Endothelial Cell Loss

In this chapter, it has been shown that MICS is associated with decreased phaco time, decreased inflammation and less ocular trauma; in theory, this should result in lower ECL.

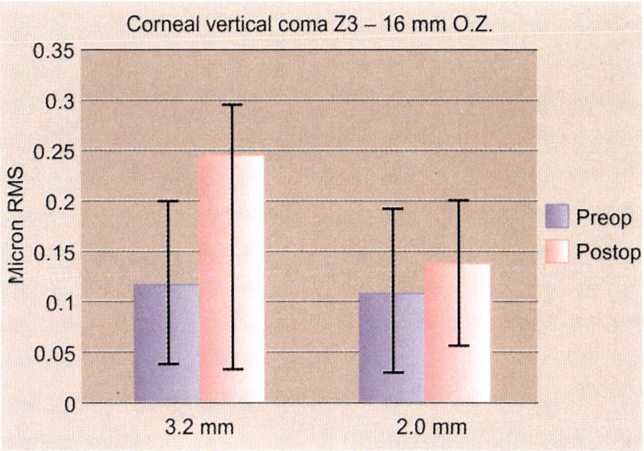

Fig. 13: Comparison of vertical corneal coma; MICS versus coaxial cataract surgery (from Bellucci R, Morselli S. Aberration control in cataract surgery with the Akreos MI60 microincision IOL. ASCRS Presentation. Chicago, 2008)

Before looking in depth into this aspect of MICS, it is important to understand the measurement of ECL. Measurements of endothelial cell counts are highly reproducible by a model of specular microscope but the results are not interchangeable between different models of specular microscopes;[23] thus in comparing ECL, it is essential that the same type of specular microscope is used. Cell loss of 10% is within confidence interval of measurement error with a specular microscope.[24] In multicentre studies, precision of only 8-10% can be expected; improved precision of 2% can be anticipated only if one centre and experienced staff are employed for interpretation of the data.[25] In standard coaxial phaco, ECL of 6.4–8.8% at 90 days postcataract surgery has been reported. To be determined that MICS is safe, it must be shown that at least comparable ECL occurs. A number of studies prospectively comparing coaxial phaco to MICS have confirmed this (Beiko GHH. Endothelial cell loss with micro-incisional cataract surgery. Presented ASCRS Annual Meeting. Washington, 2005.)[6,7,26-30] (see Figure 14 for summary of the data).

The amount of ECL is proportional to the density of cataract being emulsified, and this is also true for MICS, as has been reported by Tsuneoka et al.[16] (Fig. 15).

Corneal damage as assessed by ECL is similar whether coaxial phaco or MICS is employed to remove cataracts.

Infection

Endophthalmitis in cataract surgery has been proposed to be associated with many factors including incision construction; incision location; preoperative, intraoperative,

	No. of eyes	Endothelial cell loss (%) 3 mos	
		Coaxial	MICS
Crema 2007	60	4.7 ± 6.1	4.5 ± 5.1
Cavalini 2007	100	10.1 ± 11.7	11.9 ± 15.2
Mencucci 2006	80	6.5	6.3
Kurz 2006	70	4.7 ± 6.1	4.5 ± 5.1
Kahraman 2006	66	3.1 ± 6.2	6.2 ± 5.1
Alio 2005	100	11.7 ± 16.0	7.4 ± 9.2

Fig. 14: Comparison of endothelial cell loss between MICS and coaxial phaco

and postoperative use of antibiotics; surgical trauma and patient health. Some authors have claimed that clear corneal incisions compared to scleral incisions are at increased risk of endophthalmitis due to decreased integrity of the incision and delayed incision healing.[31-34] Scleral and near limbal incisions are thought to have decreased infection due to the ability of the conjunctiva to cover the wound and allow for faster incision sealing. The causal nature of clear corneal incisions in endophthalmitis is controversial and no clear connection has been made.

It has been proposed that as MICS incisions are smaller than coaxial and microcoaxial incisions, there may be potential features of the incisions which would make them prone to allowing ingress of infectious fluids.

In a comparison study of clear corneal incisions in cadaver eyes, looking at MICS, microcoaxial and coaxial phaco, it has been suggested that MICS incisions are prone to leakage. The authors used India ink to determine if there was penetration into the eyes and found that both MICS eyes allowed India ink into the incision compared to one standard coaxial and none of the microcoaxial eyes

Cataract grade	Endo Cell Loss %
1	4.6 +/– 12.8
2	6.9 +/– 16.5
3	10.8 +/– 12.4
4-5	15.6 +/– 13.7

Fig. 15: Endothelial cell loss related to cataract density in MICS[16]

(Figs 16A and B). They hypothesized that MICS incisions would be prone to allowing ingress of fluid and infection.

In a rabbit study of MICS and microcoaxial phaco, in which 0.5 cc of *Staphylococcus epidermidis* culture was placed on the cornea for 2 minutes, following surgery, it was found that there was greater penetration of bacteria into the MICS eyes (1358.1 vs. 250.9 CFU per 0.1 mL of aqueous fluid).[35] The authors proposed that oar locking of the irrigating and phaco tips in the MICS wound might cause distortion of the wound, resulting in wound leakage and allowing for hypotony and ingress of extraocular fluid.

In these studies, incisions with parallel sides were constructed which facilitate greater damage from oar locking than if trapezoidal incisions had been made. With trapezoidal incisions, the oar locking only occurs at the internal lip of the incision and thus trauma is minimized (personal communication, H Fine).

Despite these laboratory studies suggesting greater risk of endophthalmitis with MICS, there have been no reports of any epidemics of infection with MICS. In fact, a literature search found mention of one case report, in which endophthalmitis developed on day 4 postoperatively. Clinically, there was fibrin present at the 7 o'clock incision, which was in contact with the inferior fornix. This infection grew alpha-hemolytic streptococcus.[36] It is this

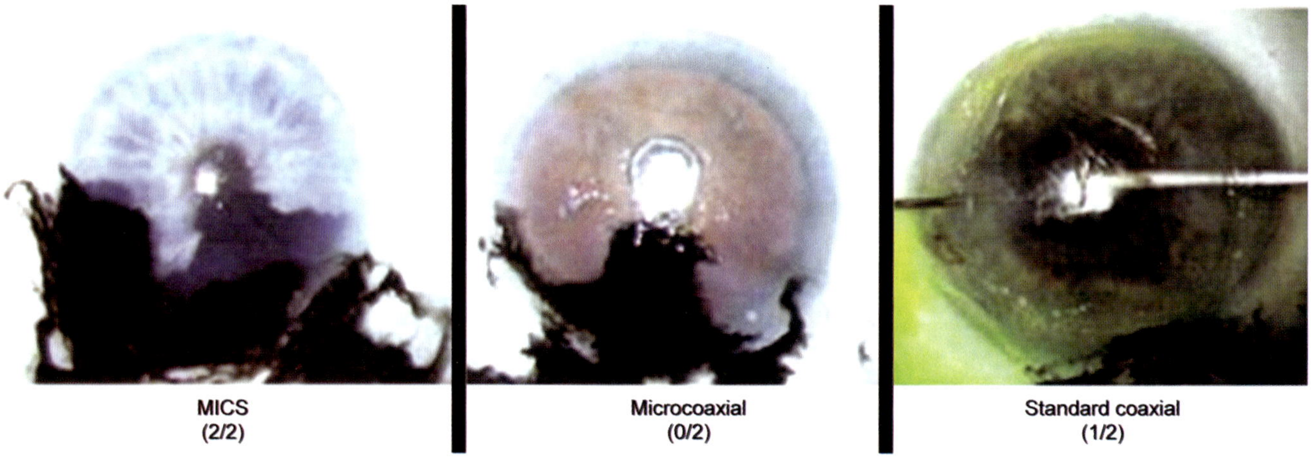

Fig. 16A: India ink penetration. Clear corneal incisions after phacoemulsification in cadaver eyes[11]

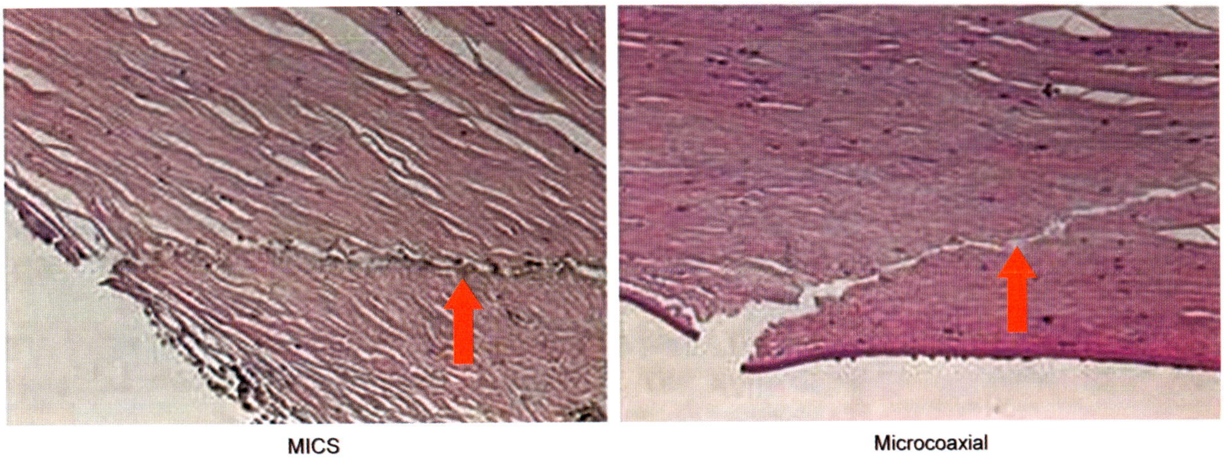

Fig. 16B: India ink penetration. Clear corneal incisions after phacoemulsification in cadaver eyes[11]

author opinion that the lack of clinical correlation to the laboratory findings is that the smaller MICS incisions, if properly hydrated at the end of the case, are closed tighter than larger coaxial incisions. This would explain the lack of increased endophthalmitis.

Summary

This author has been performing exclusively MICS for the past 6 years. All of the reasons stated at the beginning of the chapter were the appeal in transitioning to MICS. There has been no safety concerns related to MICS. The control during surgery and the visual outcomes are the main reasons for author's continued implementation of this technique.

Take Home Messages

1. Visual outcomes and rehabilitation with MICS superior than coaxial surgery.
2. Incision damage minimal and comparable to coaxial phaco.
3. No increase in corneal incision burn despite use of sleeveless phaco tip.
4. Superior vision with MICS than coaxial due to less induced astigmatism and higher order aberrations.
5. Endothelial cell loss comparable to coaxial phaco.
6. No increase in infection with MICS compared to coaxial phaco.

References

1. Shock JP. Removal of cataracts with ultrasonic fragmentation and continuous irrigation. Trans Pac Coast Otoophthalmol Soc Annu Meet. 1972; 53:139-44.
2. Girard LJ. Ultrasonic fragmentation for cataract extraction and cataract complications. Adv Ophthalmol. 1978; 37:127-35.
3. Shearing SP, Relyca RL, Louiza A, et al. Routine phacoemulsification through a one millimeter non-sutured incision. Cataract. 1985;2:6-11.
4. Alio JL. What does MICS require? In: Alio JL, Rodriquez-Prats JL, Gala A, (Eds). MICS Micro-incision Cataract Surgery. Miami: Highlights of Ophthalmlogy; 2004.
5. Fine IH, Hoffman RS, Packer M. Why we prefer bimanual microincisional phacoemulsification. Cataract Ref Surg Today. 2004;9:43-6.
6. Kurz S, Krummenauer F, Gabriel P, et al. Biaxial microincision versus coaxial small incision clear corneal cataract surgery. Ophthalmology. 2006;113(10):1818-26.
7. Alio J, Rodriguez-Prats JL, Galal A, et al. Outcomes of microincision cataract surgery versus coaxial phacoemulsification. Ophthalmology. 2005;112(11):1997-2003.
8. Fine IH, Hoffman RS, Packer M. Optimizing refractive lens exchange with bimanual microincision phacoemulsification. J Cataract Refract Surg. 2004;30:550-4.
9. Braga-Mele R, Lui E. Feasibility of sleeveless bimanual phacoemulsification with the Millenium microsurgical system. J Cataract Refract Surg. 2003;29:2199-203.
10. Agarwal A, Agarwal A, Agarwal S, et al. Phaconit: phacoemulsification through a 0.9 mm corneal incision. J Cataract Refract Surg. 2001;27(10):1548-52.
11. Berdahl JP, DeStafeno JJ, Kim T. Corneal wound architecture and integrity after phacoemulsification. Evaluaiton of coaxial, micorincisional coaxial and microincisional bimanual techniques. J Cataract Refract Surg. 2007;33(3):510-5.
12. Sporl E, Genth U, Schmalfuss K, et al. Thermomechanical behaviour of the cornea. Ger J Ophthalmol. 1997;6:322-7.
13. Goldblatt WS, Finger PT, Perry HD, et al. Hyperthermic treatment of rabbit corneas. Invest Ophthalmol Vis Sci. 1989;1778-83.
14. Donnenfeld E, Olson RJ, Solomon R, et al. Efficacy and wound-temperature gradient of WhiteStar phacoemulsification through a 1.2 m incision. J Cataract Refract Surg. 2003;29(6):1097-100.

15. Soscia W, Howard JG, Olson RJ. Microphacoemulsification with WhiteStar: a wound-temperature study. J Cataract Refract Surg. 2002;28:1044-6.
16. Tsuneoka H, Shiba T, Takahashi Y. Ultrasonic phacoemulsification using 1.4 mm incision: clinical results. J Cataract Refract Surg. 2002;28:81-6.
17. Pesudovs K, Dietze H, Stewart OG, et al. Effect of cataract surgery incision location and intraocular lens type on ocular aberrations. J Cataract Refract Surg. 2005;31:725-34.
18. Tsuneoka H, Shiba T, Takahashi Y. Feasibility of ultrasound cataract surgery with a 1.4 mm incision. J Cataract Refract Surg. 2001;27:934-40.
19. Ke Yao, Xiajing Tang, Panpan Ye. Corneal Astigmatism, Higher Order Aberrations, and Optical Quality After Cataract Surgery: Microincision Versus Small Incision. J Refract Surg. 2006;22(9 Suppl): S1079-82.
20. Elkady B, Alió JL, Ortiz D, et al. Corneal aberrations after microincision cataract surgery. J Cataract Refract Surg. 2008;34(1):40-5.
21. Marcos S, Rosales P, Llorente L, et al. Change in corneal aberrations after cataract surgery with two types of aspherical intraocular lenses. J Cataract Refract Surg. 2007;33(2):217-26.
22. Alió JL, Schimchak P, Montés-Micó R, et al. Retinal image quality after microincision intraocular lens implantation. J Cataract Refract Surg. 2005;31(8):1557-60.
23. Landesz M, Siertsema JV, Van Rij G. Comparative study of three semiautomated specular microscopes. J Cataract Refract Surg. 1995;21(4):409-16
24. Probst LE, Hakim OJ, Nichols BD. Phacoemulsification with aspirated or retained Viscoat. J Cataract Refract Surg. 1994;20(2):145-9.
25. Edelhauser HF, Sanders DR, Azar R, et al. ICL in treatment of myopia study group. Corneal endothelial assessment after ICL implantation. J Cataract Refract Surg. 2004;30(3):576-83.
26. Crema AS, Walsh A, Yamane Y, et al. Comparative study of coaxial phacoemulsificaiton and microincisonal cataract surgery. One-year follow-up. J Cataract Ref Surg. 2007;33:1014-8.
27. Mencucci R, Ponchietti C, Virgili G, et al. Corneal endothelial damage after cataract surgery: MICS versus standard technique. J Cataract Ref Surg. 2006;32: 1351-4.
28. Mathys K, Cohen KL, Armstrong BD, et al. Determining factors for corneal endothelial cell loss by using bimanual microincisional phacoemulsification and power modulation. Cornea. 2007;26(9):1049-55.
29. Cavallini GM, Campi L, Masini C, et al. Bimanual microphacoemulsification versus coaxial miniphacoemulsification: prospective study. J Cataract Refract Surg. 2007;33(3): 387-92.
30. Kahraman G, Amon M, Franz C, et al. Intraindividual comparison of surgical trauma after bimanual microincision and conventional small-incision coaxial phacoemulsification. J Cataract Refract Surg. 2007;33(4):618-22.
31. McDonnell PJ, Taban M, Sarayba M, et al. Dynamic morphology of clear corneal cataract incisions. Ophthalmology. 2003;110:2342-8.
32. Taban M, Rao B, Reznik J, et al. Dynamic morphology of sutureless cataract wounds-effect of incision angle and location. Surv Ophthal. 2004;49(supp 2):S62-72.
33. Taban M, Sarayba MA, Ignacio TS, et al. Ingress of India Ink into the anterior chamber through sutureless clear corneal cataract wounds. Arch Ophthal. 2005;123:643-8.
34. John ME, Noblitt R. Endophthalmitis: Scleral tunnel versus clear corneal incision. In: Buzzard K, Friedlander MH, Febbraro JL, (Eds). The Blue Line Incision and Refractive Phacoemulsification. New Jersey: Slack Inc; 2001.
35. Gajjar D, Praveen MR, Vasavada AR, et al. Ingress of bacterial inoculum into the anterior chamber after bimanual and microcoaxial phacoemulsification in rabbits. J Cataract Refract Surg. 2007;33(12):2129-34.
36. Chee SP, Bascal K. Endophthalmitis after microincisional cataract surgery. J Cataract Refract Surg. 2005;31:1834-5.

10 Biaxial Phaco Surgical Tools

Luis Felipe Vejarano-Restrepo (Colombia)

Since the beginning of microincision cataract surgery in 1998 by Dr Amar Agarwal when he started with a needle and an anterior chamber maintainer, the instrumentation has changed enormously, since the knives until the intraocular lenses (IOLs)[1-4], in every step of the procedure turns critical the use of the precise instruments to obtain the best results.[5]

Incision

As in any kind of phacoemulsification technique (biaxial or coaxial) the incision is one of the key points for the successful of the procedure, mainly in microincision because the fluidics[6-9], plays a very important role in the stability of the anterior chamber during the whole surgery, if the incision is too small, the manipulation of the instruments produce corneal damage causing troubles for the self sealing of the incision either in the main incision as the side port one, also difficult the normal maneuverability of the instrument into the eye for the disassembling and emulsification of the nucleus; instead if the incision is too large, it causes excessive of leakage causing instability of the anterior chamber with collapse of it and endothelial damage; not only the size of the incision is important but also the tunnel length, it has to be at least 1.5 mm and its length is contingent on the needle diameter.

Based on this, surgeons have to know the diameter of the tip of phaco needle to calculate the size of their main incision and also the diameter of their irrigation instrument (chopper most of the time) for the side port one; remember, the needle and the chopper are a metallic rigid circumference and the incision is a longitudinal elastic line, calculating the circumference length of the instrument, using the formula $2 \pi r$, where r means radius of the instrument in millimeter; but since each lip of the incision covers a half, not the whole length of the instrument's circumference is needed, so you have to divide the result by two. Moreover, the cornea is an elastic tissue and so, surgeons have to take in account the tissue compliance, which author has calculated in approximately 20%. Thus the final formula to decide upon the right length of the incision is:

$$(2 \pi r/2) - 20\%, \text{ that is to say: } \pi \times r \times 0.80.$$

As an example, if surgeons are going to use a 1.067 mm outer diameter needle or irrigating chopper (19 gauge), the calculation for the main and side port incision will be as follows:

$$(\pi \times 0.533 \text{ mm} \times 80) = 1.674 \text{ mm} \times 0.80 = 1.33 \text{ mm}$$

If surgeons are going to use an irrigating chopper or microtip 20 gauge (0.9 mm outer diameter), their side port and main incision length must be:

$$(\pi \times 0.45 \text{ mm} \times .8) = 1.396 \text{ mm} \times 0.80 = 1.11 \text{ mm}$$

Finally if surgeons are going to use a 0.7 mm outer diameter needle (nanotip) or irrigating chopper (22 gauge), the calculation for the main and side port incisions will be as follows:

$$(\pi \times 0.35 \text{ mm} \times 0.80) = 1.11 \text{ mm} \times 0.80 = 0.89 \text{ mm}$$

The most common gauge of phaco needles/irrigating choppers and applying the previous formula to them is in the Table 1.

At the beginning of this technique when most of the authors of this book started to make microincision, author of this chapter had to use instruments that exist at that time as MVR blades or asking to the manufacturers to make diamond blades in standard or trapezoidal shape for the right size depending on the needle diameter, author started with 1.5 mm diamond blade (Natural Clear Cornea Vejarano's Microincision Knife; AK6018 Accutome, Malvern, USA)

TABLE 1 Gauge of phaco needles and size of incision

Gauge	*Millimeters*	*Incision*
18	1.245	1.50 mm
19	1.067	1.33 mm
20	0.889	1.11 mm
21	0.759	0.91 mm
22	0.711	0.89 mm

(Figs 1A and B) because at that time author used the Storz Premiere machine with the microflow needle 19 gauge but his irrigating chopper was 20 gauge (Accutome, Malvern, USA) (Figs 2A and B) for the technique "Vejarano's Safe Chop"[10-19], so also author had to order to make a trapezoidal knife with 0.9/1.2 mm (Accutome, Malvern, USA) (Figs 3A to C) which gives 1.1 mm internal incision (precise to any 20 gauge); right now because of the spread of this technique many manufacturers have in their catalogs many of these knives, in diamond, sapphire or metallic, lately with micro-biaxial technique author started to use the nanotip (Figs 15A and B) and the Vejarano's Irrigating Chopper (Figs 4A and B) both 22 gauge (Du 02357; MicroSurgical Technology, Redmond, USA) using a 1 mm diamond knife (Accutome, Malvern, USA) (Figs 5A and B). So, again depending on instruments diameter (phaco needle and irrigation device) surgeons need to construct their incision size to achieve a good architecture, if may be the cost of the diamonds is too high and microincision is not yet their technique of choice, then is possible to use a 20 gauge vitreoretinal blades (any manufacture) or 1.2/1.4 mm steel blades (MicroSurgical Technology, Redmond, USA) in Biaxial (Figs 6A and B) or could use a 1 mm steel lancet too (Alcon, Fort Worth, Texas, USA) or the 0.8 mm knife (SK 080A; MicroSurgical Technology, Redmond, USA) (Fig. 7) in micro-biaxial.

The way how to construct the correct architecture of the incision will be explained in the different sections regarding surgical techniques, as a part of this book.

Viscoelastics

In this technique (microincision), one of its great advantages is that surgeons can use any kind of viscoelastic; whichever cohesive, dispersive or viscoadaptative, because through the small size of the incision it is very difficult to remove the visco agent from the anterior chamber maintaining a stable space during the whole rhexis, so this gives surgeons the safety to try to avoid or diminish the incidence of anterior capsular tear (Argentinian flag) in the capsulorhexis and to solve any problem in its construction even to avoid a tear to periphery, remove any fibrosis or enlarge it in a case where it was too small.

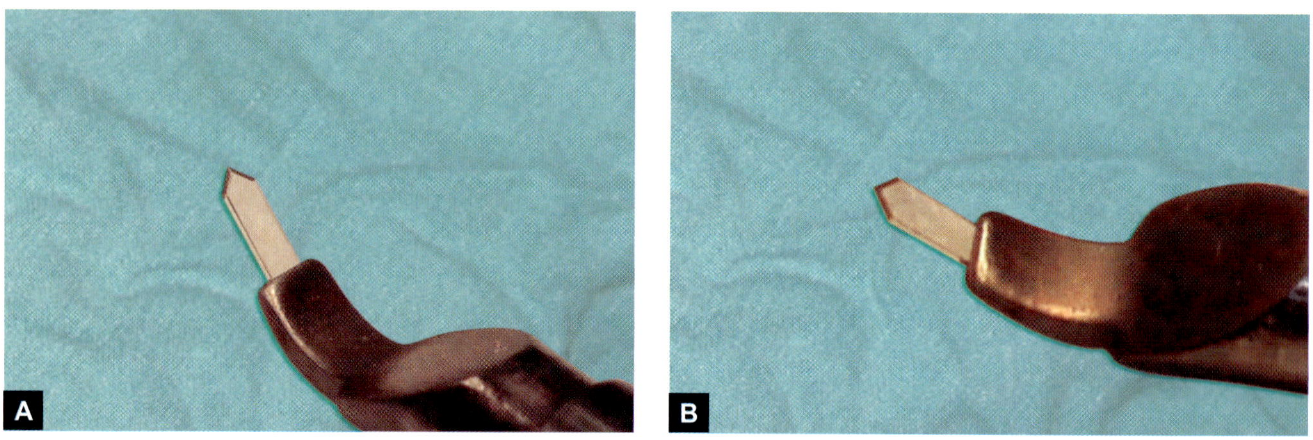

Figs 1 A and B: Natural clear cornea Vejarano's microincision knife. AK6018 Accutome, Malvern, USA

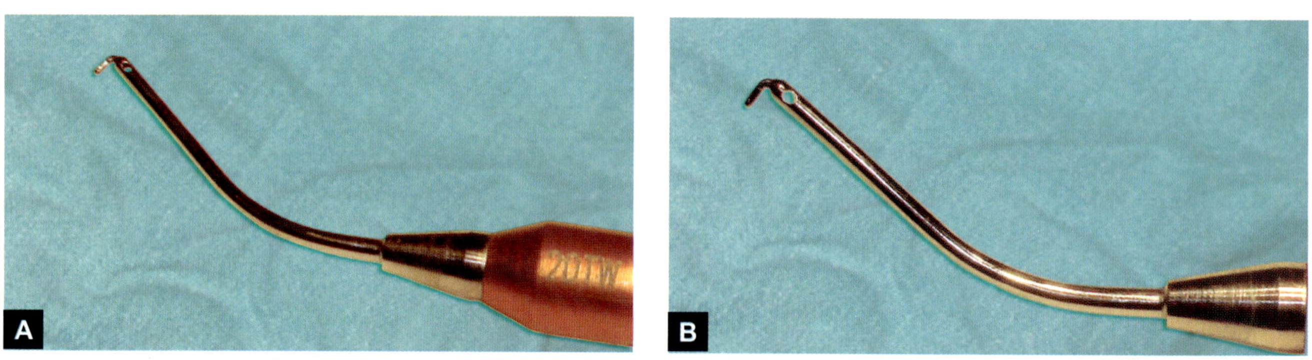

Figs 2 A and B: Irrigating chopper 20 gauge (Accutome, Malvern, USA)

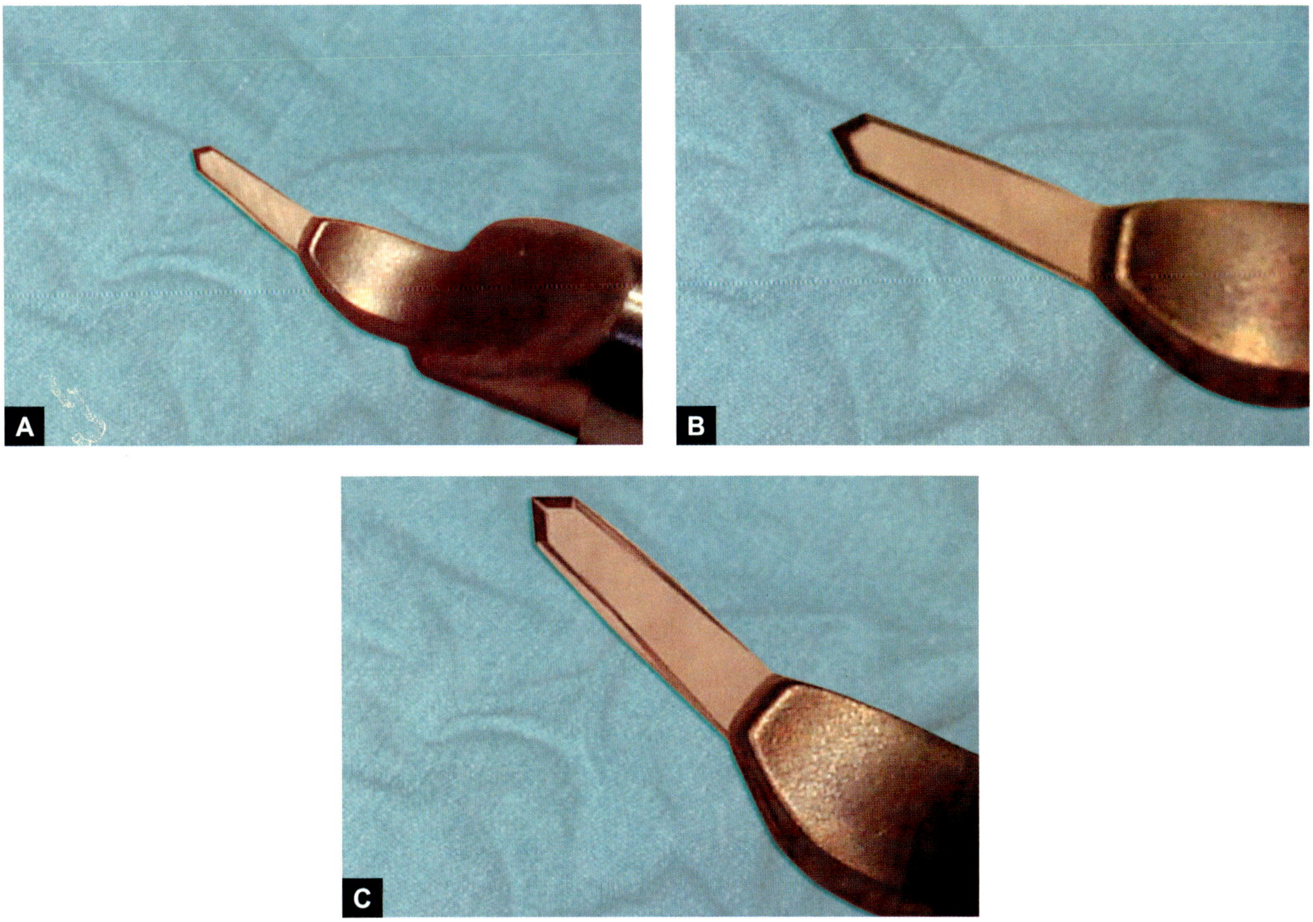

Figs 3 A to C: Trapezoidal knife with 0.91 to 2 mm (Accutome, Malvern, USA)

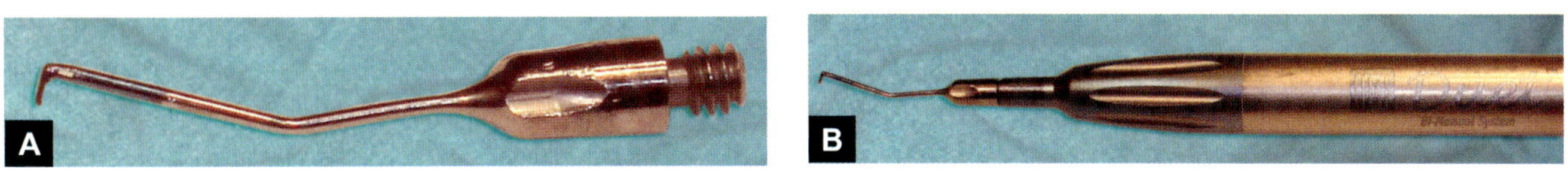

Figs 4 A and B: Vejarano's irrigating chopper

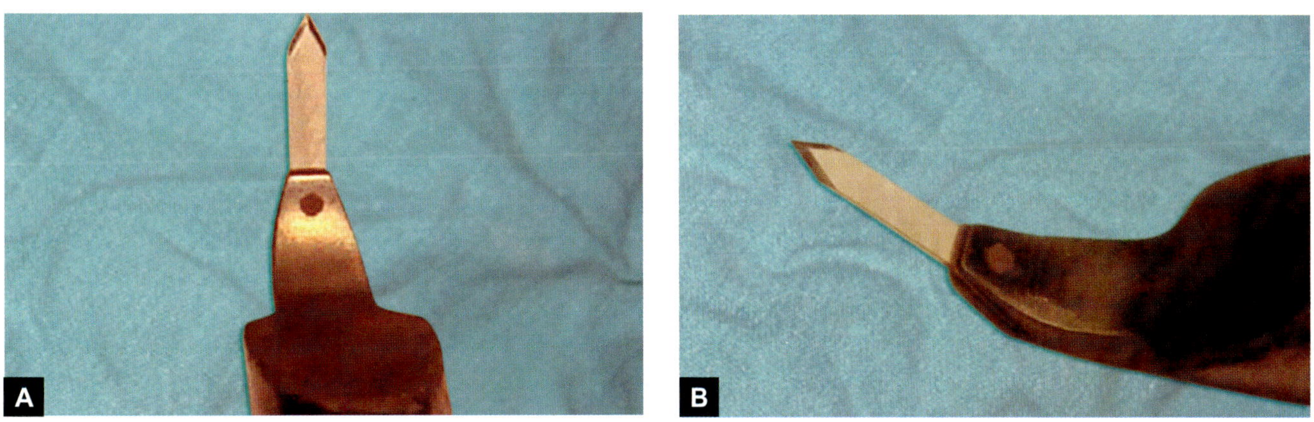

Figs 5 A and B: 1 mm diamond knife (Accutome, Malvern, USA)

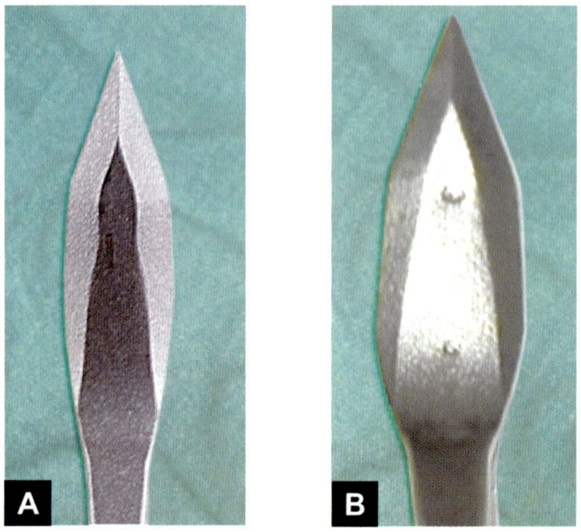

Figs 6 A and B: 1.2 to 1.4 mm steel blades (MIcro Surgical Technology, Redmond, USA)

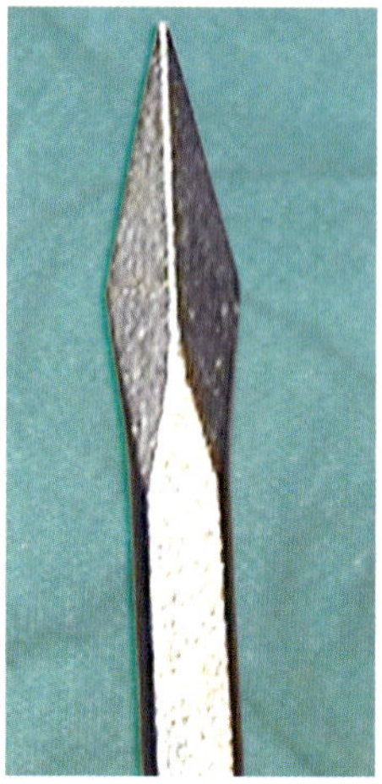

Fig. 7: 0.8 mm knife (SK - 080A MicroSurgical Technology, Redmond, USA)

For the injection of the ophthalmic viscosurgical device (OVD) always use thin cannula 27 gauge (Fig. 8) to avoid incisional trauma as focal descemet tear trying to go into the eye.

Capsulorhexis

Like in coaxial phaco this is the most important step in the whole surgery, so you have to try to avoid any complication or rupture of the anterior capsule with a tear toward the periphery even more if you are beginning with this technique, other big advantage of this technique is that you can switch the hands and use the microutrata forceps through the main or through the side port incision, to facilitate the successful in this step.

To assure surgeon better maneuverability, the incision size again is vital because of the its size any movement brings surgeon to move the whole eye, so surgeons have to counteract their movements making contralateral pressure at the incision (between internal and external edge), this means that the friction between the forceps and the walls of incision tunnel will move the eye but also help to maintain the eye at the center the microutrata forceps has to be smaller than incision size, then surgeons have to use 21 or 23 gauge (with or without the rhexis ruler) (MicroSurgical Technology, Redmond, USA) (Figs 9A to C). There are also a lot of other models of Microutrata forceps from many other commercial manufactures but always surgeons have to look for some specific features, like, the axis of direct action, the curve arm and the small tips at the end of the forceps, even they are open or closed. These features help to avoid the lock at the internal lip of the incision with the join between the cylinder of the forceps and its tips causing focal descemet detachment. Maybe another important feature of these forceps can be the sharp end tips, that help to facilitate the tear of the anterior capsule giving you an easy grasp of the first flap of the Rhexis.

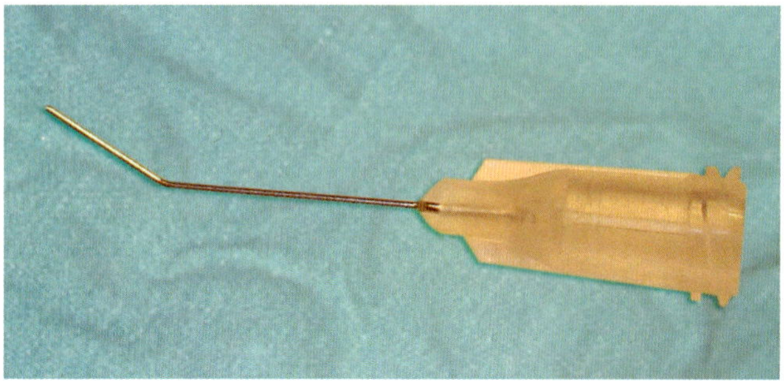

Fig. 8: Cannula 27 gauge

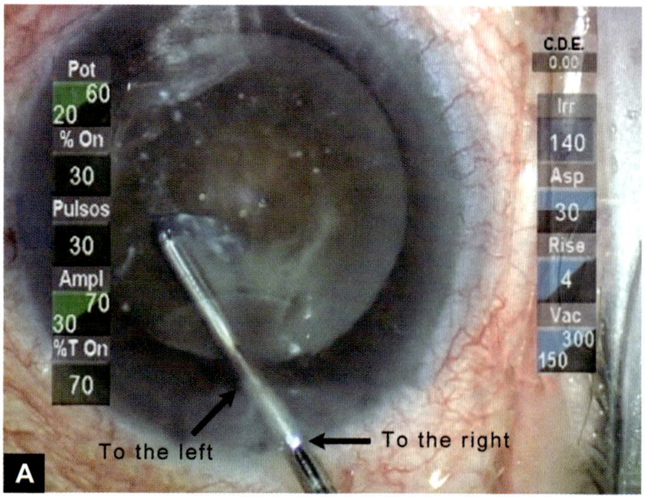

Fig. 9 A: Performance of contralateral pressure at the incision (between internal & external edge)

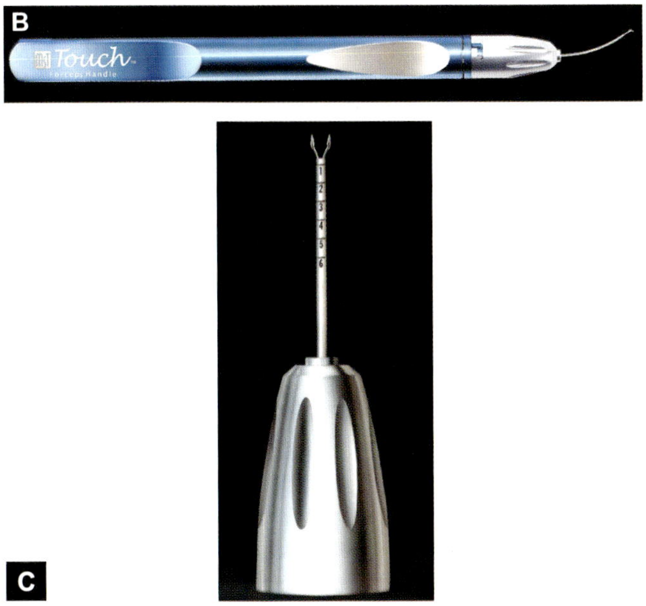

Figs 9 B and C: Microutrata forceps

With respect of the rhexis technique in Microincision also will be explained deeply in the different sections regarding the surgical technique as a part of this book.

If surgeons had a small diameter of the rhexis they can also use the microscissors (MicroSurgical Technology, Redmond, USA) (Figs 10A and B) 21 or 23 gauge to cut an edge of the rhexis and switch to microutrata forceps and enlarge it (because the handle (Fig. 9A) can be used for both utrata and scissors), the advantage of microincision is the possibility of use any of these microinstruments through any of the incisions (main and lateral), whether there is a fibrosis or a tight and old synechia surgeons can used the microscissors but if surgeons find a membrane then use a microforceps (MicroSurgical Technology, Redmond, USA) (Fig. 11); all of these microinstrumentations not only are useful at the rhexis, also are helpful removing a foreign body or grasping an IOL or making a knot inside of the anterior chamber so the investment worth it.

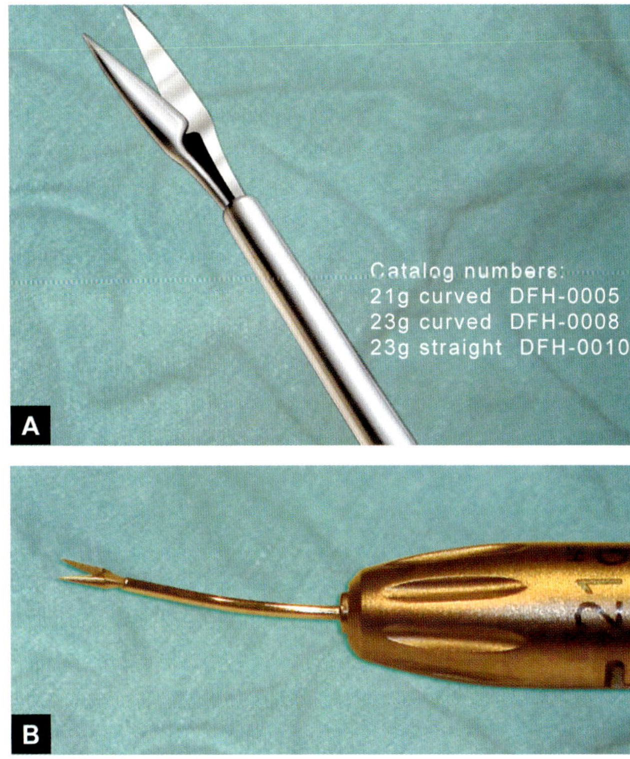

Figs 10 A and B: Microsissors (Microsurgical Technology, Redmond, USA)

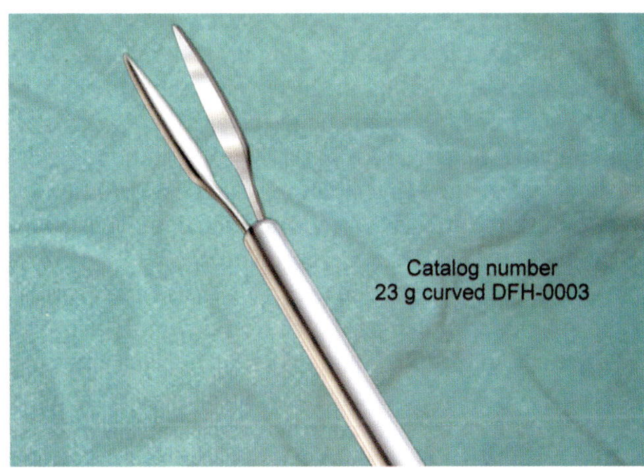

Fig. 11: Microforceps (Microsurgical Technology, Redmond, USA)

Hydrodissection

Before this step, surgeons have to remove some viscoelastic from the anterior chamber to avoid excess of pressure and rupture of the posterior capsule with nuclear drop, always surgeons have to remember that now they are working in a small space, so the cannula has to be the smallest gauge possible with enough flow, like 26 or 27 gauge, but also easy to maneuver so it is better curved or angled cannula, author uses in his regular cases the Chang cannula (Katena, Denville, New Jersey, USA) 27 gauge (Fig. 12) and in his very frequent hypermature cases, the Gimbel cannula (Katena, Denville, New Jersey, USA) 26 gauge (Fig. 13) because its end is totally blunt avoiding any damage of the capsule or equator of the bag, but these ones are not the only cannulas that surgeons can use, also the angled viscoelastic cannula can be used in this step of the procedure (Fig. 8),

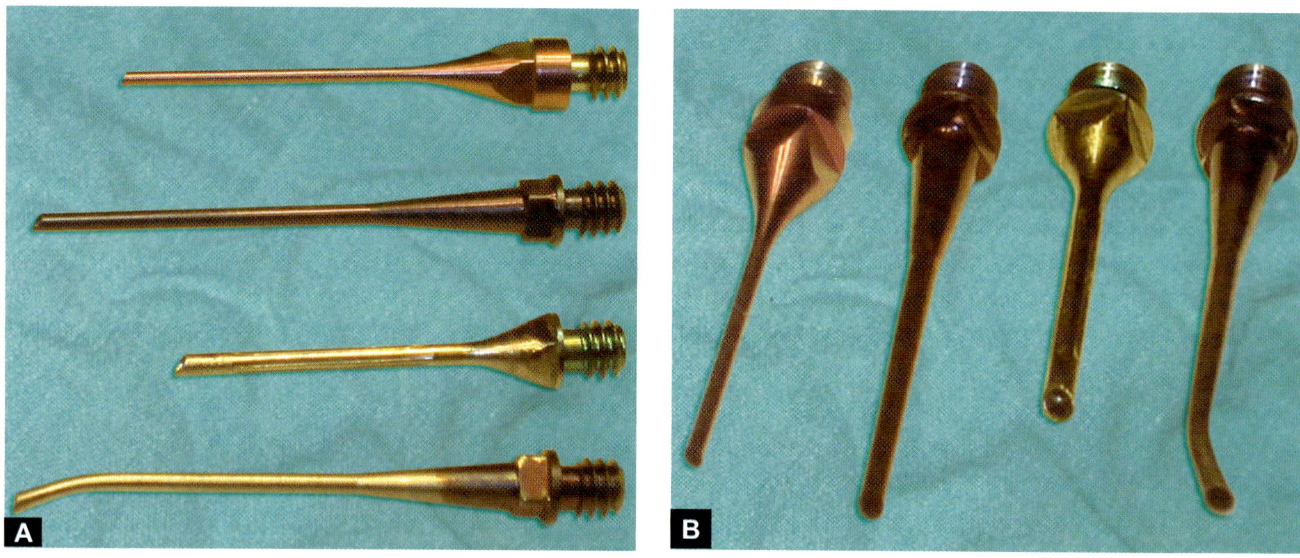

Figs 18 A and B: Comparison of tip diameters

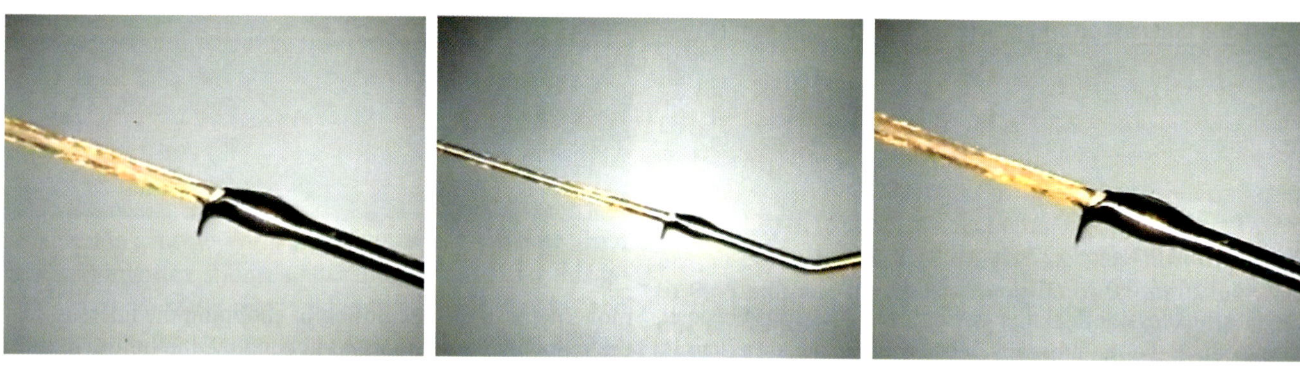

Fig. 19 A. Frontal opening irrigating chopper

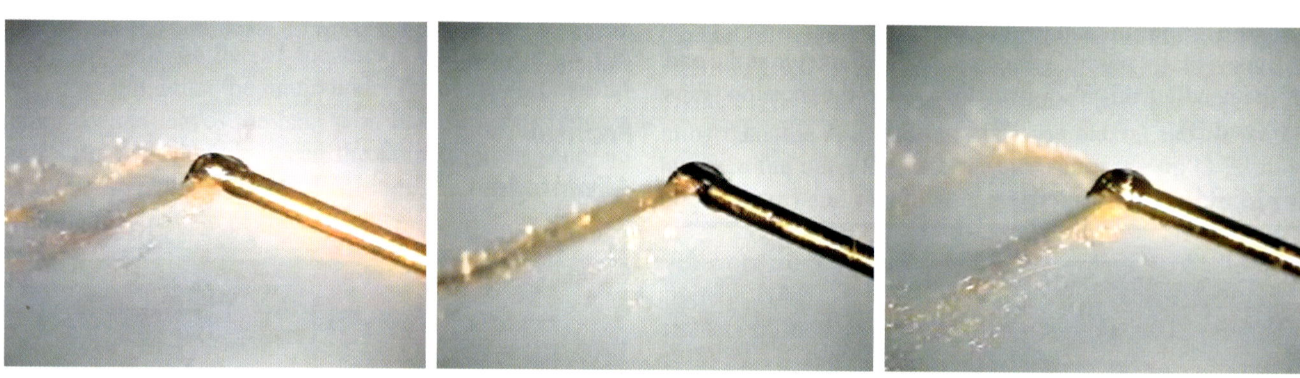

Fig. 19 B. Inferior opening irrigating chopper

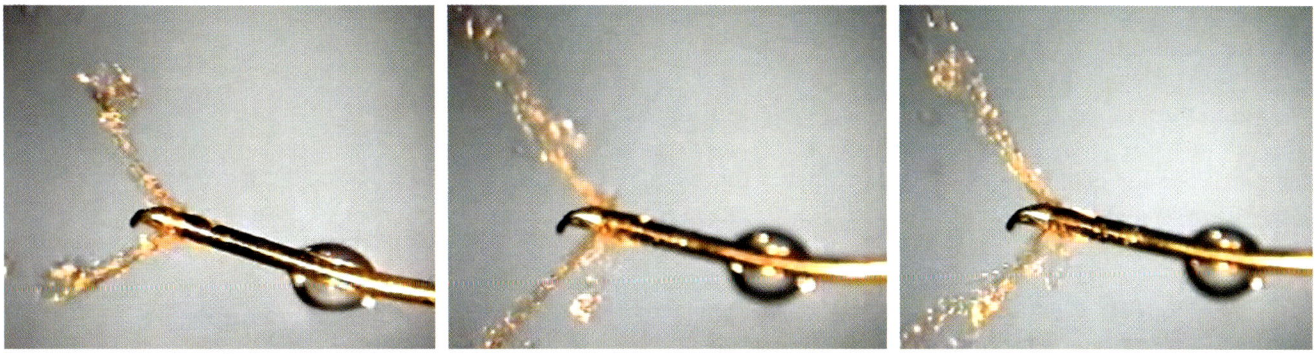

Fig. 19 C. Lateral opening irrigating chopper

Inferior

Advantages

Best fluid circulation in the anterior chamber

Disadvantages

- Lowest inflow related with gauge
- Biggest gauge to improve inflow
- Big side port incision
- Introduction technically difficult

Lateral

Advantages

- Enough inflow
  - 70–77% compared to frontal
  - 75–85% compared to inferior (biggest gauge)
- Good gauge
- Good size of the side port incision
- Minimal turbulence
- Good fluid circulation in the anterior chamber
- Better stability of the anterior chamber

Disadvantages

Very high vacuum has insufficient inflow

Depending of the irrigation chopper of surgeons' choice in design and in direction of the stream, they have to know the inflow of each one which depends on its own internal diameter (thickness of the walls). To select the right flow and vacuum settings in their phaco machine, here is a table (Table 2) which compares the most known choppers in the market with different designs, trends and flow.

Author usually uses in my regular cases micro-biaxial (smaller incisions less than 1 mm) technique, so his incisions have 0.9 mm length, but in his hypermature cases the author uses biaxial (bigger incisions between 1.1 mm and 1.5 mm) technique with bigger instruments to obtain better inflow and holding power, so his incisions have

TABLE 2 Comparison of different designs irrigating choppers

Irrig. Chopper	Gravity 2 Extenders	IOP 100 mm Hg	AVGFI 120 mm Hg
Coaxial	114 cc/min	142 cc/min	131 cc/min
Tsuneoka	74 cc/min	88 cc/min	75 cc/min
Olson I-II	73 cc/min	81 cc/min	77 cc/min
Nagahara	74 cc/min	84 cc/min	75 cc/min
Braga-Mele	60 cc/min	68 cc/min	61 cc/min
Vejarano HOR.	57 cc/min	66 cc/min	60 cc/min
Vejarano INF.	44 cc/min	55 cc/min	45 cc/min
Vejarano 22 GA.	44 cc/min	55 cc/min	54 cc/min
Irrig. 20 GA.	58 cc/min	67 cc/min	64 cc/min
Irrig. 22 GA.	46 cc/min	58 cc/min	53 cc/min

1.1 mm; 22 gauge and 20 gauge (Vejarano's Irrigating Chopper) (Figs 20A and B) even in irrigation chopper and phaco needles respectively.

With respect of the best Phacoemulsification technique in Microincision, this topic will be explained in detail by the different authors of the chapters of this book. Author's uses called Vejarano's Safe Chop Technique[10-18]. With these tips, now you can choose based in your fluidic settings and Phaco technique the better design of the irrigating chopper also depending on your vertical or horizontal chopping technique.

Irrigation/Aspiration

Here in biaxial or micro-biaxial (microincision) also based on the side port and the main incision length surgeons have to select the adequate gauge of their bimanual irrigation/aspiration (I/A) instruments, there are a lot of them in the market called long time ago "Burato Bimanual I/A hand piece", but also there are a lot in sizes and manufactures, the most common in biaxial are 20 gauge and in micro-biaxial is 22 gauge (Figs 21A to C), in some of them the aspiration hand piece has a polish tip to help to clean the posterior capsule and the epithelial cells from the anterior capsule (MicroSurgical Technology, Redmond, USA), with those instruments surgeons can set their machine with the usual settings when surgeons make coaxial and aspirate the residual cortex with bimanual instruments, surgeons don't need any additional skill.

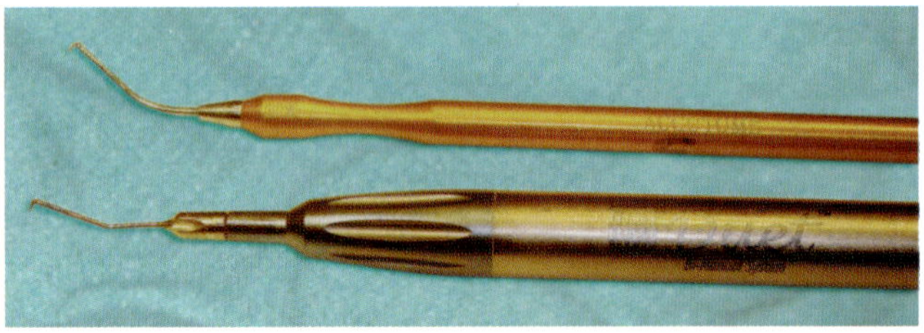

Fig. 20 A: 19G Vejarano's irrigating chopper

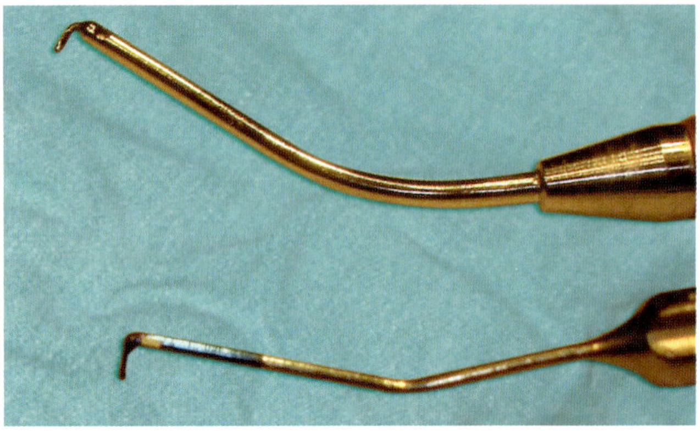

Fig. 20 B: 20G Vejarano's irrigating chopper

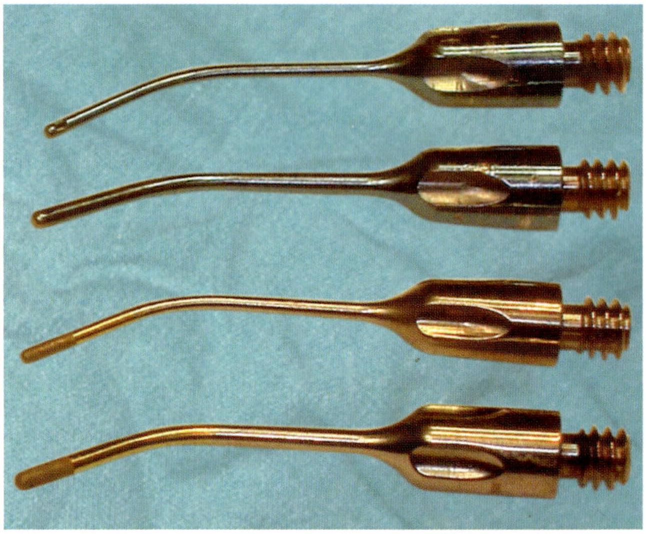

Fig. 21A. 20 & 22 gauge bimanual I/A handpieces

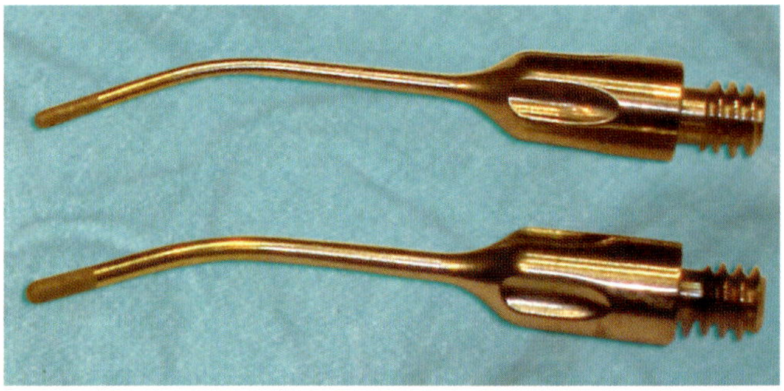

Fig. 21B. 20 & 22 gauge bimanual aspirating handpieces

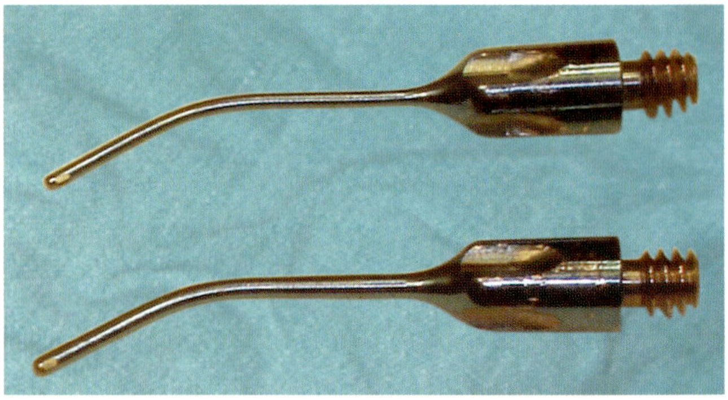

Fig. 21C. 20 & 22 gauge bimanual irrigating handpieces

Intraocular Lens

Because this chapter is only about instruments and of course not about techniques, author just wants to talk about the two preferred ways to introduce in biaxial or micro-biaxial the IOL, some of the authors of this book prefer to make a third incision, but others including author prefer to enlarge the main incision a little bit. Author uses a sapphire blades trapezoidal shape of 1.8/2.2 mm (Fig. 22), it gives author an internal incision of 2.0 mm and other of 2.0/2.4 mm (Fig. 23) (both Epsilon, Borivli, Mumbai, India) which gives author 2.2 mm internally; author uses them based on the power of the IOL, that means that with power less than 20 diopter. Author introduces it through 2.0 mm or less and if the power is higher, then he uses the 2.2 mm knife, but also surgeons can use a single metal blade for all of the cases from multiple manufacturers (Fig. 24); as you will see in the different sections regarding Microincision Lenses in this book, the advance in its technology even optical and in foldability is amazing. That's why only with small enlarging of about 0.8–1 mm from the initial main incision surgeons can introduce a very modern IOL with aspheric profile even more multifocal with correction of presbyopia, also the way how to introduce them (injector and cartridge) through such a small incision will be touch in that section of the book.

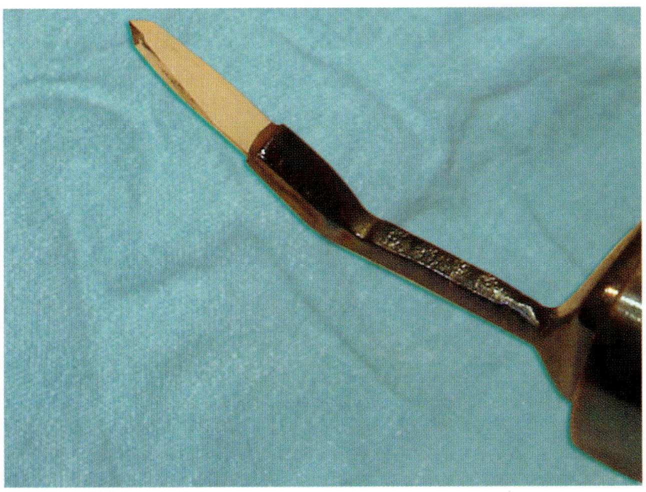

Fig. 22. Sapphire blades trapezoidal shape of 1.8 to 2.2 mm

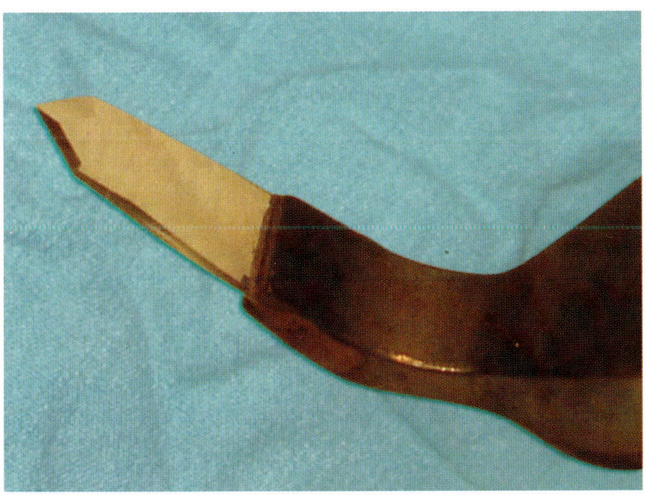

Fig. 23. Sapphire blades trapezoid 2.0 to 2.4 mm

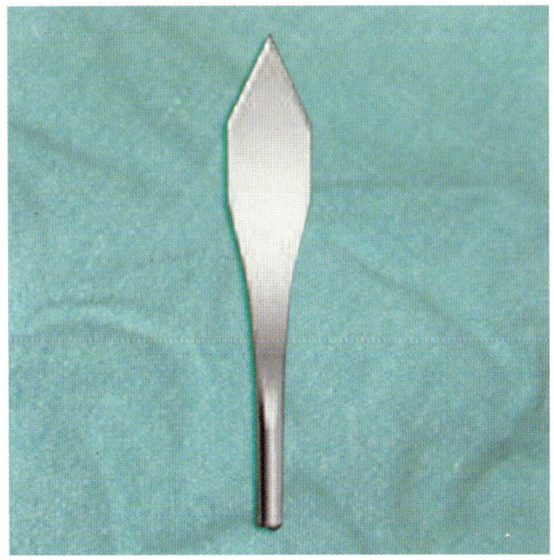

Fig. 24. Metal blade

Note: Author does not have any financial interest in any of the products mentioned in this chapter.

References

1. Tsuneoka H, Shiba T, Takahashi Y. Ultrasonic phacoemulsification using a 1.4 mm incision: clinical results. J Cataract Refract Surg. 2002;28:81-6.
2. Blumenthal M, Assia E. Using an anterior chamber maintainer to control intraocular pressure during phacoemulsification. J Cataract Refract Surg. 1994;20:93-6.
3. Agarwal A, Agarwal S, Agarwal A. Antichamber collapse. J Cataract Refract Surg. 2002;28:1085.
4. Agarwal S, Chaudhry R, Chaudhry S. Bomba Anticolapso de Cámara. In: Fako (Eds). Fakonit y Fako con láser. Panamá: Highlights of Ophthalmology International; 2002.
5. Vejarano L Felipe, Fine I Howard, Packer Mark, et al. MICS instrumentation growing in versatility, variety. Ocular Surgery News. 2004;22(11):26-7.
6. Vejarano L Felipe, Tello Alejandro. Fluidics in bimanual phaco. In: Amar Agarwal (Eds). Bimanual Phaco: Mastering the Phakonit/MICS Technique. Thorofare: Slack Inc; 2004.
7. Vejarano L Felipe, Vejarano Alberto, Tello Alejandro. Fluidics in phakonit. In: Ashok Garg (Eds). Mastering the Art of Bimanual Microincision Phaco (Phaconit/MICS). New Delhi: Jaypee Brothers Medical Publishers; 2005.
8. Fluidics in phakonit and microphakonit. In: Ashok Garg (Eds). Mastering the Phacodynamics (Tools, Technology and Innovations). New Delhi: Jaypee Brothers Medical Publishers; 2007.
9. Vejarano Luis Felipe, Vejarano Alberto, Tello Alejandro, et al. Fluidics in biaxial lens surgery. In: Arturo Perez-Arteaga (Eds). Step by Step Biaxial Lens Surgery. New Delhi: Jaypee Brothers Medical Publishers; 2008.

10. Vejarano L Felipe, Tello Alejandro, Vejarano Alberto, et al. The safer and most effective techniques in cataract surgery. Highlights of Ophthalmology. 2004;32(2):10-6.
11. Vejarano L Felipe, Tello Alejandro, Vejarano Alberto, et al. La técnica más segura y efectiva de Microincisión en cirugía de catarata. Highlights of Ophthalmology. 2004;32(2):13-9.
12. Vejarano L Felipe, Vejarano Alberto, Vejarano Manuel, et al. Faconit, Una técnica de microincisión segura y efectiva en cirugía de cataratas. Franja Ocular. 2004;5(31):10-6.
13. Vejarano L Felipe, Tello Alejandro. Vejarano Safe Chop makes transition to chopping easier. Ocular Sugery News. 2005;23(5):10-1.
14. Vejarano L Felipe, Tello Alejandro. Vejarano's Safe Chop Technique: A Safer Chopping. Techniques in Ophthalmology. 2005;3(3):109-15.
15. Safe chopping in bimanual phaco. In: Amar Agarwal.(Eds). Bimanual Phaco: Mastering the Phakonit/MICS Technique. Thorofare: Slack Inc; 2004.
16. Vejarano L Felipe, Vejarano Alberto, Tello Alejandro. Implantation techniques in microphaco: Vejarano's safe chop in phakonit. In: Ashok Garg (Eds). Mastering the Art of Bimanual Microincision Phaco (Phaconit/MICS). New Delhi: Jaypee Brothers Medical Publishers; 2005.
17. Safe Chop: a safer technique in phaco chop. In: Samuel Boyd, Jack Dodick (Eds). Highlights Collection, vol. I New Outcomes in Cataract Surgery. Panamá: Highlights of Ophthalmology; 2005.
18. Using Safe horizontal Chopping to prevent ruptures. In: Amar Agarwal. Phaco Nightmares. Thorofare: Slack Inc; 2006.
19. Barrett GD. Improved fluid dynamics during phacoemulsification with a new (MicroFlow) needle design, ASCRS meeting, Symposium on Cataract, IOL and Refractive Surgery, Washington, USA, 1996

11 MICS and the Abbott Medical Optics (AMO) Platform

George HH Beiko (Canada)

Microincisional cataract surgery (MICS) is an important innovation in ophthalmic surgery. The term MICS was first coined by Jorge Alio in 2001 to describe sub 2.0 mm incisions performed with a bare phaco needle. In the years since there has been growing interest in MICS, particularly as phacoemulsification, intraocular lens, and instrumentation manufacturers have advanced technologies to the point that microincisional cataract surgery is truly safe and viable.

Bimanual MICS allows the surgeon to use almost completely closed fluid system; fluid enters the eye from one side and exits from the other. Separating the irrigation and phacoemulsification handpieces allows the surgeon to direct the flow from one to the other, using both instruments independently to efficiently engage and emulsify nuclear fragments. This flow of fluid also minimizes competing currents in the anterior chamber of the eye.

The advantages of MICS, which are discussed in other chapters in this textbook in much greater detail, include maintaining an extremely stable anterior chamber throughout the case and reducing trauma to the eye. Smaller incisions have been shown to reduce the potential for induced cylinder[1] and higher-order aberrations, and to improve refractive outcomes.[2]

MICS would not be possible at all without the considerable advancements in ultrasound power modulation first introduced with the WhiteStar Sovereign phaco system, from Allergan Inc., Santa Ana, USA (later, Advanced Medical Optics Inc., Santa Ana, USA and now Abbott Medical Optics Inc., Santa Ana, USA).

AMO WhiteStar Micropulse Technology

The first generation phacoemulsification machines employed continuous 100% ultrasound power. The first innovation was the advent of the foot pedal, which allowed for linear control of the power, but still delivered power in a continuous fashion.

To understand the subsequent innovations, some definitions must be reviewed. "Pulse mode" refers to the energy being delivered for a period of time followed by a rest period. The on and rest periods are of equal duration. For example, a setting of 4 pulses per sec (pps) represents a pulse of 125 msec followed by a rest of 125 msec; thus, each cycle is 250 msec. In pulse mode, the foot pedal controls the amount of power. "Burst mode" results in a preset amount of energy being delivered; depression of the foot pedal determines the number of bursts per unit time.

A "duty cycle" consists of a period of energy delivery followed by an energy-free or rest period. The duty cycle refers to the percentage of time that ultrasound is on; it is calculated by dividing the amount of time that ultrasound is on by the total time of on and off periods. Thus, continuous ultrasound has a duty cycle of 100% while conventional pulse phaco has a duty cycle of 50%.

The primary impediment to bare needle MICS with continuous phacoemulsification was the potential for wound burn. Continuous phaco with a bare needle results in friction between the needle and the wound, an increase

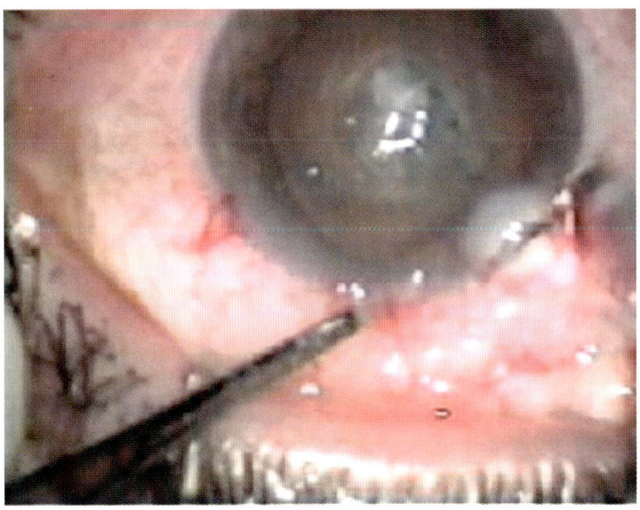

Fig. 1: Corneal wound burn

Sovereign WhiteStar v.6.0 Settings

Setting	On Pulse Time	Off Pulse Time	Duty Cycle
B/L	4	24	14%
C/N	6	28	18%
C/L	6	24	20%
C/I	6	18	25%
D/I	8	18	31%
B/D	4	8	33%
C/F	6	12	33%
C/D	6	8	43%
C/B	6	4	60%
D/B	8	4	67%

Fig. 2: AMO WhiteStar Settings. The duty cycle is represented by alphabet designations, each letter progression being equivalent to 2 msec. For example, a duty cycle of "CF" means an energy period of "C" or 6 msec and a rest period of "F" or 12 msec (Source: AMO, Santa Ana, USA)

in wound temperature and collagen coagulation leading to wound burn and its consequences including wound distortion, wound leak and induced corneal astigmatism (Fig. 1).

The introduction of AMO WhiteStar "cold phaco" technology in 2001 for the AMO Sovereign phacoemulsification system, allowed for programmable pulse and rest durations. This technology made it possible to vary the duration of the pulse and of the rest period, independently. Pulses and rests as short as 4 msec could be utilized, and the ultrasound on/off cycle could occur in 2 msec increments. An example is a 33% duty cycle with a 6 msec of applied energy followed by a 12 msec rest period resulting in 55 pps (Figs 2 and 3).

By increasing the rest period and decreasing the pulse period, fluid flowing from the irrigation handpiece to the phaco tip in bimanual MICS effectively increases the amount of time that a nuclear fragment is in contact with the phaco tip. Thus, a low duty cycle (increased rest period) facilitates holding of the nuclear fragment. By contrast, increasing the energy period and decreasing the rest period (high duty cycle) results in better cutting of the cataract.
Corneal wound burn (Fig. 1) will occur at a temperature of 60°C and can occur at lower temperatures of 45°C if the temperature is sustained.[3] With AMO WhiteStar technology, Steinert and Schafer showed that AMO WhiteStar's micropulsing or hyperpulsing reduced the temperature rise at the phaco tip by as much as 20°C.[4] Laboratory studies demonstrated that the maximum wound temperature using AMO WhiteStar ranged from 21°C to

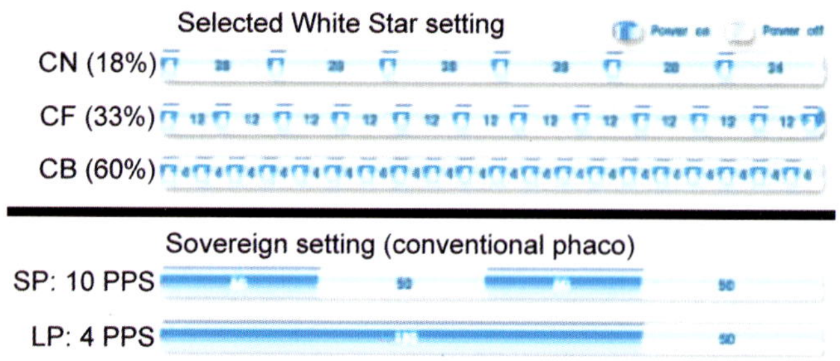

Fig. 3: Comparison of WhiteStar to conventional phaco duty cycles (Source: AMO, Santa Ana, USA)

37°C,[3,5,6] well below the 45–50°C threshold for thermal collagen damage. In fact, the energy needed to obtain a wound burn during bimanual phaco with a bare aspiration needle in human cadaver eyes was extremely high—well beyond anything one would see in a normal clinical setting.[3] Donnenfeld and colleagues provided confirmation of this in a clinical study in which temperature gradients, measured directly adjacent to the wound in 10 patients undergoing MICS, never exceeded 34°C.[7]

Taken together, these studies showed that the phaco sleeve was superfluous and that microincisional phaco with a bare needle could be safely performed in human eyes.

AMO WhiteStar micropulsing enables a surgeon to employ variable pulse-to-rest ratios; the duration of the pulse and of the rest can be programmed for a set time in the duty cycle. In this author experiences, the micropulse period is set for 4, 6 or 8 msec and the rest period for 4, 8, 12 or 24 msec. The duty cycle consists of combinations of these microbursts and rests, depending on whether the goal is emulsification or attraction of the nuclear fragments. Figure 4 illustrates the comparison between continuous power, traditional pulse and micropulse with a 1:2 duty cycle ratio.

Earlier pulse/burst modes allowed some modulation of continuous wave phaco energy, controlled by the surgeon with the foot pedal. But these were not as effective as AMO

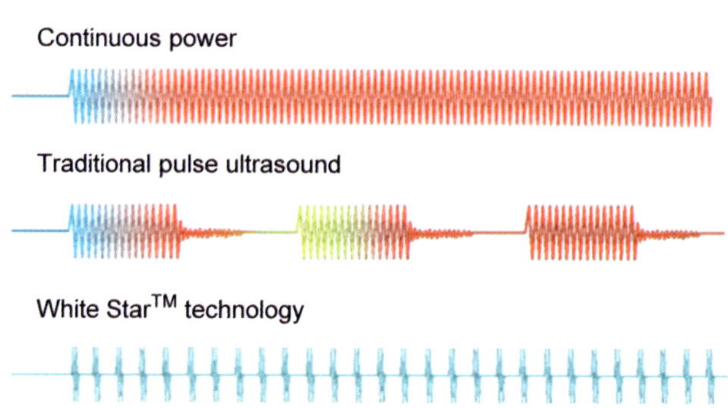

Fig. 4: Comparison of energy modes (Source: AMO, Santa Ana, USA).

WhiteStar in allowing safe MICS.[8,9] The automated rapid ultrasound pulsing in AMO WhiteStar functions much like a fluorescent lightbulb, with the rapid on/off cycling allowing the phaco tip to stay cold. This technology reduced the total energy into the eye by 50–70%.[10]

Moreover, the reduction in energy was accomplished without sacrificing cutting efficiency. Several studies demonstrated that even very hard nuclei (3+ and harder) could be safely and effectively removed through microincisions using the AMO WhiteStar system.[9,11,12] Later, performance in hard nuclei was further improved with AMO Variable WhiteStar, which permitted the surgeon to adjust the duty cycle based on the cutting requirements of the case.

In addition to virtually eliminating the risk of thermal damage, AMO WhiteStar micropulse technology has had other benefits, as well. Because it is more efficient and requires less ultrasound energy, the effective phaco time (EPT) is shorter, turbulence and chatter of nuclear material in the eye is limited, and trauma to the trabecular meshwork and endothelium is reduced. Less damage to the trabecular meshwork minimizes postoperative intraocular pressure spikes.[13] Less endothelial damage results in less endothelial cell loss.

AMO WhiteStar pulsing draws nuclear fragments to the phaco tip, optimizing transient cavitational energy (which produces a momentary "water jet" that breaks up nuclear fragments through high-energy, localized implosions) and minimizing stable cavitational energy (vibration of cavitation bubbles which has no effect on nuclear material). Maximizing selective transient cavitational energy and minimizing stable cavitational energy optimizes cutting performance and reduces overall energy input and heat production at the wound.

When researchers compared turbulence with and without AMO WhiteStar using high-resolution color digital ultrasound imaging, increased fluid velocity away from the phaco tip as continuous phaco power increased, was demonstrated, while the amount of such turbulence with AMO WhiteStar was much more limited (Fig. 5).[4] This explains why conventional phaco pushes away nuclear fragments and accounts for the better followability reported with AMO WhiteStar. High-speed digital photography also showed that the brief rest periods in AMO WhiteStar's on-off pulses diminished the repelling force of the vibrating phaco tip, reducing chatter and turbulence.[14]

For patients, the result may be a healthier endothelium. Fishkind and colleagues reported less endothelial cell loss at three months with AMO WhiteStar compared to standard AMO Sovereign phaco (319.6 cells/mm^2 vs. 430.3 cells/mm^2).[15]

Turbulence

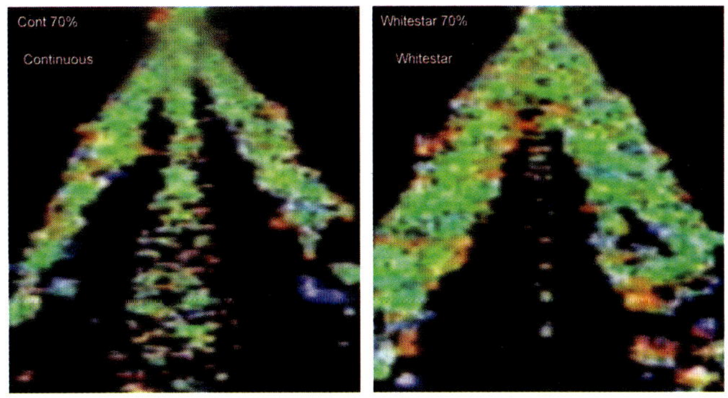

Fig. 5: Experimental simulation of turbulence, comparing AMO WhiteStar to continuous phaco. Continuous phaco has increased fluid velocity away from the phaco tip, resulting in a repulsion of the nuclear fragments. (Steinert RF, Schafer ME. Thermal energy and turbulence with WhiteStar and conventional phacoemulsification. Presented at ASCRS Annual Meeting. 2003)

With previous phaco systems, when phacoemulsification of a nuclear fragment resulted in an occlusion break, there was a transient inability of flow to keep up with vacuum, the intraocular pressure in the anterior chamber dropped, and the chamber swallowed; this is the phenomenon of "surge". The other innovation with AMO WhiteStar for the AMO Sovereign System was surge control via "smart pump" strategy; this relies on sensors which measure the vacuum 50 times per sec. When the phaco tip is occluded, the vacuum rises to half the preset value and aspiration flow decreases slowly to 0 ml/min. This strategy avoids the momentary overaspiration that occurs with postocclusion surge. Minimizing surge minimizes complications of posterior capsular rupture and phaco induced iris damage.

AMO Variable WhiteStar

The introduction of "AMO Variable WhiteStar" allows a surgeon to have linear control of AMO WhiteStar energy delivery. With this software, a surgeon can choose and tailor the AMO WhiteStar duty cycles. Up to four duty cycles can be programmed into position 3 on the footpedal; depression of the footpedal allows for linear progression through these cycles. Thus, each phaco setting can have increased flexibility as there is the potential to have four duty cycles available in footpedal position 3. This allows the surgeon to maneuver through various densities of nuclear fragments, to optimize the delivery of energy to the cataract and to maintain followability (Fig. 6).

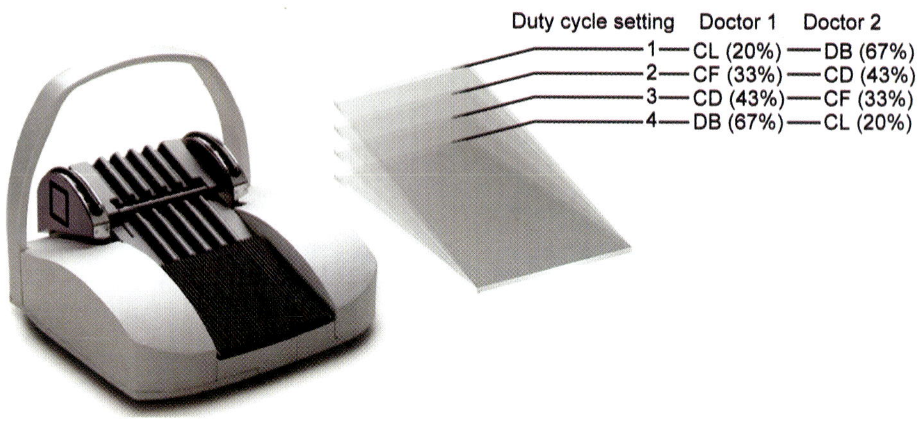

Fig. 6: An example of AMO Variable WhiteStar Settings in foot position 3. This software allows programing of up to 4 duty cycles, and also of the amount of up/down excursion of the foot pedal for each duty cycle (Source: AMO, Santa Ana, USA)

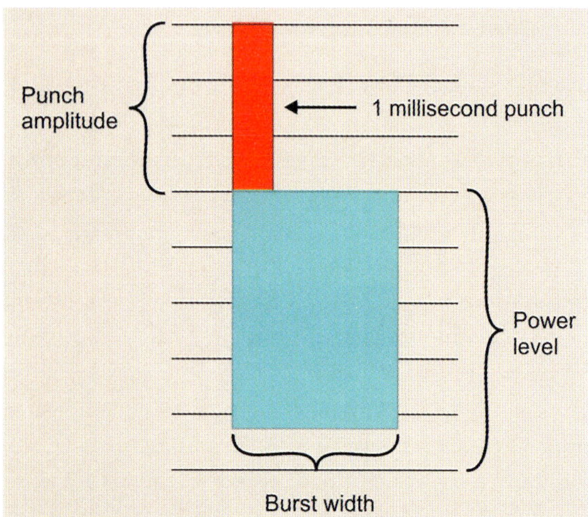

Fig. 7: ICE Pulse created by AMO WhiteStar ICE Technology (Source: AMO, Santa Ana, USA)

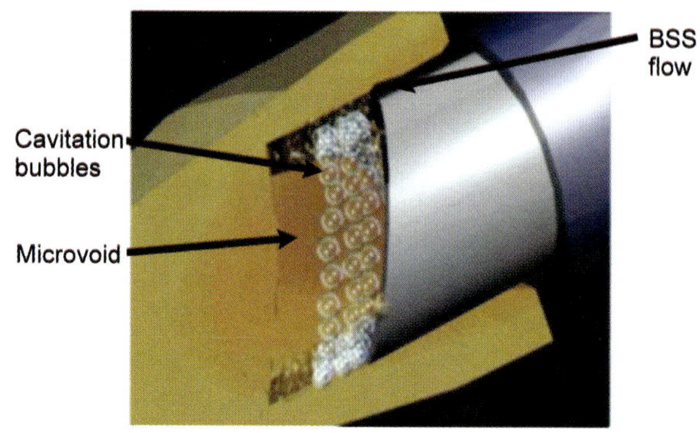

Fig. 8: Artist rendering of ICE pulse (Source: AMO, Santa Ana, USA)

AMO WhiteStar Ice

Several additional features were introduced with the second-generation micropulse technology for Sovereign. AMO WhiteStar ICE (increased control and efficiency) included the foot-pedal controlled variable duty cycles mentioned above for better efficacy in hard nuclei, advanced pulse shaping and an automated chamber stabilization algorithm known as CASE.

The pulse shaping is probably the best known feature of AMO WhiteStar ICE. Engineers added a microburst at the beginning of each pulse to maximize cavitational energy (Fig. 7). The microburst physically separates the nuclear material from the phaco tip, allowing the creation of a "microvoid" between the occluded tip and the nuclear material. Fresh balanced salt solution (BSS) can get into the microvoid, between the tip and the nuclear material, where it interacts with the ultrasound power to accelerate cavitational emulsification and increase the ultrasound efficiency (Fig. 8). The pulse amplitude can be customized to increase, decrease or remain steady throughout the phaco procedure (Fig. 9).

AMO WhiteStar ICE pulse shaping reduced EPT. Dewey reported that his EPT with ICE for a 3+ cataract was down from 4.63 s to 3.70 s—about a 20% reduction.[16] ICE prevents full occlusion but keeps the nuclear particle adjacent to the tip for magnetic followability. This reduced the surgeon's reliance on mechanical manipulation in the eye, paralleling the accomplishments with MICS. With the flow directed from the other side of the chamber in a bimanual MICS procedure, the surgeon has tremendous control over nuclear fragments.

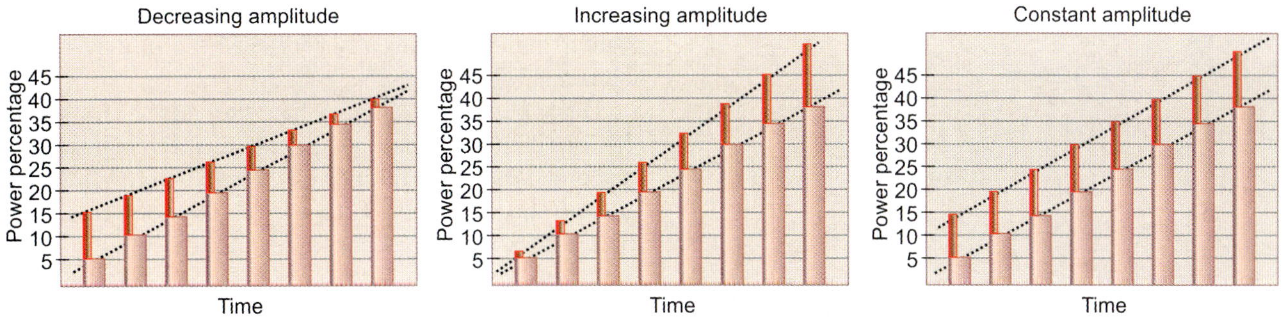

Fig. 9: The amplitude of the ICE pulse can be increased, decreased or maintained at a constant level, depending on surgeon preference (Source: AMO, Santa Ana, USA)

AMO Chamber Automated Stabilization Environment

Of the AMO WhiteStar ICE advances, Chamber Automated Stabilization Environment (CASE) was probably the most important, as it dramatically increases safety and enhances the role of fluidics in phacoemulsification. CASE dramatically reduces surge. Prior to CASE, the power modulation or occlusion modes of various phaco systems were only able to regulate the rising portion of the vacuum curve. CASE significantly reduces postocclusion surge by automating control of the descending vacuum curve, where the sudden drop in vacuum is most likely to break the posterior capsule. CASE constantly monitors the anterior chamber, begins to recognize occlusion even before it happens (when vacuum levels have crossed a predetermined "up threshold") and then proactively reverses the pump to step down the vacuum to predetermined levels before the occlusion break occurs (Fig. 10). This essentially duplicates what an experienced surgeon might be able to do with the foot pedal—but does it much faster (within 26 msec of the occlusion with previous versions of AMO WhiteStar; down to just 20 msec with CASE).

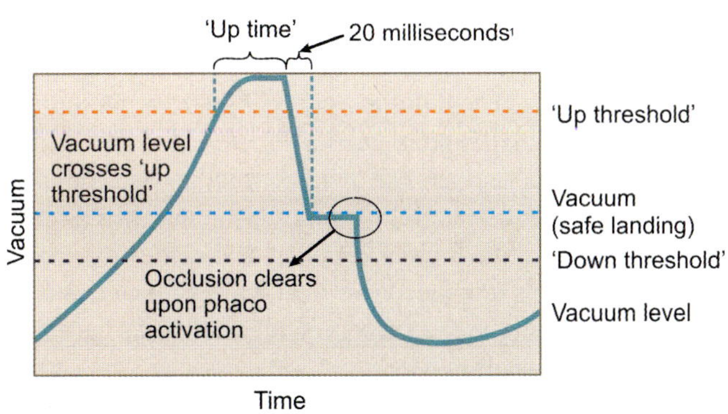

Fig. 10: AMO WhiteStar Signature System with fusion fluidics proactive vacuum adjustment (Source: AMO, Santa Ana, USA)

According to some reports, CASE reduces surge by 56% (Fig. 11). Regardless of the surgeon's preferred technique (MICS or standard coaxial) and instrumentation, this technology improves the safety of phaco by maintaining an extremely stable chamber.

AMO WhiteStar Signature

The latest-generation phacoemulsification system from AMO is the AMO WhiteStar Signature System with fusion fluidics. Existing technology has been strengthened in this system and a number of key innovations have been added.

Fusion Fluidics encompasses both the CASE vacuum-regulating algorithms as well as automated adjustments to the aspiration rate and phaco power/mode settings. Reaction time to preocclusion vacuum "up time" is even faster, as noted previously. Additionally, rise—the speed at which the pump stops and starts—can be controlled as

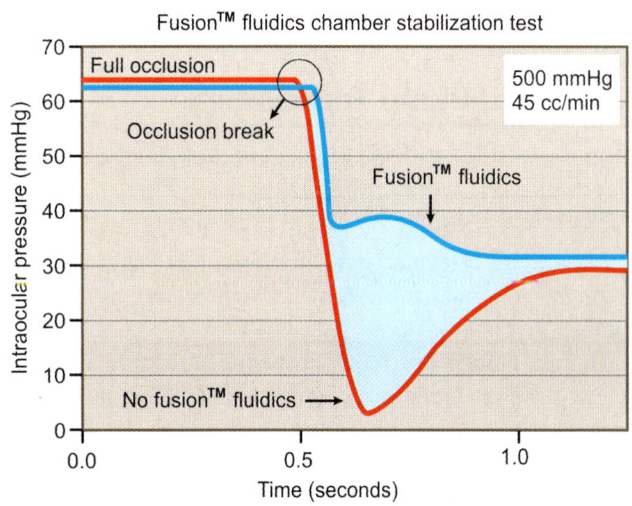

Fig. 11: Chamber stability with AMO WhiteStar Signature System with fusion fluidics demonstrating approximately 56% less surge with a 20 gauge tip. (data on file, AMO)

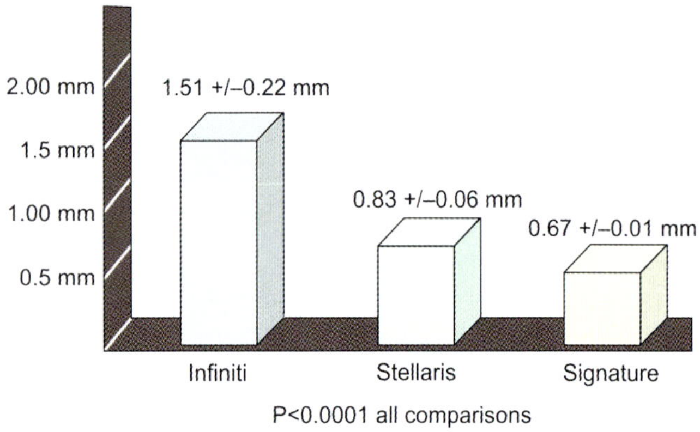

Fig. 12: Postocclusion surge comparison with various phaco systems

an independent variable. Surgeons can adjust rise time according to their own technique and the hardness of the nucleus in a particular case, further enhancing surgeon comfort and chamber stability.

In MICS cases, the separation of flow and vacuum increases one's flexibility to primarily use the fluidics to remove soft nuclei with minimal or no ultrasound power at all.

The peristaltic pump is also more powerful, which helps to compensate for any disadvantages of a smaller phaco tip for MICS. There is a 20% increase in the peristaltic flow rate, up to 60 cc/min, and a 30% increase in peristaltic vacuum, up to a maximum of 650 mm Hg. CASE is really a prerequisite to use these higher parameters safely.

The Signature system is an extremely stable platform with considerable advantages. When tested against other manufacturers' devices, Signature had both the lowest postocclusion surge and the lowest unoccluded flow vacuum[17,18] (Fig. 12).

AMO Dual-Pump Technology

In addition to its advanced peristaltic pump with all the Fusion Fluidics features, AMO Signature also has a high-quality Venturi pump. Surgeons can switch on the fly between peristaltic and Venturi pumps and the system can be preprogrammed to switch between pumps as needed within a given procedure.

Venturi pumps are more powerful and more reliable in low-vacuum situations, while peristaltic pumps have typically offered greater control and safety for anterior segment surgery. There are limited data thus far on the advantages of one pump style versus another for MICS. In a recent study from Turkey, the authors found that a Venturi pump significantly shortened the surgery time in bimanual MICS cases.[19]

Dual pump technology has the added advantages of enabling a surgeon to use the Venturi high-vacuum performance and holding power, if desired, and the flexibility of both modalities for multi-surgeon environments where preferences may vary from surgeon to surgeon.

AMO Ellips

Non-longitudinal phaco modes are another important innovation in cataract surgery. Alcon's OZil (Alcon, Fort Worth, USA) torsional phaco handpiece for the Alcon Infiniti system (Alcon, Fort Worth, USA) was the first to add a horizontal direction to the in-and-out motion of longitudinal phaco. AMO's version, ELLIPS Transversal Phaco, was introduced in 2008. With this handpiece, the needle moves simultaneously in an elliptical and longitudinal pattern, making it the first technology to simultaneously blend longitudinal and nonlongitudinal modes, and the first that can be used with a straight-tip needle.

AMO ELLIPS transversal phaco offers increased cutting power, especially in brunescent nuclei, because it is constantly emulsifying in all directions. It also reduces the amount of energy in the eye. These modes are the least likely of any phaco technique to cause a wound burn, so they make sleeveless MICS even safer to contemplate, provided one continues to utilize the WhiteStar pulse modality. Finally, the transversal mode limits the jackhammering action of longitudinal phaco, thereby enhancing followability. This may also make MICS easier to perform through small incisions with smaller instrumentation.

All in all, the AMO Signature System greatly reduces the surgeons' anxiety level by reducing routine trauma, endothelial cell loss and chamber swallowing, and greatly reducing the risk of capsular rupture and vitrectomy. It permits great customization and individualization for the surgeons' preferred techniques and parameters, including for complex or challenging cases.

These benefits accrue regardless of whether one chooses to perform standard coaxial phaco or bimanual MICS, but they make MICs much more efficient and safe. Moreover, AMO Signature's advanced Surgical Media Center, while perhaps not critical to the surgery itself, facilitates learning new techniques such as MICS.

Personal Technique

Anesthesia

Author routinely uses topical anesthesia for all of his cases. Author has used 0.75% bupivacaine, amethocaine and lidocaine gel, with comparable efficacy. Author currently uses a lidocaine gel preparation; the mixture is formulated by the clinic pharmacy and consists of 5 mL 2% xylocaine (20 mg/mL) and 4 drops of each of 10% epinephrine, 1% cyclopentolate, 1% tropicamide, Ocuflox and Acular (reference: Ophthal Times June 15, 2002, letter to editor). The mixture is administered 0.3 mL via a tuberculin syringe, 1 hour and 10 min preoperatively.

Intraoperatively, author uses 1% unpreserved xylocaine to hydrodissect and/or hydrodelineate the nucleus. This provides additional anesthesia to the ciliary body; it also may decrease posterior capsule opacification (PCO) (personal communication, R. Menapace).

Incisions

Author routinely sits at the head of the patient for both right and left eyes. He places his incisions at the 10 and 2 o'clock positions. The incisions are as small as possible so as to prevent leakage of irrigating fluid through these wounds during implementation of instruments. Preventing leakage ensures a stable chamber. Author employs a trapezoidal blade; the goal is to make the internal opening smaller than the external, so as to minimize oar locking. Since author uses 19 gauge irrigating and phaco tips, he uses a blade design of 1.2 mm more than 1.4 mm.

Author prefers a diamond blade because of the increased control in incision construction; however, he does use metal blades at one surgical center without significant problems. These blades are available from any number of ophthalmic instrument manufacturers.

In order to minimize astigmatic induction, author makes a three-plane, Langerman's type of incision at the 10 o'clock position. The initial groove is in the posterior limbus, through conjunctiva but as anterior as possible. This groove is longer than the wound, so as to minimize conjunctival ballooning. Author makes the incision in the posterior limbus as he prefers to have conjunctival covering of the incision so as to promote a faster seal of the incision and decrease the risk of endophthalmitis. The entry into the anterior chamber with the 1.2 mm more than 1.4 mm trapezoidal blade is made through this incision, with a tunnel of 1.5–2.0 mm. Following phacoemulsification and cortical cleanup, this incision is enlarged to 2.8 mm for IOL insertion.

Author makes a Wong pocket anterior to the 10 o'clock incision. This pocket is hydrated at the end of the cataract surgery so as to seal the wound more effectively. Author uses BSS solution to hydrate, but see no objection to using steroid or antibiotics, as advocated by some authors who believe these drugs act as a reservoir.

The incision at the 2 o'clock position, also made with the 1.2 mm more than 1.4 mm trapezoidal blade, is a two-plane incision without the benefit of a groove, also in the posterior limbus. No groove is made as this incision is not enlarged.

Instruments

Author uses a 19 gauge straight phaco tip with a 30 degree bevel. He uses the phaco tip with the bevel down for phacoemulsification. This tip is introduced through the 10 o'clock incision.

The irrigating handpiece is a straight 19 gauge cannula, with a Sinskey hook at the tip. The tip also has two side ports for irrigation. This device is custom-made for author by Katena. He finds it is versatile because the round Sinskey tip allows him to not only to manipulate and chop the nucleus but also to be able to touch delicate tissues such as the iris or capsule. This is used at the 2 o'clock incision (Fig. 13).

Author uses a microforceps for capsulorhexis creation. Any number of instrument companies currently make these, with a 23 gauge design for easy manipulation through the small incisions employed in bimanual MICS. Author's preference is for the MST capsulorhexis microforceps with Seibel Rhexis ruler. This device allows for accurate rhexis sizing, something that is becoming a critical issue for the implantation of some premium IOLs.

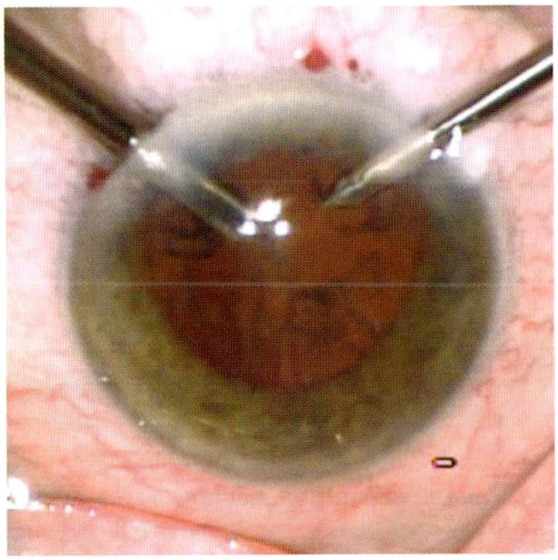

Fig. 13: Straight 19 gauge phaco tip at 10 o' clock incision and irrigating handpiece (Katena Instruments, USA) at 2 o'clock incision

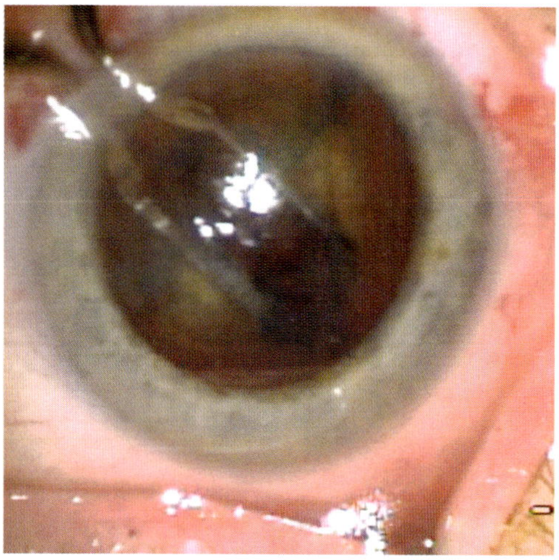

Fig. 14: Akahoshi combo prechopper (Asico Instruments, USA) being employed to break up the nucleus into quadrants

Author also uses the Akahoshi Combo prechopper (Asico Instruments, USA) in the majority of his cases. In 1–3+ nuclear sclerosis cases, he employs it directly to break up the nucleus into either four quadrants (if there is easy rotation of the hydrodissected nucleus) or three segments with a "V" configuration (if the nucleus is difficult to rotate). Author has found that this device reduces the amount of phaco energy by 45% in my cases. In 4+ or brunescent cataracts, author will phaco a central groove, making it so deep that the red reflex begins to come through. Author will then place the prechopper into the groove and separate the halves of the nucleus, with minimal force and manipulation; author finds that this strategy even works with the dense leathery cataracts (Fig. 14).

OVDs

Author uses Healon 5 (AMO, Santa Ana, USA) in all his cases. For capsulorhexis creation, he will inject enough Healon 5 to block the incision at the 10 o'clock position. Typically, he will fill the chamber half with viscoelastic, using the viscoelastic to tamponade the anterior capsule. The remainder of the chamber will be BSS.

Healon 5 is used to manipulate the tissues in the eye. The pupil is enlarged with this OVD (termed "viscomydriasis"), and it is particularly useful for floppy iris cases or cases where there has been damage to the iris. Healon 5 also can be useful for tissue separation, such as cases of anterior or posterior synechia.

Author finds that the Healon 5 provides excellent control for capsulorhexis creation, as the leading flap remains in the position in which it is placed. Capsulorhexis microforceps are used to create the capsulorhexis. In difficult cases such as intumescent or brunescent cataracts, author will purposefully overfill the anterior chamber with Healon 5 so as to push back on the anterior capsule; author finds this maneuver creates a dimple in the capsule which facilitates capsulorhexis and minimizes the risk of run out of the rhexis.

If using Vision Blue, author will instill the Vision Blue into the anterior chamber to paint the anterior capsule, then use BSS to wash out the Vision Blue. Healon 5 is then placed into the anterior chamber as previously described for intumescent cataracts.

During IOL implantation, author again injects enough Healon 5 to block the incision. Author uses BSS to fill the capsular bag and the remaining anterior chamber. Because of its retentive properties, the Healon 5 does not leave the eye, even during IOL injector insertion.

Finally and importantly, author finds that Healon 5 remains in the eye throughout the phacoemulsification, unlike dispersive or cohesive viscoelastic which tend to leak out of the wound with even the least amount of wound manipulation. This protects the endothelium and reduces endothelial damage and loss.

Typical Case

After incision creation, author places the phaco tip through the 10 o'clock incision and the irrigation tip through the 2 o'clock position. For 1–3+ nuclei, author uses Phaco Two settings (See Addendum), after hydrodissection and prechopping. Author finds that he is able to remove most nuclei with an EPT of 1–3. There is great chamber stability and minimal turbulence.

For remaining epinucleus or soft nuclei, author uses Phako One settings.

For dense segments, author briefly employs Phaco Three settings to debulk the nucleus, the revert to Phaco Two settings for the remainder of the nuclear removal.

For 4+ or brunescent nuclei, author uses Phaco Four settings for creation of the central groove. He then uses the Akahoshi Prechopper to separate the nucleus, and Phaco Three settings to debulk the nucleus. Author then uses Phaco Two settings for removal of the remaining nuclear fragments.

For aspiration of the remaining cortex, author uses irrigation/aspiration (I/A) One settings. Author uses the same irrigating cannula that he used for bimanual phaco, and a curved aspiration tip. Author employs both wounds for either handpiece to ensure that he removes any subincisional cortex. Author uses I/A Two settings for polishing of the posterior capsule.

Prior to OVD removal, author hydrates the Wong pocket and 2 o'clock incision with BSS. He finds that this helps to maintain chamber stability once the OVD is removed. I/A Three settings are used for OVD removal. Author places the aspiration tip posterior to the optic, to remove any OVD in the capsular bag. He then lets the IOL fall into the bag, and uses the rock-and-roll technique to ensure that he has aspirated all of the viscoelastic.

Intraocular Lens Choice

Author's preference is for the Tecnis 1-piece (AMO, Santa Ana, USA). He is convinced by his studies which have demonstrated the superiority of aspheric IOLs over standard IOLs, and in particular of the Tecnis over the Alcon IQ.[20] Author also encouraged by the work of U Mester who has found that the one piece design takes up a position in the capsular bag with tilt and decentration comparable to a young phakic individual.[21]

The Tecnis 1-piece is a hydrophobic acrylic lens with a 360° square edge and three point fixation which provides constant backward and outward pressure. Both of these features are designed to prevent PCO. This acrylic material is free of calcifications and glistenings, and has minimum chromatic aberration, ensuring optimal visual performance.

Author will enlarge the 10 o'clock wound with a 2.8 mm keratome so as to allow for IOL insertion at this site. Author uses the AMO cartridge and injector. The lens is loaded with the leading haptic in the tip of the cartridge, and the following haptic folded into the "taco" of the optic. The lens is delivered in a planar fashion into the bag, and quickly unfolds. There is no haptic-optic sticking or adhesion.

- Sovereign/Sovereign WhiteStar
  - Equivalent phaco time-26% decrease
  - Endothelial cell loss (3 months) decrease-30%
- Sovereign WhiteStar/Sovereign WhiteStar with ICE
  - 2 + 48% decrease EPT
  - 3 + 36% decrease EPT
  - 4 + 56% decrease EPT
- Vitrectomy rate
  - Before Micro-pulse 1.18%
  - After Micro-pulse 0.66%

Fig. 15: Benefits of the AMO phacoemulsification technology (Source: AMO, Santa Ana, USA).

Summary of Advantages of AMO Technology

Figure 15 highlights the advantages of AMO technological advances for phacoemulsification. These advantages are for both standard coaxial phaco and bimanual MICS.

References

1. Yao K, Tang XJ, Huang XD, et al. Clinical evaluation of the bimanual microincision cataract surgery. Zhonghua Yan Ke Za Zhi. 2008;44(6):525-8.
2. Saeed A, O'Connor J, Cunnife G, et al. Uncorrected visual acuity in the immediate postoperative period following uncomplicated cataract surgery: bimanual microincision cataract surgery versus standard coaxial phacoemulsification. Int Ophthalmol. 2008.
3. Soscia W, Howard JG, Olson RJ. Microphacoemulsification with WhiteStar: a wound-temperature study. J Cataract Refract Surg. 2002;28(6):1044.
4. Steinert RF, Schafer ME. Thermal energy and turbulence with WhiteStar and conventional phacoemulsification. Presented at ASCRS Annual Meeting. 2003.
5. Soscia W, Howard JG, Olson RJ. Bimanual phacoemulsification through 2 stab incisions: a wound-temperature study. J Cataract Refract Surg. 2002;28(6):1039-43.
6. Jiang Y, Liu Y, Cao Q. An experimental wound-temperature study of bimanual microphacoemulsification using the WhiteStar system. Yan Ke Xue Bao. 2005;21(2):122-5.
7. Donnenfeld E, Olson RJ, Solomon R, et al. Efficacy and wound-temperature gradient of WhiteStar phacoemulsification through a 1.2 mm incision. J Cataract Refract Surg. 2003;29:1097-100.
8. Olson RJ, Jin Y, Kefalopoulos G, et al. Legacy AdvanTec and Sovereign WhiteStar: a wound temperature study. J Cataract Refract Surg. 2004;30(5):1109-13.
9. Liu Y, Jiang Y, Wu M, et al. Bimanual microincision phacoemulsification in treating hard cataracts using different power modes. Clin Experiment Ophthalmol. 2008;36(5):426-30.
10. Data on file, AMO.
11. Assaf A, El-Matassem Kotb AM. Feasibility of bimanual microincision phacoemulsification in hard cataracts. Eye. 2007;21(6):807-11.
12. Olson RJ. Clinical experience with 21-gauge manual microphacoemulsification using Sovereign WhiteStar technology in eyes with dense cataract. J Cataract Refract Surg. 2004;30(1):168-72.
13. Vasavada AR, Mamidipudi PR, Minj M. Relationship of immediate intraocular pressure rise to phaco-tip ergonomics and energy dissipation. J Cat. Refract Surg. 2004:30;137-43.
14. Miyoshi T. Ultra high speed images of phaco tip. ASCRS Video presentation.

15. Fishkind W, Bakewell B, Donnenfeld ED, et al. Comparative clinical trial of ultrasound phacoemulsification with and without the WhiteStar system. J Cataract Refract Surg. 2006;32(1):45-9.
16. Dewey S. Increased control and efficiency; the next evolution of micropulse phaco. Presented at ASCRS. 2006.
17. Georgescu D, Payne M, Olson RJ. Objective measurement of postocclusion surge during phacoemulsification in human eye bank eyes. Am J Ophthalmol. 2007;143(3):437-40.
18. Georgescu D, Kuo AF, Kinard KI, et al. A fluidics comparison of Alcon Infiniti, Bausch & Lomb Stellaris, and Advanced Medical Optics Signature phacoemulsification machines. Am J Ophthalmol. 2008;145(6):1014-7.
19. Karaguzel H, Karalezli A, Aslan BS. Comparison of peristaltic and venturi pumps in bimanual microincisional cataract surgery. Int Ophthalmol. 2008.
20. Beiko G. Targeting spherical aberration correction in cataract surgery: Comparison of 0.00 and 0.10 microns. Presented at WOC Meeting. 2008.
21. Mester U. Comparison of decentration and tilt in the Tecnis ZCB00 IOL Vs. the young, phakic eye. Presented at ESCRS. 2008.

Addendum

Bimanual Settings for Dr Beiko
(Incorporating Variable WhiteStar Software)

Software Version Version 2.033

Surgeon Dr Beiko
Program Bi- Manual

PHACO 1 Soft Nuclei

Active Yes
Occluded Mode Off
Case Mode Off
Pump Type Peristaltic
Bottle Height 66 cm

Unoccluded Settings

Aspiration 10 cc/min Panel
Vacuum 200 mmHg Linear
Power 10% Linear
Mode Continuous
Pump Ramp 70
WS 6/12 (33%, 55 pps)

WS Settings

Continuous 6/12 (33%, 55 pps)
Variable WS 1
FootPedal Position 3: 0 - 25% 6/24 (20%, 33 pps)
FootPedal Position 3: 26 - 50% 6/12 (33%, 55 pps)
FootPedal Position 3: 51 - 75% 6/8 (43%, 71 pps)
FootPedal Position 3: 76 - 100% 8/4 (67%, 83 pps)
Variable WS 2
FootPedal Position 3: 0 - 25% 8/4 (67%, 83 pps)
FootPedal Position 3: 26 - 50% 6/8 (43%, 71 pps)
FootPedal Position 3: 51 - 75% 6/12 (33%, 55 pps)
FootPedal Position 3: 76 - 100% 6/24 (20%, 33 pps)

Pulse Shaping Settings

Active NO
Percent Kick: Low End of Range 5
Percent Kick: High End of Range 5
Low Power Limit 0
High Power Limit 80

Occlusion Mode Settings

Aspiration 18 cc/min
Vacuum 25 mmHg
Power 40% Linear
Mode Continuous
Pump Ramp 85
WS 6/12 (33%, 55 pps)

WS Settings

Continuous 6/12 (33%, 55 pps)
Variable WS 1
FootPedal Position 3: 0 - 25% 6/24 (20%, 33 pps)
FootPedal Position 3: 26 - 50% 6/12 (33%, 55 pps)
FootPedal Position 3: 51 - 75% 6/8 (43%, 71 pps)
FootPedal Position 3: 76 - 100% 8/4 (67%, 83 pps)
Variable WS 2
FootPedal Position 3: 0 - 25% 8/4 (67%, 83 pps)
FootPedal Position 3: 26 - 50% 6/8 (43%, 71 pps)
FootPedal Position 3: 51 - 75% 6/12 (33%, 55 pps)
FootPedal Position 3: 76 - 100% 6/24 (20%, 33 pps)

Pulse Shaping Settings

Active NO
Percent Kick: Low End of Range 5
Percent Kick: High End of Range 5
Low Power Limit 0
High Power Limit 80

Case Mode Settings

Down Threshold 70 mmHg
CASE Vacuum 85 mmHg
Up Threshold 100 mmHg
Up Time 300 msec
One Touch Standard

PHACO 2 Standard Nuclei (up to 3+ NS)

Active Yes
Occluded Mode On
Case Mode Off
Pump Type Peristaltic
Bottle Height 76 cm

Unoccluded Settings

Aspiration 22 cc/min Panel
Vacuum 250 mmHg Linear
Power 10% Linear
Mode Continuous
Pump Ramp 65
WS Variable WS 1

WS Settings

Continuous 6/12 (33%, 55 pps)
Variable WS 1
FootPedal Position 3: 0 - 25% 6/24 (20%, 33 pps)
FootPedal Position 3: 26 - 50% 6/24 (20%, 33 pps)
FootPedal Position 3: 51 - 75% 4/8 (33%, 83 pps)
FootPedal Position 3: 76 - 100% 6/8 (43%, 71 pps)
Variable WS 2
FootPedal Position 3: 0 - 25% 8/4 (67%, 83 pps)
FootPedal Position 3: 26 - 50% 6/8 (43%, 71 pps)
FootPedal Position 3: 51 - 75% 6/12 (33%, 55 pps)
FootPedal Position 3: 76 - 100% 6/24 (20%, 33 pps)

Pulse Shaping Settings

Active Yes
Percent Kick: Low End of Range 10
Percent Kick: High End of Range 10
Low Power Limit 0
High Power Limit 80

Occlusion Mode Settings

Aspiration 20 cc/min
Vacuum 200 mmHg
Power 15% Linear
Mode Continuous
Pump Ramp 65
WS Variable WS 1

WS Settings

Continuous 6/12 (33%, 55 pps)
Variable WS 1
FootPedal Position 3: 0 - 25% 6/24 (20%, 33 pps)
FootPedal Position 3: 26 - 50% 6/24 (20%, 33 pps)
FootPedal Position 3: 51 - 75% 4/8 (33%, 83 pps)
FootPedal Position 3: 76 - 100% 6/8 (43%, 71 pps)
Variable WS 2
FootPedal Position 3: 0 - 25% 8/4 (67%, 83 pps)
FootPedal Position 3: 26 - 50% 6/8 (43%, 71 pps)
FootPedal Position 3: 51 - 75% 6/12 (33%, 55 pps)
FootPedal Position 3: 76 - 100% 6/24 (20%, 33 pps)

Pulse Shaping Settings

Active Yes
Percent Kick: Low End of Range 10
Percent Kick: High End of Range 10
Low Power Limit 0
High Power Limit 80

Case Mode Settings

Down Threshold 109 mmHg
CASE Vacuum 144 mmHg
Up Threshold 176 mmHg
Up Time 1020 mSec
One Touch Standard

PHACO 3 Hard Nuclei (3-4+ NS)

Active Yes
Occluded Mode On
Case Mode On
Pump Type Peristaltic
Bottle Height 76 cm

Unoccluded Settings

Aspiration 22 cc/min Panel
Vacuum 300 mmHg Linear
Power 35% Linear
Mode Continuous
Pump Ramp 65
WS Variable WS 1

WS Settings

Continuous 6/12 (33%, 55 pps)
Variable WS 1
FootPedal Position 3: 0 - 25% 6/24 (20%, 33 pps)
FootPedal Position 3: 26 - 50% 6/12 (33%, 55 pps)
FootPedal Position 3: 51 - 75% 6/8 (43%, 71 pps)
FootPedal Position 3: 76 - 100% 6/8 (43%, 71 pps)
Variable WS 2
FootPedal Position 3: 0 - 25% 4/8 (33%, 83 pps)
FootPedal Position 3: 26 - 50% 4/8 (33%, 83 pps)
FootPedal Position 3: 51 - 75% 6/8 (43%, 71 pps)
FootPedal Position 3: 76 - 100% 8/4 (67%, 83 pps)

Pulse Shaping Settings

Active	Yes
Percent Kick: Low End of Range	10
Percent Kick: High End of Range	10
Low Power Limit	0
High Power Limit	80

Occlusion Mode Settings

Aspiration	24 cc/min
Vacuum	150 mmHg
Power	50% Linear
Mode	Continuous
Pump Ramp	65
WS Variable	WS 2

WS Settings

Continuous 6/12 (33%, 55 pps)

Variable WS 1

FootPedal Position 3:	0 - 25%	6/24 (20%, 33 pps)
FootPedal Position 3:	26 - 50%	6/12 (33%, 55 pps)
FootPedal Position 3:	51 - 75%	6/8 (43%, 71 pps)
FootPedal Position 3:	76 - 100%	8/4 (67%, 83 pps)

Variable WS 2

FootPedal Position 3:	0 - 25%	8/4 (67%, 83 pps)
FootPedal Position 3:	26 - 50%	6/8 (43%, 71 pps)
FootPedal Position 3:	51 - 75%	6/12 (33%, 55 pps)
FootPedal Position 3:	76 - 100%	6/24 (20%, 33 pps)

Pulse Shaping Settings

Active	Yes
Percent Kick: Low End of Range	10
Percent Kick: High End of Range	10
Low Power Limit	0
High Power Limit	80

Case Mode Settings

Down Threshold	200 mmHg
CASE Vacuum	235 mmHg
Up Threshold	270 mmHg
Up Time	1060 msec
One Touch	Standard

PHACO 4 Brunescent Cataract

Active	Yes
Occluded Mode	Off
Case Mode	Off
Pump Type	Peristaltic
Bottle Height	76 cm

Unoccluded Settings

Aspiration	20 cc/min Panel
Vacuum	30 mmHg Linear
Power	45% Linear
Mode	Continuous
Pump Ramp	70
WS	6/8 (43%, 71 pps)

WS Settings

Continuous 6/8 (43%, 71 pps)

Variable WS 1

FootPedal Position 3:	0 - 25%	6/24 (20%, 33 pps)
FootPedal Position 3:	26 - 50%	6/12 (33%, 55 pps)
FootPedal Position 3:	51 - 75%	6/8 (43%, 71 pps)
FootPedal Position 3:	76 - 100%	8/4 (67%, 83 pps)

Variable WS 2

FootPedal Position 3:	0 - 25%	8/4 (67%, 83 pps)
FootPedal Position 3:	26 - 50%	6/8 (43%, 71 pps)
FootPedal Position 3:	51 - 75%	6/12 (33%, 55 pps)
FootPedal Position 3:	76 - 100%	6/24 (20%, 33 pps)

Pulse Shaping Settings

Active	NO
Percent Kick: Low End of Range	5
Percent Kick: High End of Range	5
Low Power Limit	0
High Power Limit	80

Occlusion Mode Settings

Aspiration	24 cc/min
Vacuum	30 mmHg
Power	40% Linear
Mode	Continuous
Pump Ramp	85
WS	6/12 (33%, 55 pps)

WS Settings

Continuous 6/12 (33%, 55 pps)

Variable WS 1

FootPedal Position 3:	0 - 25%	6/24 (20%, 33 pps)
FootPedal Position 3:	26 - 50%	6/12 (33%, 55 pps)
FootPedal Position 3:	51 - 75%	6/8 (43%, 71 pps)
FootPedal Position 3:	76 - 100%	8/4 (67%, 83 pps)

Variable WS 2

FootPedal Position 3:	0 - 25%	8/4 (67%, 83 pps)
FootPedal Position 3:	26 - 50%	6/8 (43%, 71 pps)
FootPedal Position 3:	51 - 75%	6/12 (33%, 55 pps)
FootPedal Position 3:	76 - 100%	6/24 (20%, 33 pps)

Pulse Shaping Settings

Active	No
Percent Kick: Low End of Range	5
Percent Kick: High End of Range	5
Low Power Limit	0
High Power Limit	80

Case Mode Settings

Down Threshold	200 mmHg
CASE Vacuum	250 mmHg
Up Threshold	300 mmHg
Up Time	300 msec
One Touch	Standard

IA 1 IA 1

Active	Yes
Aspiration	30 cc/min Panel
Vacuum	300 mmHg Linear
Pump Type	Peristaltic
Bottle Height	43 cm
Pump Ramp	80

IA 2 IA 2

Active	Yes
Aspiration	6 cc/min Linear
Vacuum	10 mmHg Panel
Pump Type	Peristaltic
Bottle Height	50 cm
Pump Ramp	80

IA 3 IA 3

Active	Yes
Aspiration	40 cc/min Linear
Vacuum	500 mmHg Panel
Pump Type	Peristaltic
Bottle Height	50 cm
Pump Ramp	80

VIT 1 VIT 1

Active	Yes
Aspiration	30 cc/min Panel
Vacuum	300 mmHg Panel
CUT	800 IAC, Panel
Pump Type	Peristaltic
Bottle Height	30 cm
Pump Ramp	100

VIT 2 VIT 2

Active	Yes
Aspiration	12 cc/min Panel
Vacuum	225 mmHg Panel
CUT	450 IAC, Linear
Pump Type	Peristaltic
Bottle Height	30 cm
Pump Ramp	100

DIA 1 DIA 1

Active	Yes
Power	30 Linear

DIA 2 DIA 2

Active	Yes
Power	30 Burst

Footpedal Settings

PHACO

Switch Right	Next Sub Mode
Switch Left	Previous Sub Mode
Switch Config	1 Off
Switch Config	2 Next Major Mode

IA

Switch Right	Next Sub Mode
Switch Left	Previous Sub Mode
Switch Config	1 Off
Switch Config	2 Next Major Mode

VIT 1

Switch Right	Reflux
Switch Left	Off
Switch Config	1 Off
Switch Config	2 Off

VIT 2

Switch Right	Reflux
Switch Left	Off
Switch Config	1 Off
Switch Config	2 Off

DIA

Switch Right Off
Switch Left Off
Switch Config 1 Off
Switch Config 2 Off

Thresholds

Center 5%, 30%, 60%
Feedback Yes

Sounds Settings

Vacuum 6
Diathermy 6
Phaco Power 0
Error 6
Irrigation 3
Key Press 6
Speech 6
High Vacuum Sound On
Mode Change Voice
Submode Change Voice
Value Change On
Activity Confirmation On

12 MICS with the Infinity Surgical System (Alcon)

George HH Beiko (Canada)

Introduction

As highlighted in an earlier chapter, the advantages of microincisional cataract surgery (MICS) to the patient and surgeon are safety, astigmatic neutrality and faster recovery from surgery. However the over-riding concern when using a sleeveless phaco needle are corneal wound burn. Incision burns occur as a result of thermal damage to corneal collagen, and this occurs when tissue temperatures exceed 60°C.[1,2] Factors which contribute to an increase in wound temperature include occlusion of the phaco tip, decreased flow of fluid along the phaco needle and shaft friction of the phaco needle against the incision.

Corneal wound burns are a reportable event, and the FDA Maude Database reveals that it is a major concern with the Alcon Infinity Vision system (Fig. 1). One must consider that Alcon is the market leader in terms of supplying phaco machines, and that the FDA data may be representative of this market position. It is difficult to know the exact number of cases performed with each machine, but during the first three months of 2008, Market Scope published a report saying 65% were done with Alcon's machines, 16% by AMO and 19% by Bausch & Lomb; wound burns reported during the same time period were proportionately higher at 81% with the Alcon phaco systems (Fig. 2).

A laboratory thermal analysis of the characteristics of the phaco needle has suggested that the reason that incision burns occur with the Alcon Infinity Vision System is that the torsional action causes heat to build up in the needle shaft compared to in the hub of the needle with the longitudinal system (Devine T, Schafer ME. Analysis of Thermal Characteristics in Alternative Phaco Needle Designs. ASCRS Annual Meeting, 2009). The needle shaft is in direct contact with the corneal incision, while the hub is outside the eye.

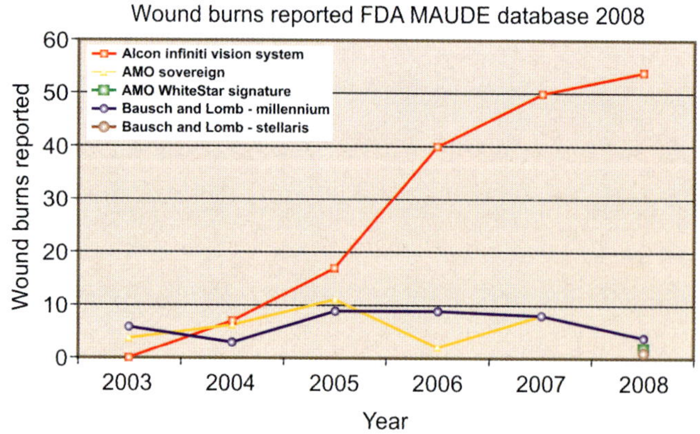

Fig. 1: Corneal wound burns reported to FDA (source: http://www.accessdata.fda.gov/scripts/cdrh/cfdocs/cfMAUDE/search.CFM)

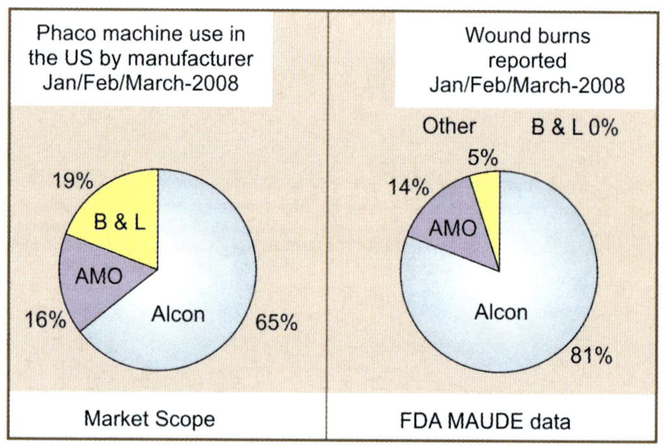

Fig. 2: Comparison of phaco system use and reported corneal wound burns during the same time period in 2008. (Source: Dr. Carolyn Bates)

The challenge for this author was to adapt the settings of the Alcon Infinity Vision System for MICS. The author has been using the system for the past year, and the current chapter reflects his experience in preventing corneal wound burns with this system.

Introduction to the Alcon Infinity System

Torsional Ultrasound

Longitudinal ultrasound was first introduced by Dr Charles Kelman for the extraction of cataracts, in the late 1960s. Longitudinal ultrasound consists of a forward and backward motion of the phacoemulsification needle; different systems use different frequencies, ranging from 28,000 to 40,000 times per second (or Hz). In the years since then, despite many innovations into phacoemulsification systems, there was little change in the motion of the phacoemulsification needle.

Torsional motion (Alcon NeoSoniX technology), the first innovation to needle movement, was introduced by Alcon at the turn of this century. Alcon NeoSoniX consists of the addition of an oscillatory motion to the forward and backward motion of the ultrasonic phacoemulsification tip. To the usual longitudinal ultrasonic tip movement of 40,000 Hz (40 kHz), there is the introduction of a sonic oscillation to the right and left. This occurs at 100 Hz (ultrasound is greater than 20,000 Hz) and is limited to 2° of amplitude, for a 4° maximal displacement. The oscillatory motion is so effective, it alone is sufficient for the removal of an epinucleus and even soft nuclei. The simultaneous use of longitudinal and torsional motions is needed to remove moderate to hard nuclei.

The introduction of torsional technology also solved a problem often seen with longitudinal phacoemulsification. Phacoemulsification needles, especially straight tips, tend to "core through" (or puncture) nuclear material. While phacoemulsifying a cataract, the surgeon has to anticipate when the needle will core through the nucleus, resulting in an occlusion break and risking a rupture of the posterior capsule. Unfortunately, visibility can be limited if the needle is drilling a hole into a large segment. The oscillatory movement induces a spinning motion to the nuclear material, which makes occlusion break with its inherent chamber fluctuation less likely. With proper settings and foot pedal control, the surgeon can see the nuclear material rotate on the phaco tip, becoming smaller as emulsification progresses. Thus, the torsional movement aids in minimizing ultrasonic power which results in less chatter and less repulsion of nuclear pieces.

The jackhammer effect of longitudinal phaco tends to push nuclear pieces away. Surgeons have compensated for this action by increasing vacuum levels so as to pull the nuclear material towards the phaco tip. Although high vacuum is effective in this regard, it also creates a powerful negative pressure, or void, at occlusion break, which increases the risk of posterior capsular contact by the phaco tip, resulting in capsular rupture. This negative pressure can be addressed by the surgeon either by lifting his foot back to foot pedal position 1 (the irrigation position), or by forcing the phacoemulsifier to bleed (or vent) this negative pressure. The reality is that, because of either repulsion of a piece or core through emulsification of a piece, the occlusion break occurs while the surgeon still has the pedal in position 2 (irrigation and aspiration) or 3 (irrigation, aspiration and phacoemulsificaiton). The compensation of the high vacuum levels and negative pressure does not occur, and Balanced Salt Solution (BSS) is sucked out of the anterior chamber. This rapid removal of anterior chamber fluid, combined with the possible reactivation of the pump (if the surgeon remains in foot position 2 or 3) can lead to instability of the intraocular environment, and significant complications.

Recently, Alcon has introduced an improved torsional movement (Alcon OZil Torsional Ultrasound). In order to achieve ultrasonic frequencies, piezoelectric crystals are used rather than a mechanical motor; a rate of 32 kHz was adopted. Another change was the use of smaller oscillatory amplitudes of 1° in each direction, for maximal amplitudes of 2°.

These innovations in the Alcon OZil Torsional system have paved the way for a new method of cataract removal. The higher rate of oscillations, combined with a bent Kelman phaco tip, create a pendulum effect, which shears the nucleus, instead of jackhammering it into pieces. Thus, the punching action of longitudinal ultrasound, with its associated repulsion, is replaced in OZil Torsional ultrasound by a scraping motion and spinning of the free moving pieces in front of the phaco needle (Fig. 3).

Alcon OZil Torsional Ultrasound should generate less heat than continuous longitudinal ultrasound. The frequency is lower (32 kHz compared to 40 kHz) and the friction created is less due to the pendulum effect of the Kelman tip. At 100% longitudinal power, the needle moves forward and backward approximately 90 microns. Similarly, at 100% torsional amplitude, the phaco needle has a side-to-side motion of about 90 microns. However, with torsional, the movement at the wound is only in the range of 30 microns compared to the 90 microns with longitudinal. As friction generates heat, a lower frequency combined with less movement at the incision, should make heat buildup at the incision less of an issue with torsional ultrasonic phaco.

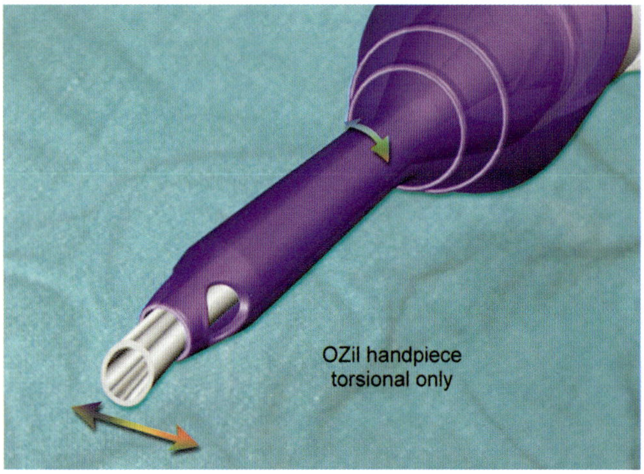

Fig. 3: With the oscillation of the needle shaft illustrated by the small blue arrow, the Kelman phaco tip moves side-to-side, shearing the nuclear material.

Alcon OZil Torsional Ultrasound compares favorably to longitudinal ultrasound.[3] In a study by Dr. Yizhi Liu et al.,[4] the mean Ultrasound Time and the Cumulative Dissipated Energy (CDE) were reduced for all densities of cataract. Corneal edema and the increase in corneal thickness were significantly less at 1 and 7 days postoperative. Endothelial cell loss was significantly less at 7 and 30 days postoperative. Finally, Best Corrected Visual Acuity (BCVA) was significantly better at 1 and 7 days postoperative.

Intelligent Phaco

Recently, Alcon added the Intelligent Phaco (IP) software to the Infiniti Vision System. This update capitalizes on the observation that the efficiency of the shearing action on the nuclear material is increased if the nuclear material is just touching the tip. Full occlusion of the tip with a nuclear fragment makes it adherent to the phaco needle or makes it become engaged in the lumen, both of these situations prevent scrapping and decrease emulsification. Full occlusion also leads to anterior chamber instability by creating changes in intraocular pressure and turbulence.

The IP software produces small bursts of longitudinal ultrasound to reduce the likelihood of getting a full occlusion. When the vacuum approaches or is at the preset threshold level, the Alcon Infiniti Vision System redirects some energy from torsional ultrasound to longitudinal ultrasound.

Setting the vacuum threshold to 90% in all cataract grades is efficient in activating some or more longitudinal motion to avoid full occlusion. For example, if the vacuum is set at 400 mm Hg and the threshold is set to 90%, upon reaching 360 mm Hg, some longitudinal ultrasound will start to be delivered (or will be added to the torsional). The machine can also be preset for a given pulse length and a ratio of powers; each cataract grade can and should be set differently. Pulses of 5 milliseconds (ms) for soft lenses are sufficient, while 10 ms is needed on Grade 3 cataracts and with Grade 4 cataracts, using 15 ms would be recommended. The IP software can be set for a ratio of torsional to longitudinal ranging from 0.7 to 1.0. At any given moment, when the vacuum reaches the level to activate the IP, the actual torsional amplitude will be multiplied by this factor, which will become the power used for the longitudinal pulse(s). If the On Time is set to 10 ms, the IP software will remove this time from the torsional impulse; the 10 ms of longitudinal ultrasound will be delivered at the ratio of the torsional amplitude at which the threshold occurred. Thus, if the ratio is set to 0.8, and if the threshold vacuum preset is achieved at 60% of the Torsional amplitude, the longitudinal ultrasound will be delivered at 48% (60% x 0.8). This will occur even if your preset longitudinal power is lower than that. Once the vacuum drops below threshold, the IP software returns the phaco settings to the original programmed ultrasound settings, as seen on the screen. IP software also disengages if the occlusion lasts longer than 200 ms of longitudinal ultrasound (20 pulses of 10 ms, as an example); this occurs in order to avoid corneal wound burn due to heat building up in the phaco shaft.

Initial experience with the IP software is that the nuclear material stays within reach of the leading sharp surface of the phaco tip, while still allowing some flow. Extended occlusion does not occur. With biaxial phaco in MICS, continuous flow through the phaco needle resulting from IP helps with chamber stability and keeps the phaco needle cooler.

Phaco Tip Selection

With torsional ultrasound, the shearing action is more effectively created by a bent Kelman tip than a straight tip. Most Kelman tips are designed with the ABS (Aspiration Bypass System) technology. This design incorporates a small port, of approximately 0.18 mm diameter, along the shaft. ABS technology allows flow through the needle upon occlusion of the distal larger port by a nuclear fragment. This flow of fluid provides cooling of the phaco tip during an occlusion, thus, decreasing the risk of corneal wound burn. It also avoids going from a fairly fast flow before occlusion to no flow when the tip is obstructed by a nuclear material; upon occlusion break, such a static situation would turn into a highly dynamic one, possibly compromising chamber stability.

Most designs for Alcon phaco tips have the ABS port on the underside of the phaco needle. In MICS, a bare phaco needle is employed in order to minimize the size of the incision. The use of a bare needle with an ABS port on the underside results in the iris being pulled into the ABS port, being caught in the port, and damage to the iris (in coaxial phacoemulsification techniques, the ABS port is covered by a flexible infusion sleeve, preventing damage to the iris, but still allowing fluid flow). In order to avoid this problem, phaco tips without an ABS port are available from Alcon; the author uses a 45°, 0.9 mm (20 gauge) Kelman tip.

More recently, phaco tip designs from Alcon have the bypass opening placed on the right side of the tip (Fig. 4). These tips can be used for MICS, provided the surgeon keeps the needle in its normal orientation or turns the bevel to the left (not to the right, as most right-handed surgeons would naturally do) when working on nuclear pieces, so as to avoid engaging the iris.

Also, attention should be taken to ensure that the ABS port is not withdrawn from the anterior chamber and out of the wound, which would result in loss of aspiration. If the backward movement allows exposure of the ABS port to air, vacuum will fall and the purchase on a fragment or quadrant will be lessened; while posing no risk, such a situation slows down the procedure.

Further discussion regarding the orientation of the Kelman tip bevel should be undertaken. In coaxial phacoemulsification, changing from bevel down for sculpting to bevel to the side for quadrant removal changes the inflow behavior significantly. The infusion sleeve will result in the infusion ports being oriented flat to the incision at times and vertical at other moments.

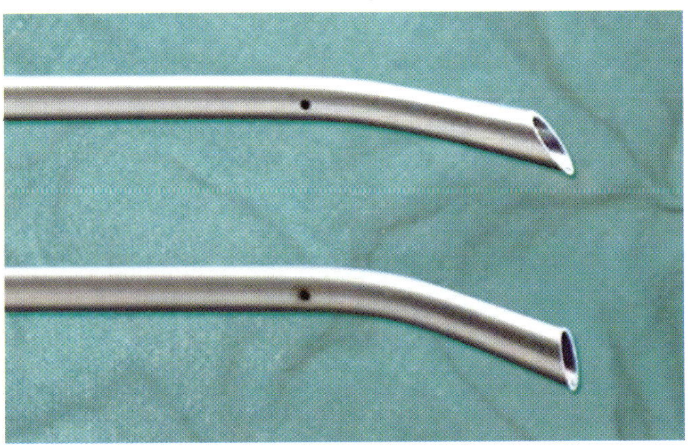

Fig. 4: 45° and 30° Kelman ABS tips, demonstrating the recent change in design to a right sided ABS port

This change from a horizontal flow to a vertical one can explain why pieces sometimes fly away from the phaco tip or spin rapidly away from the needle, being trapped in a whirlpool of BSS. Surgeons are becoming more aware of the requirement to keep the sleeve with the ports flat to the incision. It is now common for some practitioners who like to sculpt or chop with the bevel tip down, to enter the eye with the ports facing up and down, to sculpt or chop with the bevel tip down and then turn the needle to the side (so that the infusion ports are horizontal to the wound) when they engage the nuclear fragments. With MICS phaco, the flow comes from a separate irrigation cannula/handpiece and the phaco tip orientation relative to the wound does not influence nuclear fragment reaction to this flow.

Foot Pedal Control

The foot pedal is a critical component of the phacoemulsification system. The exact same settings and similar surgical techniques used by two surgeons will still look and feel different as each has his unique way of operating the system through the foot pedal. The Alcon Infinity Vision System foot pedal (Fig. 5) control allows for choice in the span of each pedal position (thus, the "sweet spot" of maximal efficiency for a particular surgeon can be placed at the level of his preference) and for the option of having a vibration to signal onset of ultrasound (so as to help surgeons who otherwise tend to apply ultrasound when not needed, or are being overly tentative).

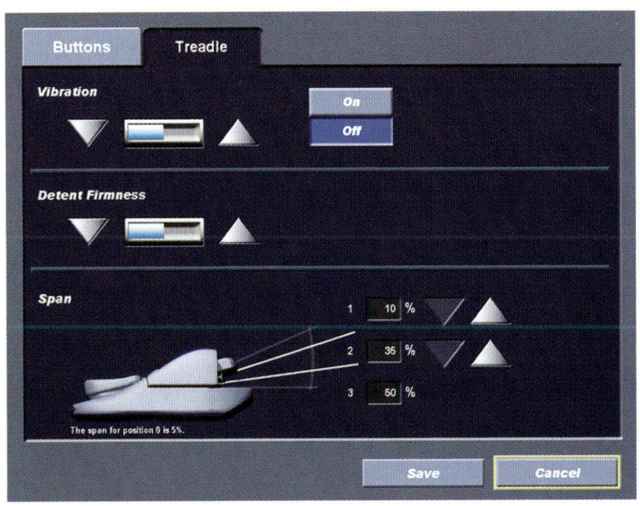

Fig. 5: The span of each footswitch position can be programmed. In this example, Position 1 (Continuous Irrigation) is shortened and position 3 is made longer to get the full benefit of the Custom Pulse power modulation.

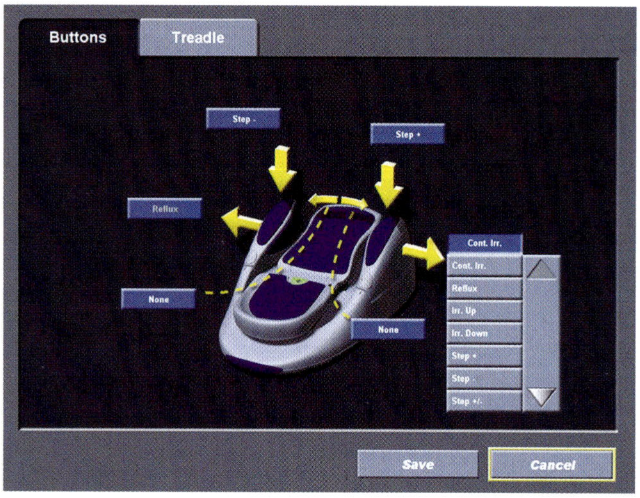

Fig. 6: Mapping of the footswitch. Each switch to the side of the main treadle as well as the rocking motion of the treadle can be assigned a function from the drop list.

The side switches surrounding the main treadle of the foot pedal can be set to control the steps of the phacoemulsification procedure. This brings speed and assurance to the surgeon when transitioning through the settings from one mode to the next. For this author, the foot pedal is set to move forward through the modes by stepping on the vertical right switch and to move backward with the left one. Continuous irrigation is an on/off switch accessible by rotating the foot to the right and reflux is attained by rotating the foot to the left (Fig. 6).

The Alcon Infiniti Vision System foot pedal works in the vertical axis only. There is no "yaw" motion as seen on some systems. Despite this, there is control over a number of variables. Titration of energy in the Infiniti system involves six variables (Fig. 12). Depression of the foot pedal results in the torsional amplitude changes and changes in the On-and-Off times. The same applies to longitudinal ultrasound. Needing only one up and down motion to control the blend of these motions is easier to learn and reproduce, for most surgeons.

Preparing the Alcon Infiniti Vision System for MICS

Sculpting

In MICS with the Alcon Infinity Vision System, this author prefers to use the PreChop technique introduced by Dr Takayushi Akahoshi. The technique employs a chopping instrument that initially bisects the nucleus; the nucleus is rotated 90°, and the nucleus is bisected again. This results in nuclear quadrants which are emulsified. The advantages of this technique are decreased use of energy (and less endothelial cell loss) and increased ease of nuclear removal (Beiko GHH. Endothelial Cell Loss with Microincisional Cataract Surgery. Paper presented at ASCRS Annual Meeting 2005). Sculpting is only used in grade 4 or denser cataracts, which are difficult to pre chop. As exemplified by Figure 7, the Sculpt mode on the Alcon Infiniti Vision System is set for the author after the Quad mode since the author normally plans to use the Quad mode for most cases.

With a dense cataract, sculpting is employed; continuous torsional ultrasound alone is suggested, and this usually results in the nucleus remaining on the phaco tip and effective creation of a central groove. Once the groove is made, then the Akahoshi prechopper can be placed at the bottom of the groove, and used to bisect the nucleus. The two fragments can then be phacoemulsified in Quad mode.

If, as the phaco tip is advanced towards the cataract, it is observed that the crystalline lens moves away from the phaco tip, then the sculpting will be ineffective. The repulsion can be minimized by backing off on the depression of the foot pedal, slowing down in the grooving and moving forward only as fast as the emulsification creates the trough. Alternatively, the settings should be changed to incorporate some longitudinal phaco, as discussed next.

With denser cataracts, it is advisable to use continuous torsional. If this is still ineffective, then longitudinal ultrasound should be added into the Sculpt mode. While the Alcon NeoSoniX mechanical handpiece allowed simultaneous back-and-forth movements and oscillations, the Alcon OZil system does not. The OZil system movements are produced by the same piezoelectric crystals in the handpiece; this design allows the crystals to produce either the longitudinal or torsional movements, and to alternate between them. There is a set pattern of alternation of the two motions; 80 milliseconds (ms) of torsional ultrasound are followed by 20 ms of longitudinal movement. This alternation is repeated ten times per second.

When longitudinal phacoemulsification is added to torsional phacoemulsification in the Sculpt mode, it is important to avoid pushing on the nucleus. In order to accomplish this, ultrasound at power levels of about 60–80% should be employed (this is comparable to the levels which would be used in sculpting with conventional longitudinal ultrasound). These power levels allow for short bursts of the jackhammer effect in dense nuclei, and more effective sculpting.

With brunescent cataracts, it is possible to increase the longitudinal phacoemulsification by going to the Pulse mode. In Pulse mode, it is possible to bypass the preassigned duty cycle of 80:20 ms (torsional/longitudinal) of the Continuous mode. By setting the On Times (torsional + longitudinal) so that they sum up to 100 %, it is possible to achieve a continuous delivery of energy with alternation of the two modalities. As an example, on a Grade 4 cataract, the Pulse Rate can be set at 5 and it is possible to opt for a 60% torsional On Time and a 40% longitudinal On Time; this would equate to 120:80 ms, and result in a larger contribution of the longitudinal stroke.

In phacoemulsification of cataracts, most of the energy used for the case is delivered during the sculpt phase of the procedure. In fact, it is not unusual to expend up to two thirds of the energy during this step of the procedure. The concern is that this expenditure of energy may result in a corneal wound burn. Additionally, the use of a bare needle in direct contact with the corneal wound in MICS increases the risk of wound burn due to friction. When using longitudinal ultrasound alone, a rapid pulse rate ("hyperpulse") with more On than Off times approximates the effectiveness of continuous motion but with a slower heat buildup and lessens the risk of a wound burn. Thus, hyperpulse is used to prevent corneal burns when using longitudinal ultrasound. It is also necessary to approximate this ideal of a rapidly pulsating needle when using torsional ultrasound. Figures 7, 8 and 9 illustrate this author settings for Sculpt mode for different degrees of cataract density.

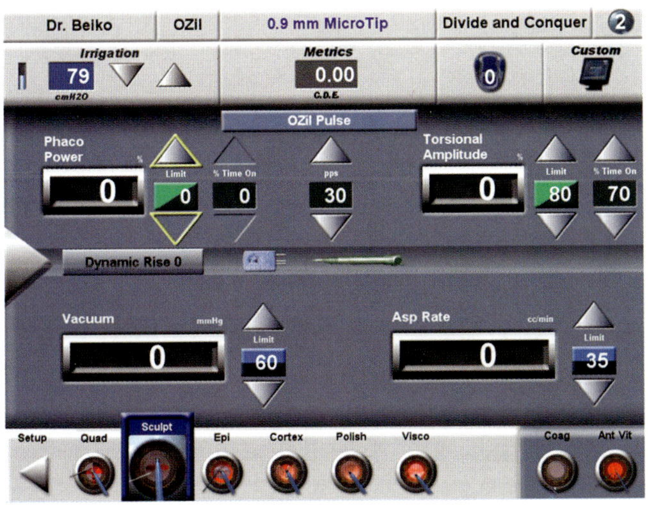

Fig. 7: Hyperpulse with short Off-Time is used on moderately dense cataracts.

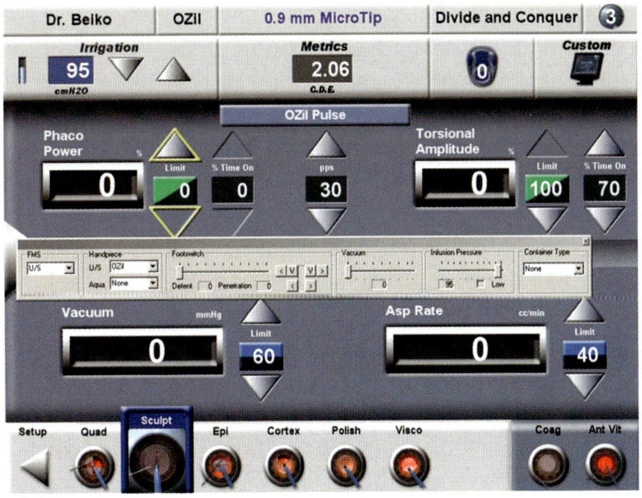

Fig. 8: Sculpting for a Grade 3 cataract; note that the torsional amplitude is increased to 100% and aspiration is increased to 40 cc/min.

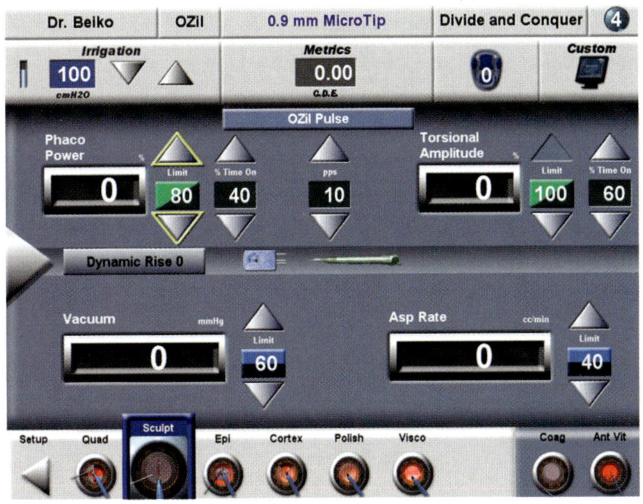

Fig 9: Sculpting for a Grade 4 cataract. Note that the Pulse mode is used but by adding the On-Times it is clear that by working 100% of the time, it is equal to delivering Continuous phaco.

Quadrant Removal

Settings in the Quad mode are used to emulsify the fragments created by prechopping either directly or in the trough created by grooving the nucleus, as described above.

One of the most important features of the Quad mode is modulation of energy input. Modulating the energy serves many functions:

Vacuum is used to hold and manipulate the quadrants, either to subdivide them with the chopper or to emulsify them as a unit; Off Times, or pauses, make it less likely that repulsion or spinning will break the occlusion.

During occlusion there is no flow through the phaco needle and subsequently no cooling of the needle; Pulse, Burst and Custom Pulse modes can be employed to minimize the heat generated by the needle movement.

Custom Pulse is a new modality that gives simultaneous linear control of the duty cycle and power, blending the benefits of Pulse and Burst modes. Modulation of the energy is multifactorial and allows for customization so that only the energy needed to emulsify the nucleus is used.

The first phacoemulsification systems delivered energy in a fixed amount; the energy delivered was either all On or Off. The first innovation was the use of a linear control of power, allowing for some titration of energy delivery. Linear control was limited; in Pulse mode, the amount of energy was varied and in Burst mode, the amount of Off time was varied (increasing power meant that rate of delivery also increased).

Pulse mode allows the modulation of energy by enabling the surgeon to control the amount of power delivered, although at a fixed repetition rate. Impaling quadrants in Pulse mode can be unproductive if the repetition rate is too fast or if the surgeon unintentionally stays in foot pedal position 3, at low power, while intending to be in position 2.

The disadvantage of the Burst mode is that the holding ability of the phaco tip can be compromised. Slowing down the pulsation to two per second, as suggested by Dr Howard Fine with his Choo-Choo Chop technique, is a valid solution. Burst mode offers the ability to have this low repetition rate at the entrance into foot position 3 and to speed up as the pedal is depressed. However, at that low rate, it can be somewhat frustrating emulsifying the nuclear fragment as the surgeon has to be aware of the foot pedal and constantly, and precisely, modulate his control of it so as to deliver optimum energy.

Custom Pulse (a concept proposed by Dr Steve Arshinoff of Toronto, Canada) is a blend of Pulse and Burst. It allows for tailoring of the Pulse and Burst modes in a variety of ways. With Custom Pulse, linear functions can be chosen that allow for proportional progress of the two variables or, alternatively, while one increases, the other can be set to decrease.

With the Alcon Infinity Vision System, this author has chosen to use Custom Pulse to manage the energy for quadrant removal. As illustrated in the following Figures, when more power is called for by depressing the foot pedal, the ON time as well as the OFF time both decrease. The strategy behind this is that the holdability (holding action of the phaco tip) of the nuclear fragments is maintained. With less dense fragments, low levels of ultrasound energy are employed to effect coring and there is minimal repulsion; the long On-Time serves this purpose. With more dense nuclei, more energy is needed; depression of the foot pedal delivers more energy at a higher repetition rate, the bursts become shorter to avoid repulsion and loss of followability.

The following (Figs 10, 11 & 12) illustrate this author's settings for quadrant removal for different densities of cataract. Please note that for any value, a horizontal division in its box means that this is a fixed, or all or nothing, parameter. A diagonal bar from bottom left ascending to the top right means that this value is linear and will increase with footswitch depression. Similarly, new to Custom Pulse, a diagonal bar from top left down to

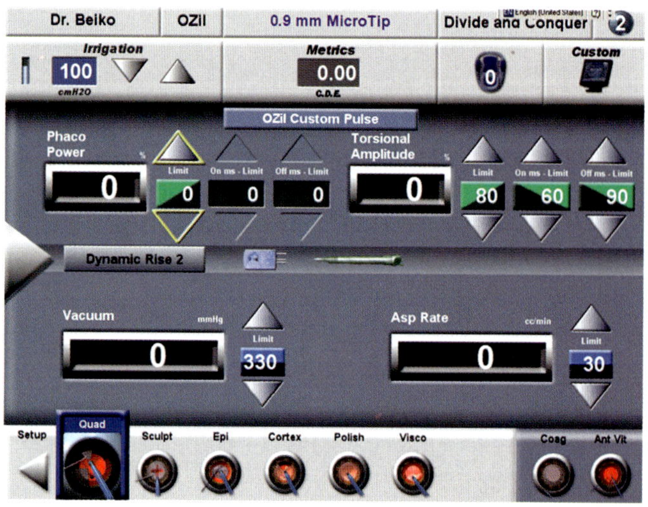

Fig. 10: Custom Pulse for a Grade 2 cataract. Only Torsional is needed and moderate energy and On-Time is required.

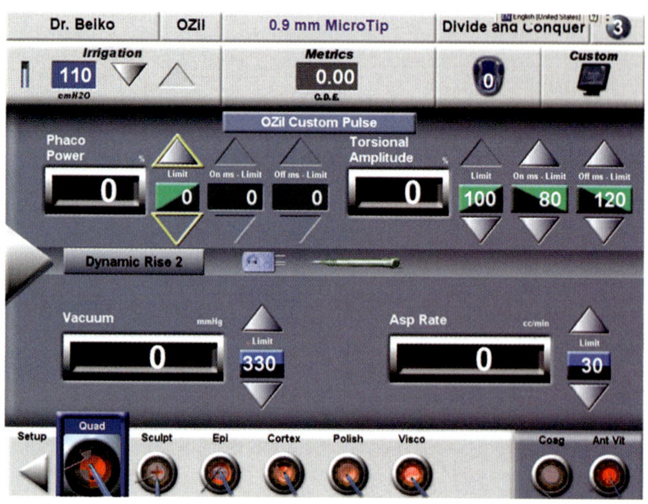

Fig. 11: Custom Pulse for Grade 3 cataracts. Maximal Torsional energy is sometimes needed and longer On-Times are used, in comparison to Grade 2.

bottom right will make the parameter decrease with pedal foot pedal depression, in a linear fashion.

Grade 4 cataracts are approached somewhat differently. As seen in Figure 12, longitudinal ultrasound is added to the torsional ultrasound. This helps to speed up nuclear emulsification and avoid possible clogging of the phaco tip. The longitudinal ultrasound is treated in a crescendo fashion. Depression of the foot pedal in position 3 results in an increase in the energy delivered, increased On-Time and shortened Off-Time. The combination of longitudinal and torsional ultrasound, using the settings demonstrated, allows for considerable efficiency. If the material can be emulsified by torsional power, longitudinal ultrasound can be minimized. If more energy is required, the foot pedal can be depressed fully to get the full benefit of the jackhammer effect of longitudinal ultrasound. Closer perusal of the On-Times in Figure 12 reveals that as the On-Time decreases for torsional ultrasound, the longitudinal On-Times increase. This blend of energy is comparable to OZil IP, although to a lesser extent. Combining Custom Pulse and IP is not only doable but likely advantageous. The author has just adopted this combination and will be able to report on results soon.

The update of the Infiniti software to version 2.03s offers threshold values for any linear parameter. With this update, it is possible to enter foot position 3 with low power and long bursts of energy. If the nuclear fragment is denser than anticipated, depression of the foot pedal results in more powerful bursts with a decreased On-Time; this rapid burst avoids chatter. For example, it is possible to set the threshold to 30%. This means that at the entrance of foot position 3, one burst of 30% amplitude and 400 ms duration will be delivered followed by a 2500 ms pause. Further depression of the foot pedal increases the amount of energy delivered; as the amplitude reaches 65%, the burst is reduced to 200 ms and the pause is now 1250 ms. At full depression of the pedal, the torsional amplitude is 100%, on for 80 ms with a pause of 120 ms. This combination is faster than Burst and offers a more controlled emulsification than Pulse for most surgeons. The advantage of this software update is analogous to the logic used with laser photocoagulation of the retina; it is possible to either set the laser at low power with a long exposure time or at a higher power with shorter exposure time.

Power modulation in quadrant removal with MICS is necessary in order to preserve wound integrity and control nuclear phacoemulsification. Power modulation is very efficient in Burst, and even more so with the Custom Pulse mode.

Cortex Removal

Linear control of the vacuum is recommended, as illustrated in Figure 12. Initial depression of the foot pedal should be to a level so as to produce just enough pulling force to free the cortical material from the bag, without going through. When the material is freed, depressing further will increase the vacuum and result in evacuation of the cortex (Fig. 13).

Epinucleus

On occasion, hydrodissection and hydrodelineation can result in a layer of epinuclear material remaining at the end of nuclear removal (Fig. 14). The strategy for removal of

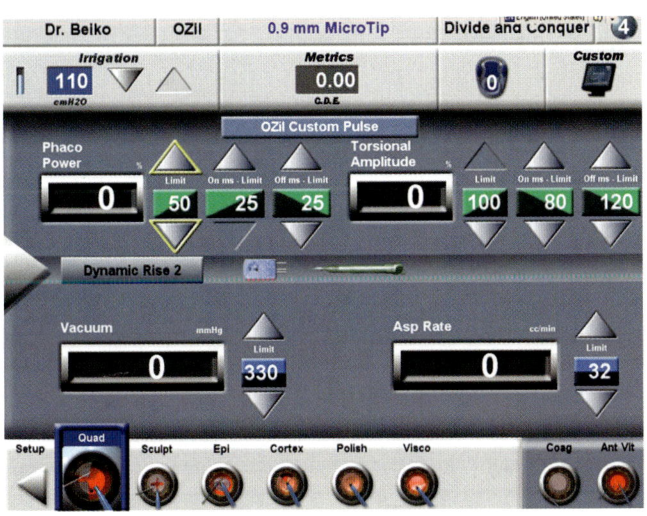

Fig. 12: Custom Pulse for a rock hard cataract. Note that six parameters are linearly controlled at the same time.

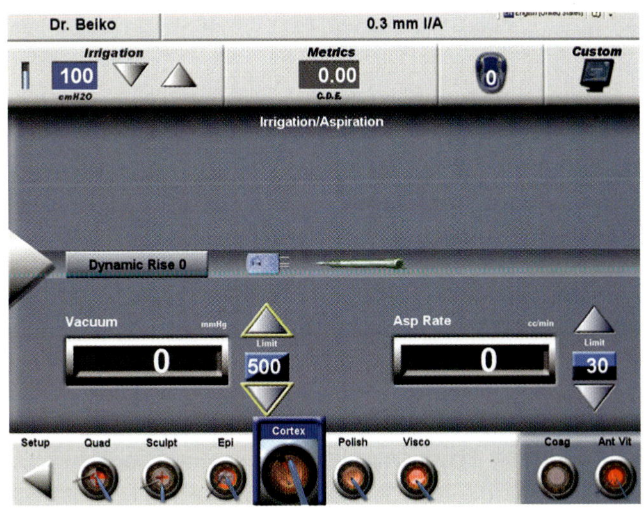

Fig. 13: Linear vacuum control is used to grasp the cortex, free it from the capsule, and evacuate it.

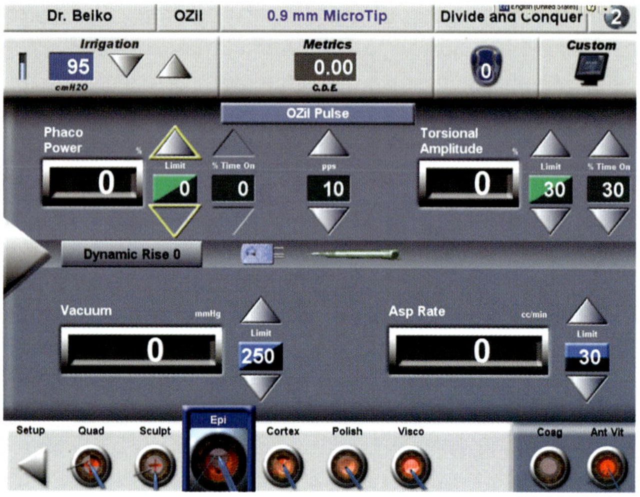

Fig. 14: Epinucleus mode. Note linear control of the vacuum in foot position 2. Low torsional amplitude available in 3 can be employed if the shell offers too much resistance for vacuum-only evacuation.

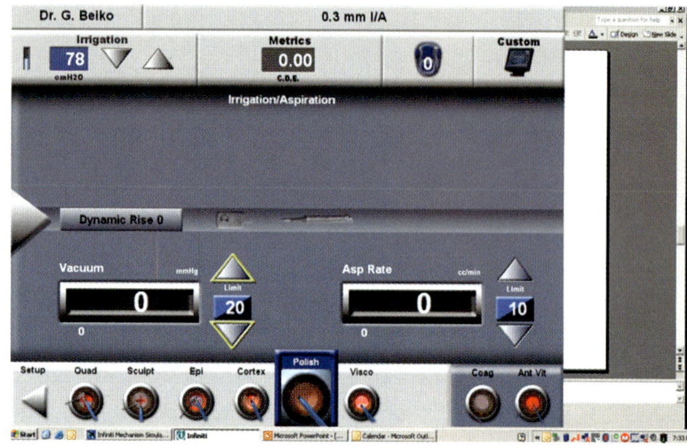

Fig. 15: Polish Mode with linear control of the vacuum and flow.

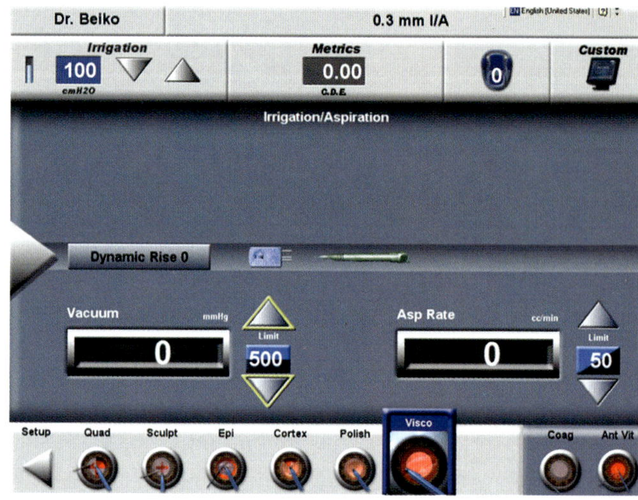

Fig. 16: Viscoelastic removal with linear control of the flow.

the epinucleus is to use vacuum and torsional ultrasound. Initially, it should be addressed similarly to cortical material; linear vacuum in foot position 2 is recommended. The epinucleus should be engaged with enough vacuum to mobilize it, without going through it, which can occur if too high of a vacuum or even worse, delivery of ultrasound energy transpires. When the epinucleus is free and in the middle of the bag, higher vacuum levels or even Torsional ultrasound can aid in speeding up its removal.

A moderate to high flow rate helps in creating enough fluid movement to float up the epinucleus to the phaco tip. This flow rate also fills the bag, avoiding contact of the capsular bag with the phaco needle.

Polishing the Capsule

This mode is programmed with a very low vacuum under linear control and a low flow rate. With a silicone I/A tip (irrigation/aspiration), a mechanical brushing of the capsule is very similar to using the Terry Squeegee (Alcon Surgical Inc., Fort Worth, Texas). Aspirating the capsule with a silicone or polymer I/A tip is unlikely to rupture the bag. If a bare metal tip is used for polishing, surgeons should be aware that burrs can be present within the aspiration port and these increase the risk of capsular tear. Notice the polishing mode of the panel in Figure 15.

Viscoelastic Removal

Control of the foot pedal allows for tailoring of the turbulence created by the flow so as to be most effective and efficient in ophthalmic viscosurgical device (OVD) removal. Once the intraocular lens is in place, removing the OVD is accomplished using linear flow. Placing the aspiration tip under the implant, with a low to moderate aspiration rate, reduces sudden movements of the lens or the posterior capsule. This is especially helpful in keeping a toric lens on its intended axis. In the anterior chamber, a faster flow is generated to mobilize the OVD. Vacuum should be set high enough to address any OVD material, typically in the range of 500 mm Hg. Notice the viscoelastic removal mode in Figure 16.

Personal Technique

Anesthesia

Author routinely uses topical anesthesia for all of his cases. Author has used 0.75% bupivacaine, amethocaine and lidocaine gel, with comparable efficacy. Author currently uses a lidocaine gel preparation; the mixture is formulated by the clinic pharmacy and consists of 5 ml 2% xylocaine (20 mg/mL) and 4 drops of each of 10% epinephrine, 1% cyclopentolate, 1% tropicamide, Ocuflox, and Acular (reference: Ophthal Times June 15, 2002, letter to editor). The mixture is administered 0.3 ml via a TB syringe, 1 hour and 10 min preoperative.

Intraoperatively, author uses 1% unpreserved xylocaine to hydrodissect and/or hydrodelineate the nucleus. This provides additional anesthesia to the ciliary body; it also may decrease PCO (personal communication, R. Menapace).

Incisions

Author routinely sits at the head of the patient for both right and left eyes. Author places his incisions at the 10 and 2 o'clock positions. The incisions are as small as possible so as to prevent leakage of irrigating fluid through these wounds during implementation of instruments. Preventing leakage ensures a stable chamber. Author prefers to employ a trapezoidal blade; the goal is to make the internal opening smaller than the external, so as to minimize oar-locking. Since author uses a 20 gauge instrumentation (irrigating cannula and phaco tip), he uses a blade design of 1.4 > 1.6 mm for the incisions.

Author prefers a diamond blade because of the increased control in incision construction; however, author does use metal blades at one surgical center without significant problems. These blades are available from any number of ophthalmic instrument manufacturers. In order to minimize surgically induced astigmatism, author makes a three-plane, Langerman's type of incision at the 10 o'clock position, where author locates the phaco handpiece. The initial groove is in the posterior limbus, through conjunctiva but as anterior as possible. This groove is longer than the wound, so as to minimize conjunctival ballooning. Author makes the incision in the posterior limbus as he prefers to have conjunctival covering of the incision so as to promote a faster seal of the incision and decrease the risk of endophthalmitis. The entry into the anterior chamber with the 1.2>1.4 mm trapezoidal blade is made through this incision, with a tunnel of 1.5 to 2.0 mm. Following phacoemulsification and cortical cleanup, this incision is enlarged to 2.8 mm for IOL insertion. Author makes a Wong pocket anterior to the 10 o'clock incision. This pocket is hydrated at the end of the cataract surgery so as to seal the wound more effectively. Author uses BSS solution to hydrate, but sees no objection to using steroid or antibiotics, as advocated by some authors who believe these drugs used in this manner will act as a reservoir. The incision at the 2 o'clock position, also made with the trapezoidal blade, is a two-plane incision without the benefit of a groove, also is located in the posterior limbus. No groove is made as this incision is not enlarged.

Instruments

Author uses an Alcon 45°, 0.9 mm (20 gauge) Kelman tip. Author uses the phaco tip with the bevel down for phacoemulsification. This tip is introduced through the 10 o'clock incision. The irrigating hand piece is a straight 20 gauge cannula, with a Sinskey hook at the tip. The tip also has two side ports for irrigation. This device is custom-made for me by Katena Instruments. Author finds it is versatile because the round Sinskey tip allows me not only to manipulate and chop the nucleus, but also to be able to touch delicate tissues such as the iris or capsule. This is used at the 2 o'clock incision (Fig. 17).

Author uses a microforceps for capsulorhexis creation. Increased numbers of instrument companies currently making these, with a 23 gauge design for easy manipulation through the small incisions employed in bimanual MICS. His preference is for the MST capsulorhexis microforceps with Seibel Rhexis ruler. This device allows for accurate rhexis sizing, something that is becoming a critical issue for the implantation of some premium IOLs. Author also uses the Akahoshi Combo prechopper (Asico Instruments,

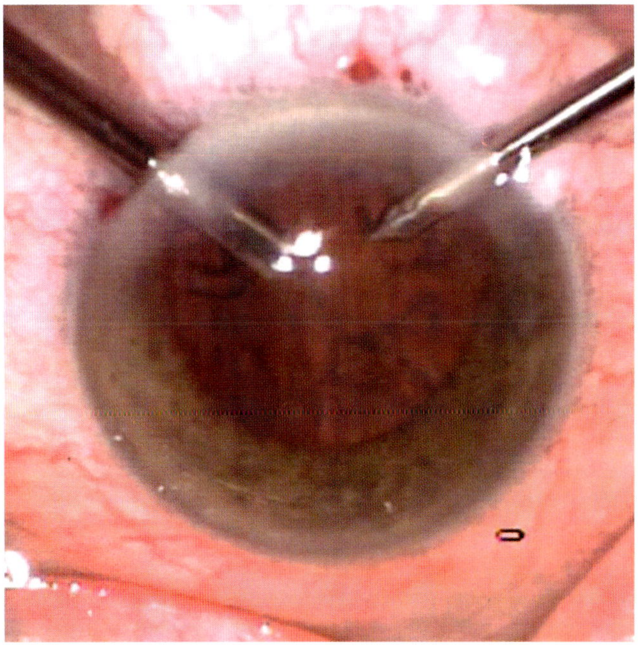

Fig. 17: Phaco tip at 10 o'clock incision, and irrigating handpiece (Katena Instruments, USA) at 2 o'clock incision.

USA) in the majority of his cases. In 1 to 3 + nuclear sclerosis cases, author employs it directly to break up the nucleus into either four quadrants (if there is easy rotation of the hydrodissected nucleus) or three segments with a "V" configuration (if the nucleus is difficult to rotate). Author has found that this device reduces the amount of phaco energy by 45% in his cases. In 4+ or brunescent cataracts, author will sculpt a central groove, making it so deep that the red reflex begins to come through. Author will then place the prechopper into the groove and separate the halves of the nucleus, with minimal force and manipulation; author finds that this strategy even works with the dense leathery cataracts (Fig. 18).

Ophthalmic Viscosurgical Devices

Author prefers to use Healon 5 (AMO, Santa Ana, USA). For capsulorhexis creation, author will inject enough Healon 5 to block the incision at the 10 o'clock position. Typically, author will fill the chamber half full with viscoelastic, using the viscoelastic to tamponade the anterior capsule. The remainder of the chamber will be BSS. Healon 5 is used to manipulate the tissues in the eye. The pupil is enlarged with this OVD (termed "viscomydriasis"), and it is particularly useful for floppy iris cases or cases where there has been damage to the iris. Healon 5 also can be useful for tissue separation, such as cases of anterior or posterior synechiae. Author finds that the Healon 5 provides excellent control for capsulorhexis creation, as the leading flap remains in the position in which it is placed. Capsulorhexis microforceps are used to create the capsulorhexis. In difficult cases such as intumescent or brunescent cataracts, author will purposefully overfill the anterior chamber with Healon 5 so as to push back on the anterior capsule; author finds this maneuver creates a dimple in the capsule which facilitates capsulorhexis and minimizes the risk of runout of the rhexis. If using Vision Blue, author will instill the Vision Blue into the anterior chamber to paint the anterior capsule, then use BSS to wash out the Vision Blue. Healon 5 is then placed into the anterior chamber as previously described for intumescent cataracts.

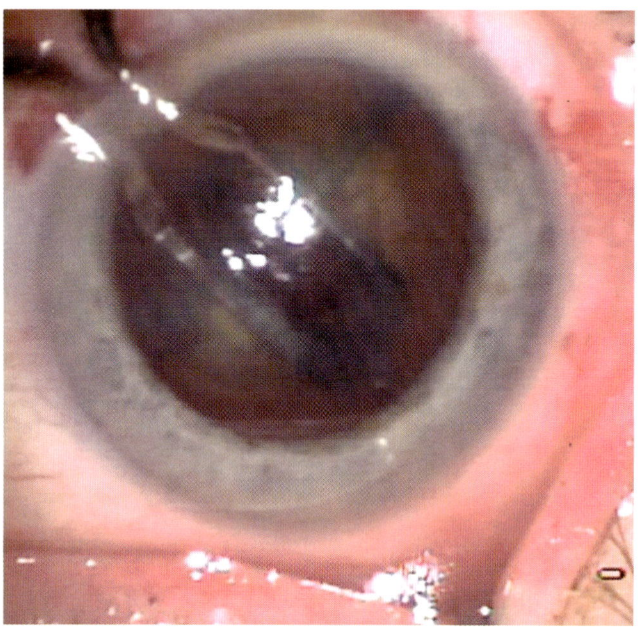

Fig. 18: Akahoshi Combo Prechopper (Asico Instruments, USA) being employed to break up the nucleus into quadrants

During IOL implantation, author again injects enough Healon 5 to block the incision. Author uses BSS to fill the capsular bag and the remaining anterior chamber. Because of its retentive properties, the Healon 5 does not leave the eye, even during IOL injector insertion.

Finally, and importantly, author finds that Healon 5 remains in the eye throughout the phacoemulsification, unlike dispersive or cohesive viscoelastics which tend to leak out of the wound with even the least amount of wound manipulation. This protects the endothelium and reduces endothelial damage and loss.

Typical Case

After incision creation, author places the phaco tip through the 10 o'clock incision and the irrigation tip through the 2 o'clock position. For 1 to 3+ nuclei, author uses Quad Mode for cataract density 2 settings (see above), after hydrodissection and prechopping. Author finds that he is able to remove most nuclei with a CDE of 4–7. There is great chamber stability and minimal turbulence.

For denser nuclei, author briefly employs Quad mode for cataract density 3 settings to debulk the nucleus, then revert to the Quad mode for cataract density 2 settings for the remainder of the nuclear removal. For 4+ or brunescent nuclei, author uses Sculpt mode for cataract density 4 settings for creation of the central groove. Author then uses the Akahoshi prechopper to separate the nucleus, and Quad mode for cataract density 3 settings to debulk the nucleus. Author then uses the Quad mode for cataract density 2 settings for removal of the remaining nuclear fragments.

For aspiration of the remaining cortex, author uses Cortex settings. Author uses the same irrigating cannula that he used for bimanual phaco, and a curved aspiration tip. Author employs both wounds for either handpiece to ensure that he removes any subincisional cortex.

Prior to OVD removal, author hydrates the Wong pocket and 2 o'clock incision with BSS. Author finds that this helps to maintain chamber stability once the OVD is removed. Visco settings are used for OVD removal. Author places the aspiration tip posterior to the optic, to remove any OVD in the capsular bag. He then lets the IOL fall into the bag, and uses the rock-and-roll technique to ensure that he has aspirated all of the OVD.

Acknowledgment

The author would like to gratefully acknowledge the invaluable assistance of Rene Cabana in the preparation of this chapter.

References

1. Berdahl JP, et al; Corneal wound architecture and integrity after phacoemulsification. Evaluation of coaxial, microincisional coaxial and microincisional bimanual techniques. JCRS. 2007; 33(3):510-5.
2. Sporl E, Genth U, Schmalfuss K,Tet al. Thermomechanical behaviour of the cornea. Ger J Ophthalmol. 1997; 6:322-7.
3. Han YK, Miller KM. Comparison of vacuum rise time, vacuum limit accuracy, and occlusion break surge of 3 new phacoemulsification systems. J Cat. Refrac. Surg. 2009; 35: 1424-9.
4. Liu Y, Zeng M, Liu X, yet al Torsional mode versus conventional ultrasound mode phacoemulsification – randomized comparative clinical study J Cat. Refract. Surg 2007;3(2): 287-92

13 Microphakonit: Cataract Surgery with a 0.7 mm Tip

Amar Agarwal (India)

History

On August 15th 1998, the author (Amar Agarwal) performed 1 mm cataract surgery by a technique called Phakonit[1-13] (Phako being done with a Needle Incision Technology). Dr Jorge Alio (Spain) coined the term MICS or microincision cataract surgery[14] for all surgeries including laser cataract surgery and phakonit. Dr Randall Olson (USA) first used a 0.8 mm phaco needle and a 21 gauge irrigating chopper and called it Microphaco.[15-18]

On May 21st 2005, for the first time, a 0.7 mm phaco needle tip with a 0.7 mm irrigating chopper was used by the authors (Amar Agarwal and colleague) to remove cataracts through the smallest incision possible as of now. This is called Microphakonit.

Microphakonit (0.7 mm) Needle Tip

When authors wanted to go for a 0.7 mm phaco needle the point which authors wondered was whether the needle would be able to hold the energy of the ultrasound. Authors gave this problem to Larry Laks from Microsurgical Technology (MST), USA, to work on. He then made this special 0.7 mm phaco needle. As surgeon will understand if authors go smaller from a 0.9 mm phaco needle to a 0.7 mm phaco needle the speed of the surgery would go down. This is because the amount of aspiration flow rate would be less.

It was decided to solve this problem by working on the wall of the 0.7 mm phaco needle. There is a standard wall thickness for all phaco tips. If authors say the outer diameter is a constant, the resultant inner diameter is an area of the outer diameter minus the area of the wall.

The inner diameter will regulate the flow rate/perceived efficiency (which can be good or bad, depending on how surgeons look at it). In order to increase the allowed aspiration flow rate from what a standard 0.7 mm tip would be, MST (Larry Laks) had the walls made thinner, thus increasing the inner diameter. This would allow a case to go, speed wise, closer to what a 0.9 mm tip would go (not exactly the same, but closer). With the gas forced infusion it would work very well. Finally authors decided to go for a 30 degree tip to make it even better.

Microphakonit (0.7 mm) Irrigating Chopper

There are two designs of 20 gauge (0.9 mm) irrigating choppers which authors have designed. One is the Agarwal irrigating chopper made by the MST company. The opening for the fluid in this is end opening. This is incorporated in the Duet system. The other irrigating chopper is made by Geuder, Germany. This has two openings in the side. Depending on the convenience of the surgeon, the surgeon can decide which design of irrigating chopper they would like to use. There are advantages and disadvantages of both types of irrigating choppers. The end opening chopper has an advantage of more fluid coming out of the chopper. The disadvantage is that there is a gush of fluid which might push the nuclear pieces away. The advantage of the side opening irrigating chopper is that there is good control as the nuclear pieces are not pushed away but the disadvantage is that the amount of fluid coming out of it is much less. That is why if one is using the side opening irrigating chopper one should use an air pump or gas forced infusion.

The MST in their irrigating chopper increased flow by removing the flow restrictions incorporated in other irrigating choppers as a by-product of their attachment method. Authors also had control of incisional outflow by having all the instruments to be of one size and created a matching knife of the proper size and geometry.

When authors decided to go smaller to using a 0.7 mm irrigating chopper authors decided to go for an end-opening irrigating chopper. The reason is as the bore of the irrigating chopper was smaller the amount of fluid coming

TABLE 1 Fluid exiting from various irrigating choppers (values in mL/minute)

Irrigating Chopper	*Without Gas Forced Infusion*	*With Gas Forced Infusion Using the Accurus Machine at 50 mm Hg*	*With Gas Forced Infusion Using the Accurus Machine at 75 mm Hg*	*With Gas Forced Infusion Using the Accurus Machine at 100 mm Hg*	*Air Pump with Regulator at Low*	*Air Pump with Regulator at High*
0.9 mm, side-opening	25	36	42	48	37	51
0.9 mm, end-opening	34	51	57	65	52	68
0.7 mm, end-opening	27	39	44	51	41	54

out of it would be less and so an end-opening chopper would maintain the fluidics better. With gas forced infusion authors thought they would be able to balance the entry and exit of fluid into the anterior chamber and that is what happened.

Authors measured the amount of fluid coming out of the various irrigating choppers with and without an air pump (Table 1). Authors also measured the values using the simple aquarium air pump (external gas forced infusion) and the Accurus machine giving internal gas forced infusion.

The microphakonit irrigating chopper which authors have designed is basically a sharp chopper which has a sharp cutting edge and helps in karate chopping or quick chopping. It can chop any type of cataract.

Air Pump and Gas Forced Infusion

The main problem in phakonit authors had was the destabilization of the anterior chamber during surgery. Authors solved it to a certain extent by using an 18 gauge irrigating chopper. Then Sunita Agarwal suggested the use of an antichamber collapse,[19] which injects air into the infusion bottle. This pushes more fluid into the eye through the irrigating chopper and also prevents surge. Thus, authors were able to use a 20/21 gauge irrigating chopper as well as solve the problem of destabilization of the anterior chamber during surgery. Now, with a 22 gauge (0.7 mm) irrigating chopper it is extremely essential that gas forced infusion be used in the surgery. This is also called external gas forced infusion.

- When the surgeon uses the air pump contained in the same phaco machine, it is called internal gas forced infusion (IFI). To solve the problem of infection authors use a millipore filter connected to the machine. The advantages of the Internal Forced Infusion over the External are: The surgeon doesn't have to incorporate an external air pump to the surgical system to obtain the advantages of the forced infusion
- The surgeon can control all the parameters (forced infusion rate, ultrasonic power modulations and vacuum settings) in the same panel of the surgical system he or she is working with
- The forced infusion rate can be actively and digitally controlled during the surgery, adjusting the parameters to the conditions and/or the surgical steps of each individual case

When authors decided to use the 0.7 mm MST Duet set authors decided to use the internal gas forced infusion of the Accurus machine to measure the pressure of air exactly. This is from Alcon. The advantage by this was that authors could regulate the amount of air entering into the infusion bottle and thus titrate the system in such a way that there is no surge or collapse of the anterior chamber. When authors are using a 0.7 mm irrigating chopper the problem is that the amount of fluid entering the eye is not enough. To solve this problem gas forced infusion is a must.

The anterior vented gas forced infusion system (AVGFI) of the Accurus surgical system helps in the performance of phakonit. This was started by Arturo Pérez-Arteaga from Mexico. The AVGFI is a system incorporated in the Accurus machine that creates a positive infusion pressure inside the eye. It consists of an air pump and a regulator which are inside the machine; then the air is pushed inside the bottle of intraocular solution, and so the fluid is actively pushed inside the eye without raising or lowering the bottle. The control of the air pump is digitally integrated in the Accurus panel. Authors preset the infusion pump at 100 mm Hg when authors are operating microphakonit.

As surgeons will notice in Table 1 if authors use the air pump at high it is equal to using the Accurus machine at about 100 mm Hg pressure and if authors use the air pump at low it is equal to using the Accurus machine at 50 mm Hg pressure. Some air pumps come with such a regulator so that one can have more air coming out of them. The regulator has a switch for low and high pressure. The cost of the air pump is about 2–10 US $ depending on the country. This can be got from an aquarium shop. If one uses an air pump one can connect a millipore filter to it to prevent any infection. Alternatively, one can use a gas forced internal infusion system using the Accurus machine. In such a case preset the pump at 100 mm Hg.

Bimanual 0.7 mm Irrigation Aspiration System

Bimanual irrigation aspiration is done with the bimanual irrigation aspiration instruments. These instruments are also designed by MST, USA. The previous set authors used was the 0.9 mm set. Now, with microphakonit authors use the new 0.7 mm bimanual I/A set so that after the nucleus removal authors need not enlarge the incision.

Duet Handles

All these instruments of the 0.7 mm set fit onto the handles of the Duet system. So if a surgeons have already got the handles and are using it for phakonit they need to get only the tips and can use the same handles for microphakonit.

Differences Between 0.9 mm and 0.7 mm Sets in Cataract Surgery

Table 2 indicates the differences between the two techniques.

Technique

Incision

The incision is made with a keratome. This can be done using a sapphire knife or a stainless steel knife. One should be careful when one is making the incision so that the incision is a bit long as one would be using gas forced infusion in microphakonit. Before making the incision, a needle with viscoelastic is taken and pierced in the eye in the area where the side port has to be made. The viscoelastic is then injected inside the eye. This will distend the eye so that the clear corneal incision can be made easily. Make one clear corneal incision between the lateral rectus and inferior rectus and the other between the lateral rectus and superior rectus. This way one is able to control the movements of the eye during surgery.

Rhexis

The rhexis is then performed of about 5–6 mm. This is done with a needle. In the left hand a straight rod is held to stabilize the eye. This is the globe stabilization rod. The advantage of this is that the movements of the eye can get controlled if one is working without any anesthesia or under topical anesthesia.

Hydrodissection

Hydrodissection is performed and the fluid wave passing under the nucleus checked. Check for rotation of the

TABLE 2 Differences between phakonit and microphakonit

Features	*Phakonit*	*Microphakonit*
Irrigating chopper	0.9 mm	0.7 mm
Phaco needle	0.9 mm	0.7 mm
Control in surgery	Good	Better control
Valve construction	Extremely important	Not very important as incision is much smaller
Iris prolapse	Can occur if valve is bad	Very rare
Intraoperative floppy iris syndrome	Can be managed	Much better to manage as incision is much smaller and there is better control
Hydrodissection	Can be done from both incisions	To be careful as very little space is there for escape of fluid
Air pump [gas forced infusion (GFI)]	Can be done without it though better with it	Mandatory; 0.7 mm irrigating choppers even with higher end machines need GFI
Flow rate	Can keep any value	Do not keep it very high. 20–24 mL/min
Bimanual I/A	0.9 mm	0.7 mm

nucleus. The advantage of microphakonit is that one can do hydrodissection from both incisions so that even the subincisional areas can get easily hydrodissected. The problem is as there is not much escape of fluid one should be careful in hydrodissection as if too much fluid is passed into the eye one can get a complication.

Microphakonit

The 22 gauge irrigating chopper (0.7 mm) connected to the infusion line of the phaco machine is introduced with foot pedal on position 1. The phaco probe is connected to the aspiration line and the 0.7 mm phaco tip without an infusion sleeve is introduced through the clear corneal incision. Using the phaco tip with moderate ultrasound power, the center of the nucleus is directly embedded starting from the superior edge of rhexis with the phaco probe directed obliquely downwards towards the vitreous. The settings at this stage are 50% phaco power, flow rate 20 mL/min and 100–200 mm Hg vacuum. Using the karate chop technique the nucleus is chopped. Thus, the whole nucleus is removed. Cortical wash-up is then done with the bimanual irrigation aspiration (0.7 mm set) technique. During this whole procedure of microphakonit gas forced infusion is used.

Summary

With microphakonit a 0.7 mm set is used to remove the cataract. At present this is the smallest one can use for cataract surgery. With time one would be able to go smaller with better and better instruments and devices. The problem at present is the intraocular lense. Authors have to get good quality intraocular lense going through sub 1 mm cataract surgical incisions so that the real benefit of microphakonit can be given to the patient.

Key Points

- On May 21st 2005, for the first time, a 0.7 mm phaco needle tip with a 0.7 mm irrigating chopper was used to remove cataracts through the smallest incision possible as of now. This is called microphakonit.
- In order to increase the allowed aspiration flow rate from what a standard 0.7 mm tip would be, MST (Larry Laks) had the walls made thinner, thus increasing the inner diameter. This would allow a case to go, speed wise, closer to what a 0.9 mm tip would go (not exactly the same, but closer).
- The microphakonit irrigating chopper is basically a sharp chopper which has a sharp cutting edge and helps in karate chopping or quick chopping. It can chop any type of cataract.
- The advantage of microphakonit is that one can do hydrodissection from both incisions so that even the subincisional areas can get easily hydrodissected.
- With microphakonit a 0.7 mm set is used to remove the cataract. At present, this is the smallest one can use for cataract surgery. With time one would be able to go smaller with better and better instruments and devices.

References

1. Agarwal A, Agarwal S, Agarwal AT. No anesthesia cataract surgery. In: Agarwal A (Ed). Textbook Phacoemulsification, Laser Cataract Surgery and Foldable IOLs, 1st edition; New Delhi: Jaypee Brothers Medical Publishers (P) Ltd.; 1998; pp. 144-54.
2. Pandey S, Wener L, Agarwal A, et al. No anesthesia cataract surgery. J Cataract Refract Surg. 2001;28:1710.
3. Agarwal A, Agarwal S, Agarwal AT. Phakonit: a new technique of removing cataracts through a 0.9 mm incision; In: Agarwal A (Ed). Textbook Phacoemulsification, Laser Cataract Surgery and Foldable IOLs, 1st edition. New Delhi: Jaypee Brothers Medical Publishers (P) Ltd.; 1998. pp. 139-43.
4. Agarwal A, Agarwal S, Agarwal AT. Phakonit and laser phakonit: Lens surgery through a 0.9 mm incision; In Agarwal A (Ed). Textbook Phacoemulsification, Laser Cataract Surgery and Foldable IOLs, 2nd edition; New Delhi: Jaypee Brothers Medical Publishers (P) Ltd.; 2000. pp. 204-16.
5. Agarwal A, Agarwal S, Agarwal AT. Phakonit. In: Agarwal A (Ed). Textbook Phacoemulsification, Laser Cataract Surgery and Foldable IOLs, 3rd edition. New Delhi: Jaypee Brothers Medical Publishers (P) Ltd.; 2003. pp. 317-29.
6. Agarwal A, Agarwal S, Agarwal AT. Phakonit and laser phakonit. In: Boyd B, Agarwal A, (Eds). Textbook Lasik and Beyond Lasik. Panama: Highlights of Ophthalmology; 2000. pp. 463-8.
7. Agarwal A, Agarwal S, Agarwal AT. Phakonit and laser phakonit: Cataract surgery through a 0.9 mm incision. In: Boyd B, Agarwal A, (Eds). Textbook Phako, Phakonit and Laser Phako. Panama: Highlights of Ophthalmology; 2000. pp. 327-34.
8. Agarwal A, Agarwal S, Agarwal AT. The phakonit Thinoptx IOL. In: Agarwal A, (Ed). Textbook Presbyopia. USA Slack; 2002. pp. 187-94.
9. Agarwal A, Agarwal S, Agarwal AT. Antichamber collapser; J Cataract Refract Surg. 2002; 28:1085.
10. Pandey S, Wener L, Agarwal A, et al. Phakonit: cataract removal through a sub 1.0 mm incision with implantation of the Thinoptx rollable IOL. J Cataract Refract Surg. 2002;28:1710.

11. Agarwal A, Agarwal S, Agarwal AT: Phakonit: phacoemulsification through a 0.9 mm incision ; J Cataract and Refractive Surgery; 2001; 27:1548-52
12. Agarwal A, Agarwal S, Agarwal AT. Phakonit with an acritec IOL. J Cataract Refract Surg. 2003;29:854-55.
13. Agarwal S, Agarwal A, Agarwal AT. Phakonit with Acritec IOL. Panama: Highlights of Ophthalmology. 2000.
14. Jorge Alio. What does MICS require in Alios Textbook MICS. Panama: Highlights of Ophthalmology; 2004. pp. 1-4.
15. Soscia W, Howard JG, Olson RJ. Microphacoemulsification with White Star. A wound-temperature study. J Cataract Refract Surg. 2002;28:1044-6.
16. Soscia W, Howard JG, Olson RJ. Bimanual phacoemulsification through two stab incisions. A wound-temperature study. J Cataract Refract Surg. 2002;28:1039-43.
17. Randall Olson. Microphaco chop. In: David Chang (Ed). Textbook on Phaco Chop; USA: Slack; 2004. pp. 227-37.
18. David Chang: Bimanual phaco chop. In: David Chang (Ed). Textbook on Phaco Chop; USA: Slack; 2004. pp. 239-50.
19. Agarwal A. Air pump. In: Agarwal A (Ed). Textbook on Bimanual Phaco: Mastering the Phakonit/MICS Technique. USA: Slack; 2005.

14 700 Micron Biaxial Phaco

Robert Weinstock (USA)

One of the most significant trends in the evolution of cataract surgery is the reduction of the incision size. In the early days of manual cataract extraction, the wound was as large as 10 mm and the risk of complications and vision loss was extremely high. As technology advanced and phacoemulsification became vogue in the 1970s and 1980s the wound quickly shrunk to a size under 4 mm and over the past twenty years we have seen a continued decrease of the cataract wound size. With the advent of hyperpulse cold phacoemulsification technology in the mid 2000s, we have again seen a trend toward smaller incision surgery. Microcoaxial phacoemulsification can now be routinely performed with incisions less than 2 mm and biaxial surgery can be performed through incisions less than 1.5 mm.

However, until recently, breaking the 1 mm barrier during cataract surgery has not been attainable. Over the past 2 years, a few pioneering surgeons from around the world have devised a way to safely and efficiently perform cataract surgery through 1 mm incisions. With the help of new 700 μm instruments designed specifically for 1 mm wounds, this ultra-small biaxial technique may be yet another step in the evolution of modern cataract surgery.

The advantages of operating through incisions less than 1 mm are fairly obvious. The decreased wound size results in a more stable intraocular environment during cataract removal with less fluid leaking through the wounds and a more consistent chamber depth. It also allows for more precise control and fine maneuvers inside the eye. In addition, with the smaller wound, there is less risk of infection, less risk of dry eye and less risk of wound induced astigmatism. It also leads to a faster visual recovery with a more stable prediction of postoperative visual results. It promises less risk of complications overall and an increase margin in safety in this delicate procedure.

The procedure is begun by making two 1 mm wounds approximately 90 degrees apart on the corneal limbus. These two wounds can be fashioned either using a 1 mm retinal (microvitreoretinal) MVR blade or a customized diamond or metal keratome that is approximately 1 mm in size (Fig. 1). After the wounds are made viscoelastic can be injected into the anterior chamber and a capsulorhexis can

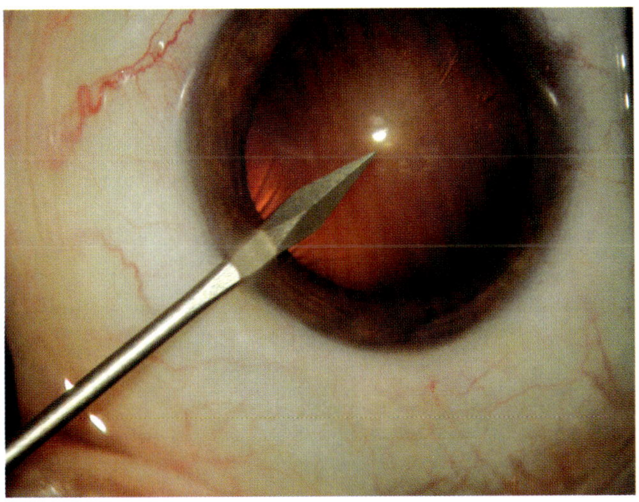

Fig. 1: A 20 gauge microvitreoretinal (MVR) blade is used to make the 1 mm limbal wounds needed for the 700 μm instrumentation

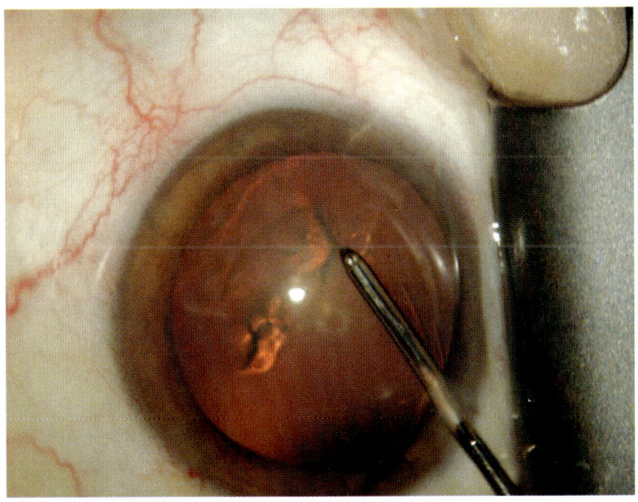

Fig. 2: A micro capsulorhexis forceps is placed easily through the 1 mm wound

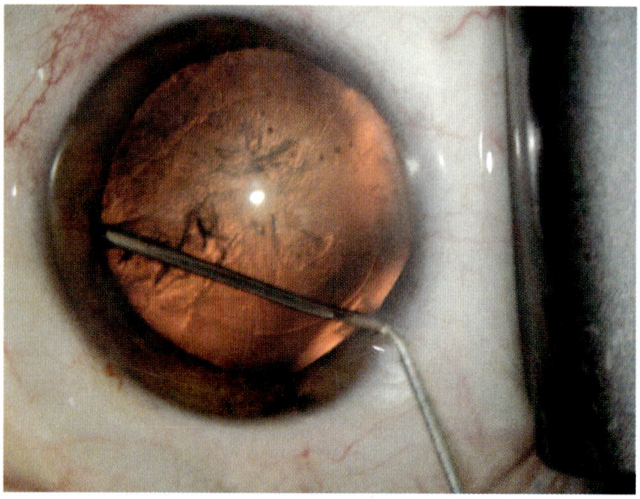

Fig. 3: Gentle hydrodissection and hydrodelineation is performed using a 27 gauge cannula

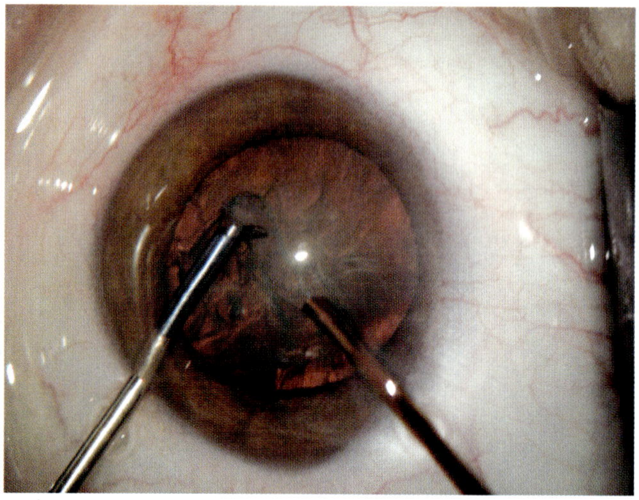

Fig. 4: The 700 µm open ended irrigating chopper and 700 µm straight 30 degree beveled phaco needle are used to remove the nucleus

be performed using a micro-capsulorhexis forceps (Fig. 2). A standard capsulorhexis forceps will not fit through this wound, however, the surgeon can use a 27 gauge bent needle cystotome to perform the capsulorhexis. After the capsulorhexis is performed, gentle hydrodissection and hydrodelineation can be executed through either one of the microwounds. In contrast to hydrodissection with a larger wound where viscoelastic can easily be prolapsed out of the eye if high pressure is achieved, it is necessary to do a more gentle technique because of these smaller wounds and the possibility of a high pressure situation inside the eye (Fig. 3). After there is ample movement of the nucleus and it is freed up from the cortex and capsule, it is time to begin phacoemulsification.

The instruments that are needed to perform this part of the procedure are found in the 700 micron biaxial instrumentation set, which is available through Microsurgical Technologies. Other companies such as Storz are also beginning to design the instruments needed. The sleeveless open-ended irrigating chopper and 700 micron phaco needle that are part of this instrument set fit well through the 1 mm wound, and there is just a little room for some fluid leak around the instruments to keep them cool and allow some movement of the instruments in the wound without oarlocking to occur. The 700 micron instrumentation set can be used with any phacoemulsification machine that has the capability to alter the phacoemulsification power with hyper-pulse software such that there is minimal to no heat generation in the phaco needle. This is paramount to avoid wound burn because the sleeveless phaco needle is in close proximity to the corneal tissue. In addition, some surgeons find it helpful to have a phacoemulsification system that allows for positive pressure infusion via an infusion pump for pressurizing the balanced salt solution bottle. On the other hand, some surgeons perform the procedure just fine with gravity fed infusion. The phacoemulsification machine settings should be similar to those used in conventional coaxial or micro-incisional phacoemulsification, however the vacuum may initially be needed to be lowered and the bottle height may need to be raised when first starting until the fluid dynamics are assessed inside the eye and then adjustments can then be made.

At first, the open-ended irrigating 700 micron chopper is introduced to the left sided wound and irrigation is commenced and then the phacoemulsification needle is introduced to the right wound and initial sculpting of the nucleus is commenced (Fig. 4). After the nucleus is sculpted then the two instruments can be used using counter-traction to crack the nucleus into two hemispheres and further sculpting can be performed to then crack distal hemisphere into two quadrants. A higher vacuum setting can then be used to pull each quadrant up into the center part of the eye and using the combination of the pulsing software plus the manual pulsing of the foot pedal, the first quadrant can be quickly evacuated from the eye and attention can be drawn to the second quadrant which is also removed in a similar fashion. Once this is complete, there is only a single hemisphere of nucleus left which is rotated around such that it is across from the surgeon and the instruments and phacoemulsification needle can be used to impale the nucleus and pull it up into the safe zone of the eye and then

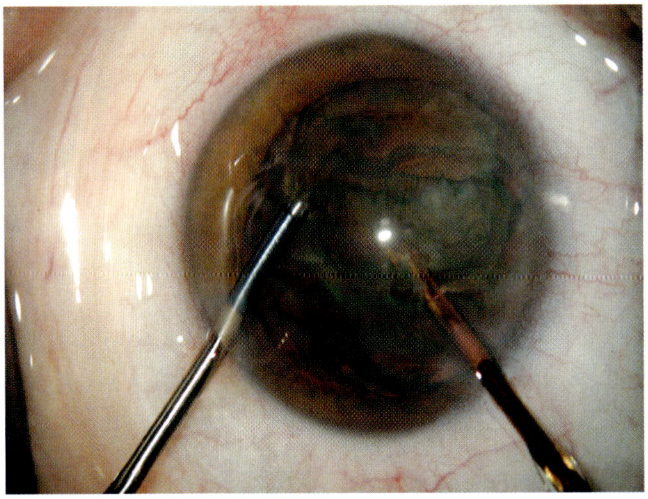

Fig. 5: A vacuum setting of 300 is used to pull nuclear quadrants up into the pupillary plane and the nuclear quadrants and rapidly evacuated

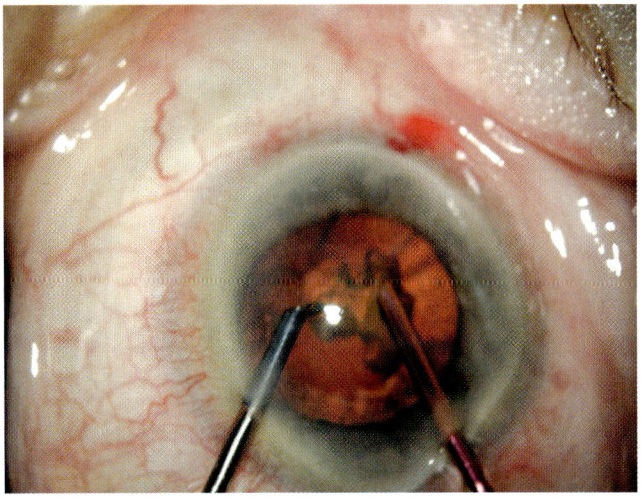

Fig. 6: A chopping technique is used to break up dense nuclear particles

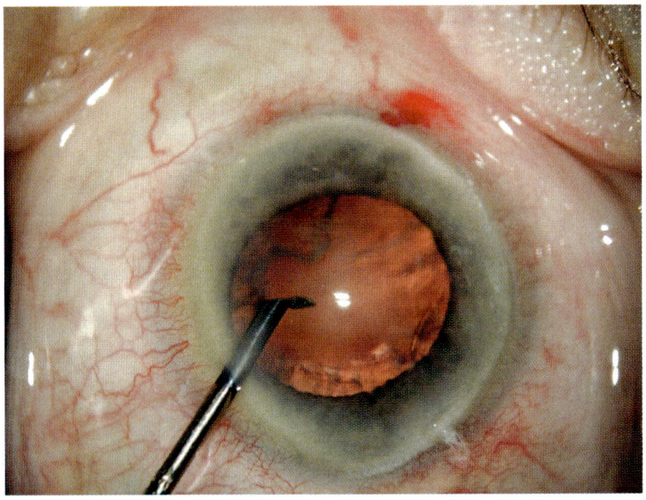

Fig. 7: After nuclear removal, the irrigating chopper can be left in the eye to maintain a deep chamber while the assistant switches the phaco needle to a 700 µm aspiration hand piece and tip

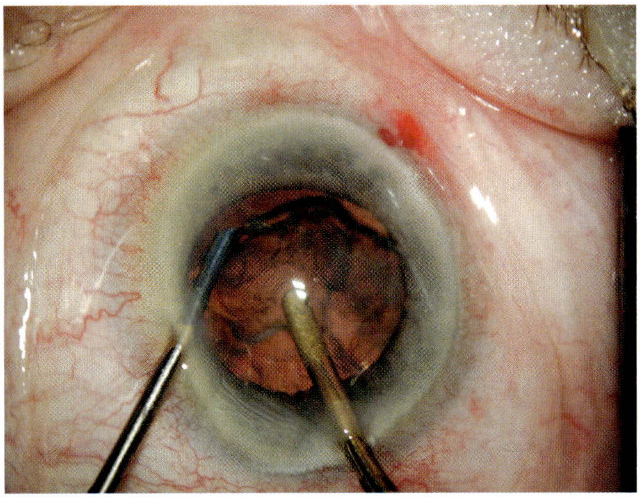

Fig. 8: 700 µm irrigation and aspiration allows for easy and controlled cortical cleanup

can rapidly be emulsified and evacuated from the eye (Figs 5 and 6). At this point the phacoemulsification needle can be removed from the eye while the irrigating chopper is left inside the eye and the assistant can switch the tubing to a 700 micron aspirating hand piece and tip (Fig. 7). This aspiration tip can also fit comfortably through the 1 mm wound and bimanual cortical cleanup, and capsule polishing can be performed using a cortical cleanup setting on the phacoemulsification machine. If there is cortex subincisionally on the aspiration side, both instruments can be removed from the eye and switched to the opposite hand to allow access to the remaining cortex (Fig. 8).

After nuclear and cortical cataract material removal both instruments can be removed from the eye while viscoelastic is then injected into the capsular bag to inflate it in anticipation of lens insertion (Fig. 9).

To date in the United States there are no implants that can be injected through a 1 mm. incision so it is necessary to enlarge the wound to at least 1.8 mm. There are several implants available outside of the United States that can go through sub 2 mm wounds and the Akreos MICS implant within the United States can go through a 1.8 mm wound. For other implants that use conventional injector systems, it is necessary to open up the 1 mm wound up to 2.8 mm.

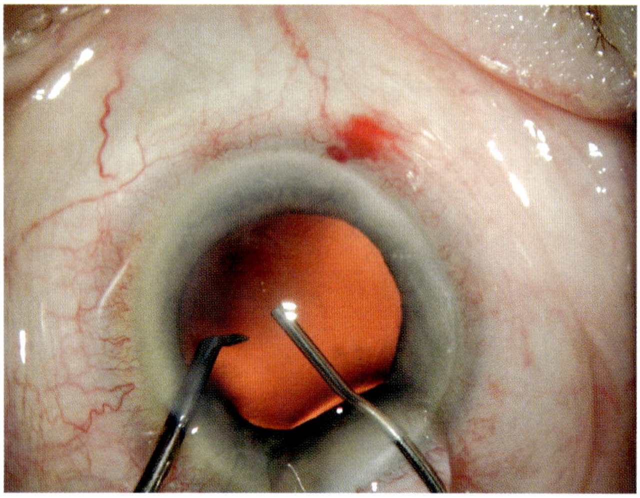

Fig. 9: After irrigation and aspiration, irrigation is stopped as viscoelastic is used to expand the capsule bag in anticipation of lens insertion

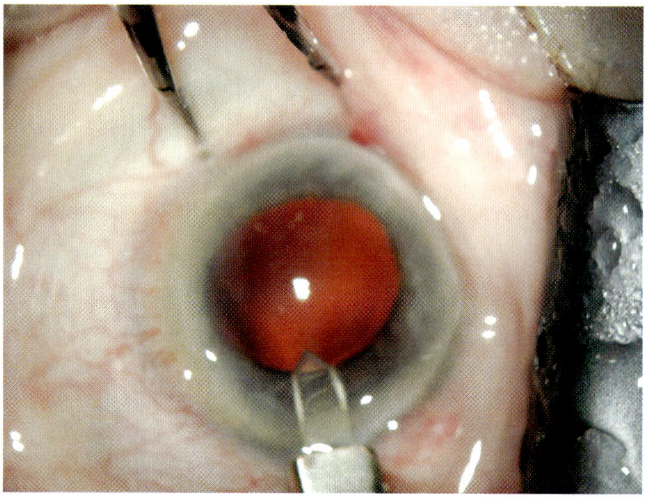

Fig. 10: Using a 1.6 mm diamond keratome, a third incision is made between the two 1 mm wounds for the implant insertion

This can be done with a diamond or metal blade. Some surgeons prefer to make a third wound between the two existing microwounds to insert the implant (Figs 10 and 11). After the implant is placed in the eye, either coaxial or bimanual irrigation and aspiration can be used to evacuate the remaining viscoelastic from the eye and to do fine positioning of the lens (Fig. 12). The two microwounds can easily be sealed with or without wound hydration and the third wound for lens insertion can also be sealed easily with hydration.

Of the few surgeons that are performing 700 micron phacoemulsification, some are reporting that the technique is especially helpful in very challenging and difficult cases. Some of these surgeons are now starting to use 700 micron surgery routinely for cases of pseudoexfoliation syndrome, floppy iris syndrome, histories of ocular trauma and other unusual conditions. It also has been reported that pediatric cases are better suited to have this ultra-small surgical technique, especially in eyes that are left aphakic.

One thing that has been noted by some surgeons using this technique is that in very dense nuclei it may take a little extra phacoemulsification energy and time to remove the dense nuclear particles. This is likely to be the case because the phaco needle has a smaller lumen and therefore

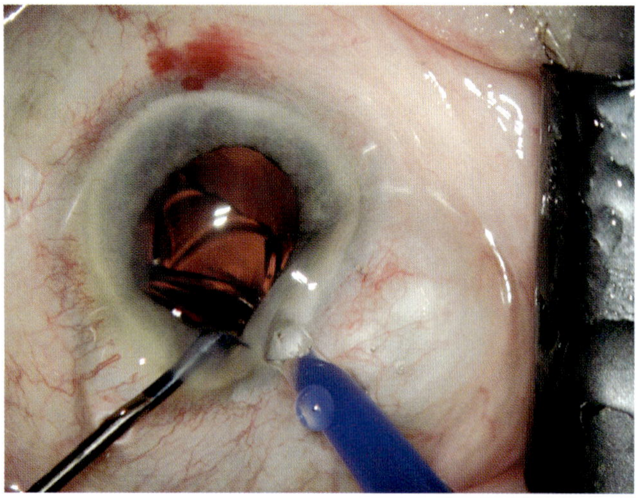

Fig. 11: Using a wound assisted technique with counter traction from the irrigating chopper, an Akreos MICS implant is injected into the capsular bag

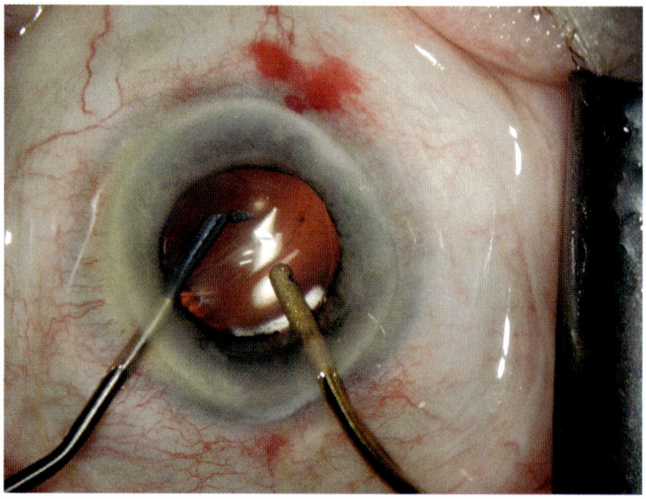

Fig. 12: After implant insertion, 700 µm bimanual irrigation and aspiration is used to remove the remaining viscoelastic

the nuclear pieces must be broken up into smaller sizes in order to evacuate them from the eye. This needs to be taken into consideration when performing the procedure on patients with compromised endothelial tissue where excessive phacoemulsification energy and power can cause postoperative edema and decompensation of the cornea. In these cases, if a surgeon does choose to use 700 micron phacoemulsification, it may be prudent to use a dispersive viscoelastic to protect the endothelium during surgery.

In conclusion, although 700 micron phacoemulsification has only been performed in recent years, it is already catching the attention of innovative surgeons and has proven itself to be an asset in the armamentarium of tools that a surgeon can use to deliver the highest quality of care possible to his or her patients. As the technique is refined, and more implants become available that can be injected through micro-incisional wounds, there will likely be a continual drift toward smaller incision cataract surgery.

15 TriMICS: A Variation of MICS

Jerome Jean-Philippe Bovet (Switzerland)

Abstract

Taking advantage of new technological advances, cataract surgery has experienced a rapid development marked by the development of new techniques that improve both the comfort of surgeon, the safety profile of patient and optical quality after surgery. This revolution deserves to be considered as refractive surgery with the ultimate goal of obtaining better uncorrected visual acuity postsurgery. The fulfillment of this requirement goes through the total control of surgical induced astigmatism (SIA). To date, the current conventional techniques of cataract removal through microincision [microincision cataract surgery (MICS)], only provide a partial answer characterized by a lower degree of SIA. This causes a problem in the prediction of postsurgery result. Authors describe TriMICS, a new technique of MICS which does not induce any astigmatism after cataract surgery and insure rapid visual rehabilitation. Cataract removal is done through two clear corneal microincisions. Afterwards, authors create a third sclerocorneal tunnel incision for implantation of intraocular lens (IOL).

Introduction and Historical Perspectives

Over the last years the cataract surgery has been evolving, always looking for how to achieve a better visual acuity associated with a better safety profile for the patient. Since the invention of phacoemulsification by Charles Kelman in 1967,[1] the evolution of the technical support has been staggering. In this process the last decade is a decade of enlightenment, marked by the development of new technologies: machinery for modern phacoemulsification, foldable IOL, IOL injector, diverse modern micro-instruments, which allowed to considerably reduce the size of incisions and the vulgarization of the biaxial microincision cataract surgery (BiMICS). MICS refers to any phacoemulsification performed through an incision smaller than 2 mm.[2,3] BiMICS has been described for the first time by Shearing et al.[4] in 1985 and made popular from the year 1998 by A Agarwal et al.,[5,6] J Alio et al.[3,7] and several other authors.[8-13] The principle of this procedure is the separation of irrigation, aspiration, during the phacoemulsification cataract removal. This contrast with traditional coaxial phacoemulsification where a single phacoemulsification handpiece provides irrigation into the eye and aspiration out of the eye.

Although the benefits of BiMICS are numerous:

- Smaller size of incisions
- Improve wound healing
- Improvement of anterior chamber fluid dynamics[14-15]
- Minimal turbulence during aspiration which leads to less invasive surgery
- Decrease risk of inflammation (including cystoïd macular edema and retinal detachment)
- High stability of the incision[2,3]
- Minimal SIA
- Easy insertion with an IOL injector
- Rapid visual rehabilitation
- Improving the comfort of the surgeon who can now use both hands

Authors also note some drawbacks which are:

- Steep learning curve
- Potential wound trauma and endothelial cell loss caused by thermal impact of the sleeveless phaco tip[15]
- Sensitive phaco dynamics
- Persistence of SIA

In total, all these innovations have enabled surgeons to achieve ever smallest incisions, encouraged by the results of studies which show that small incision causes less SIA.[3,16] The ultimate goal is to solve both the problem of cataract surgery without inducing any astigmatism and possibly that of the refraction with one unique surgery operation. This objective can be achieved only with the total control of the SIA and the predictability of the postsurgery outcomes. In the move towards this goal, authors propose the TriMICS, which is an intervention that does not induce any astigmatism after cataract surgery. What is it all about? Three microincisions cataract surgery (TriMICS) is a technique of cataract removing through two 1.0 mm microincisions, followed by the insertion of the IOL through a 2 mm sclerocorneal micro-tunnel incision.

Patients and Method

Patient Selection

This new technique cannot be applied for all patients with ocular disorders that may

- alter the reliability of corneal keratometry or biometry
- slow down the visual rehabilitation: uveitis—intraocular surgery or ocular trauma—history of serious coexisting ocular disease such as amblyopic, preexisting eye abnormality, glaucoma, optic atrophy, ocular tumor

Presurgery Ocular Examination

All selected patients should undergo clinical presurgery assessments. The same examinations have to be done during follow-up appointment after 1 day, 1 week, 1 month, 3 months and 6 months. Detailed clinical and biomicroscopic ophthalmic examination of the anterior and posterior segment have to be performed. Other measurements include:

- Visual acuity (Snellen chart).
- Ocular pressure (Goldmann applanation tonometry)
- Autorefractometry (ARK-700A, Nidek Co. Ltd., Japan)
- Biometry with IOL Master (Carl Zeiss, Meditec AG, Jena, Germany)
- Corneal toricity with Oculus Pentacam® HR (type 70900, Optikgerate GmbH, Wetzlar, Germany)
- Corneal endothelial cell count (Confoscan 4, Nidek Technologies, Italy) has to be done.

Presurgery Treatment

The day before the surgery, authors administer a preservative free eye drop Indometacin 1 drop, twice per day (0.1% Indophtal UD, Bausch & Lomb Swiss AG).

On the day at which the surgery will be carried out, 2 hours before the surgery, the pupil is dilated by administering one eye drop of tropicamide 5 mg/mL (Mydriaticum "dispersed", Omnivision, Swissmedic) every 10 minutes in the eye to be operated.

Anesthesia

The first part of surgery is performed under topical anesthesia with lidocaine hydrochloride 2% (xylocaine 2%, FO-OO3 AstraZeneca) which will be later complemented by intracamerular injection of lidocaine hydrochloride 0.2%. Before scleral microincision, authors swab the conjunctiva of the incision site for about 30 seconds, using lidocaine 2%.

Surgical Procedure

1. Authors start with two single oblique clear corneal micro-tunnel incision of 1.0 mm in width performed at 8 o'clock and 11 o'clock position for the right eye, or at 1 o'clock and 4 o'clock position for the left eye, each other separated by 90° angle step, using a 20 gauge (G) ophthalmic knife (MVR20, Mani Inc., Japan) (Figs 1 to 3).
2. Injection of viscosurgical device: Optéis 1.4% (sodium hyaluronate, Anteis SA, Geneva, Switzerland), using a 27 G standard infusion cannula (BD Visitec Viscoflow cannula 40 × 22 mm, 27 G × 7/8 in, Ref 585282 Becton, Dickinson and Company, Waltham, USA).
3. Capsulorhexis (Fig. 4): Authors practice a continuous curvilinear capsulorhexis with a MICS capsulorhexis forceps (Carl Zeiss AG, Jena, Germany). With its peak side, authors apply a pressure followed by a microincision on the front of the capsular bag. Authors pull the flap by tearing up the bag in anticlockwise direction. The diameter of the capsulorhexis should be 0.5 lower than the optic of the lens, which means about 5–6 mm.
4. Hydrodissection and hydrodelineation: In these processes, the dissection of the nucleus of lens

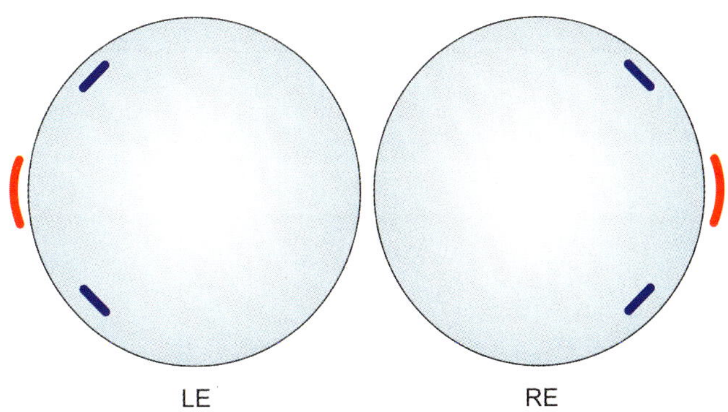

Fig. 1: Diagram of incisions sites

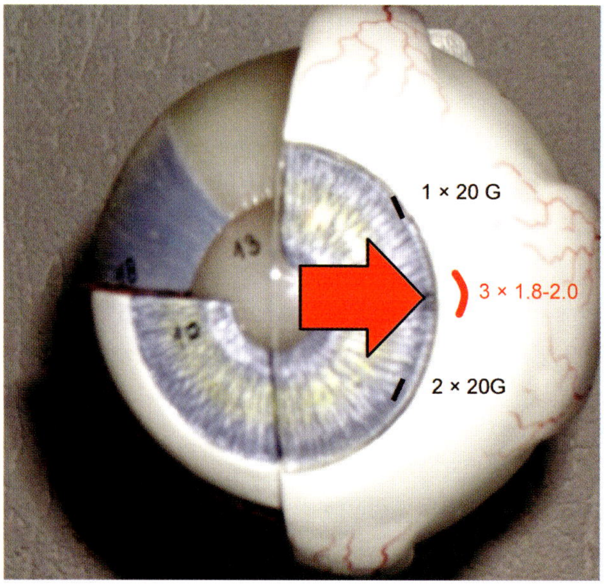

Fig. 2: Incision sites (right eye)

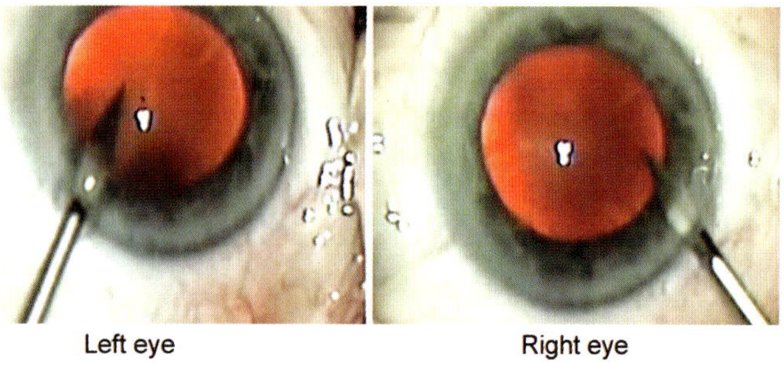

Fig. 3: Execution of the first incision using a 20 G ophthalmic knife

from the cortex is performed using a 23 G cannula, introduced through one of the paracentesis. Authors irrigate the anterior chamber (AC) with balance salt solution (BSS). Authors mobilize the lens masses until the nucleus is completely free inside the capsular bag. The objective of hydrodelineation liquid allows the nucleus to be elevated and separated from the cortical masses.

5. Preparation for phacoemulsification: Let's consider that the left eye is being handled: the incision performed in the 4 o'clock position is useful for the insertion of the irrigation sleeve (left hand): authors first place the 20 G chopper irrigating end out (Ref 85903S20, Bausch & Lomb, Heidelberg, Germany) through the 4 o'clock incision (left hand) and then introduce the 20–21 G phaco tip (Cobra Tip, Xcelens phaco-MICS Mono XMPT-B, lot 10/090, Xcelens SA, Switzerland) at the 1 o'clock incision (right hand). The 20 G irrigating end out chopper connected to the infusion line of the phaco machine is introduced with a foot pedal on position 2.
6. Phacoemulsification (Fig. 5): Authors perform their phacoemulsification with the new Stellaris Venturi Pump machine (Bausch & Lomb, Rochester, NY, USA). The nucleus is grooved by the slip and chop technique. Machine settings are shown as follows:
   - Maximum phacoemulsification power, 100 %
   - Maximum vacuum, 600 mm Hg
   - Maximum bottle height above the eye, 140 cm

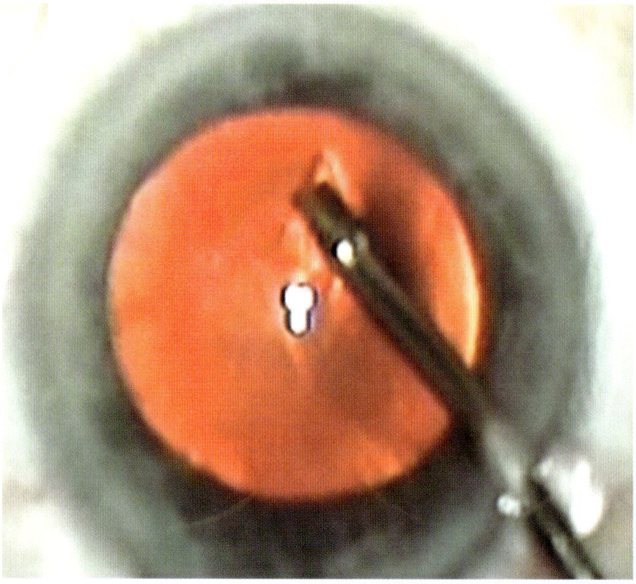

Fig. 4: Capsulorhexis. With the peak side of MICS capsulorhexis forceps, authors apply a pressure followed by a microincision

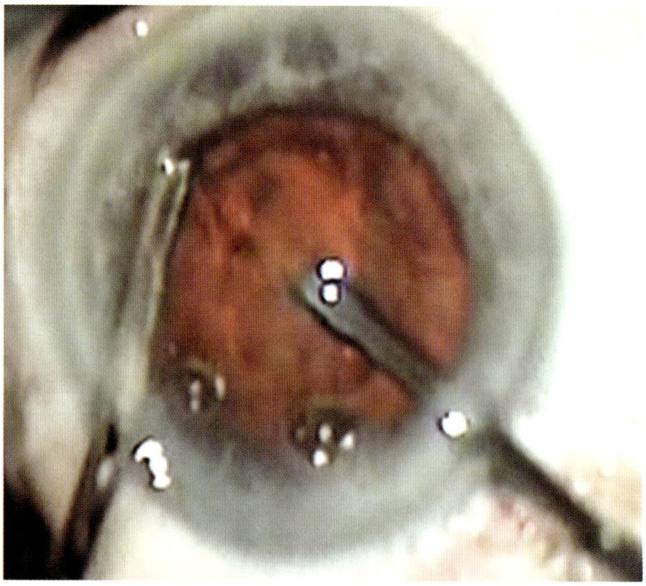

Fig. 5: Bimanual phacoemulsification performed with cobra tip

These are machine settings during phacoemulsification and aspiration of the lens nucleus.

- Maximum phacoemulsification power [(fixed ultrasound (U/S)], 30%
- Bottle height above the eye, 95 cm
- Fixed vacuum, 380
- Total phocoemulsification time, 38.43 seconds
- Total phacoemulsification intervals, 1.20 seconds
- Mean ultrasonic power, 3%
- Irrigation/Aspiration pressure, 550 mm Hg
- Phacoemulsification energy is applied in pulse mode with the pulse rate at 220 p/s (pulse/second)
- Duty cycle, 50%

Effective phaco time (TPE: amount of phaco (ultrasound) energy used) is calculated using the following formula:[17]

(phaco time) × (mean phaco power)/100

Where phaco time corresponds to TPA.

Mean ultrasound (U/S) varies according to the maturity of the cataract. When the density of the cataract is low, say grade 1–2 [Lens Opacities Classification System III (LOCS III)],[18] the mean is around 3%. For the hard cataracts, authors can reach a value of 8%.

Bimanual phacoemulsification is performed, using the Venturi Pump, a sleeveless straight cobra tip (Fig. 5) and a 20 G irrigating chopper. For normal cataracts (grade 1–2), the vacuum limit set at 380 mm Hg until the end of the phaco procedure (aspiration of epinuclear piece). Authors increase the maximum vacuum in the case of a hard cataract.

7. Bimanual irrigation/aspiration (I/A): Removal of nuclear material is now complete. Authors must switch their instruments. Firstly, authors remove the phaco tip and secondly, the chopping irrigating tip to maintain the AC depth. Then, authors introduce the irrigating handpiece followed by aspiration handpiece (disposable bimanual System 21G, Ref BSD 510, Lot HAM 15, Buerki Innomed AG, Switzerland). Residual cortex removal and posterior capsule polishing are now performed using bimanual I/A (Fig. 6).
8. Intraocular lens insertion
   - First, the capsular bag is filled up with viscoelastic material Ophtéis 1.0% (sodium hyaluronate, Anteis SA, Geneva, Switzerland), using a 27 G standard infusion cannula
   - Creation of the third scleral microincision (Fig. 7)
     - Localization: 9 o'clock position in the right eye and 3 o'clock in the left eye. The sclerocorneal tunnel microincision is made 2 mm behind the posterior limbus
     - Before scleral microincision, authors swab the conjunctiva at the incision site for about 30 seconds using lidocaine 2%
     - A slip angled ophthalmic knife is used to perform a micro-tunnel incision, which is about 2 mm long and 1.8 mm in width
   - A single piece acrylic foldable IOL (Akreos MI60, Bausch & Lomb) is implanted in the capsular bag

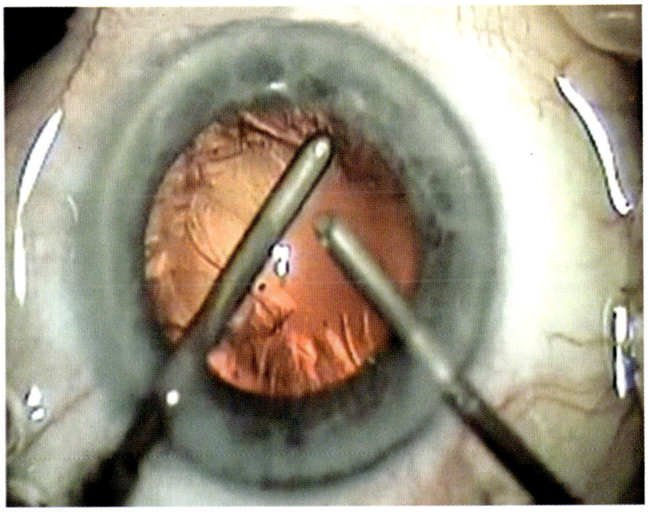

Fig. 6: Bimanual irrigation/aspiration. Residual cortex removal and posterior capsule polishing

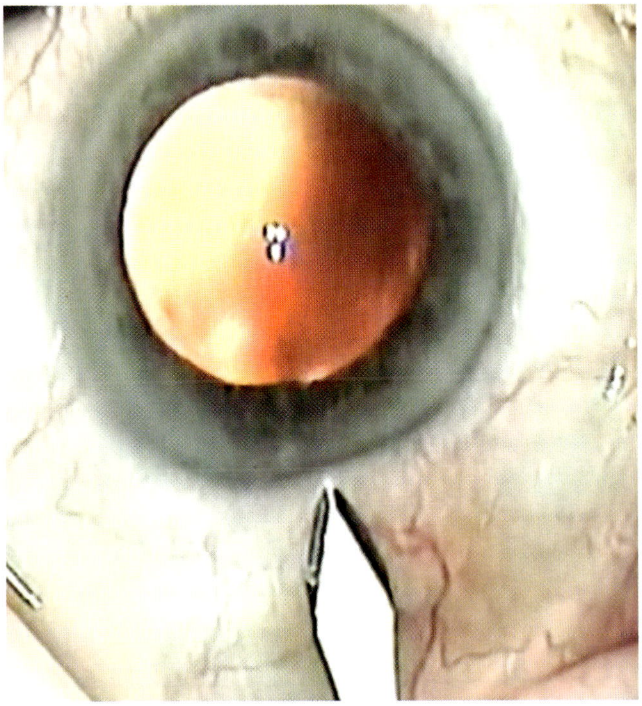

Fig. 7: Execution of sclerocorneal tunnel

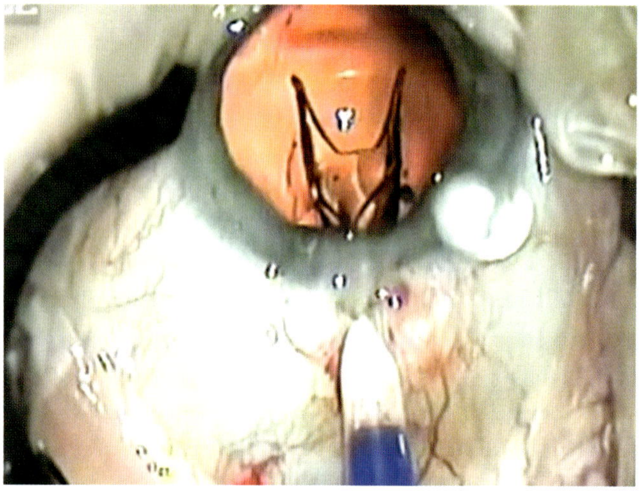

Fig. 8: Intraocular lens injection with an injector

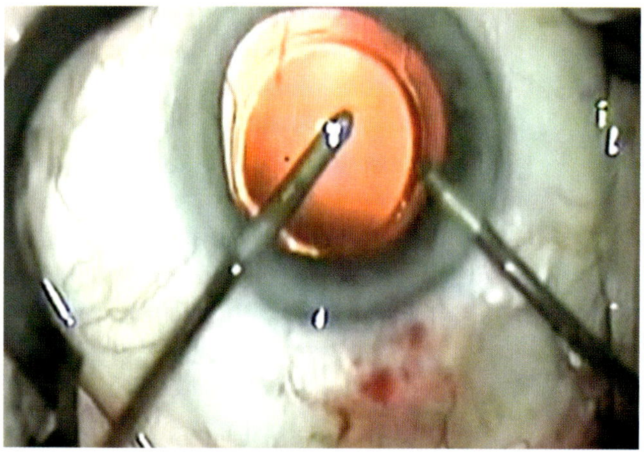

Fig. 9: Intraocular lens is now positioned in the capsular bag

through a 2 mm micro-tunnel, using a disposable one-hand injector (Viscojet, LP604350, Medical AG, Switzerland) and a wound-assisted manner with counteraction (Fig. 8). IOL is now positioned in the capsular bag (Fig. 9)

- The viscoelastic material is removed and replaced by BSS
- All wounds are checked for leakage with fluorescein and none have been found

The average total surgery time (duration of the intervention) is 12 hours 30 minutes.

At the end of the intervention, the AC is deep, the pupil is round and centered, the posterior chamber implant is in place. Authors proceed to the AC injection of lidocaine hydrochloride 0.2% (0.2% xylocaine)—diluted Cefuroxime 750 mg (Zinacef, GSK AG, Swissmedic)—Béthaméthasone 4 mg/mL (célestone 4 mg/mL, lot 0003 Schering-Plough).

The patient receives the following postsurgery treatments:

- Dexamethasone phosphate 1 mg/mL UD 0.4 mL (Dexafree 1 mg/mL, (Thea-pharma SA, Suisse): 1 eye drop, thrice per day, for a month
- Ofloxacine 3 mg UD eye drop (Floxal, Bausch & Lomb, Swiss): 1 eye drop, thrice per day, for a month

Discussion

A new generation of surgical instruments associated with recent technological innovation has led to the development of microphacoemulsification characterized by the practice of smaller and smaller microincision.[19,20] This trend was encouraged by the results of studies that shows that corneal incision of less than 1.5 mm had no impact on corneal curvature.[21-23] The smaller the incision, the lesser the SIA.[3,16,21,24] This is important because surgeons who now consider the cataract surgery as a refractive surgery are limited by the fact that it still leads to a SIA for all incisions more than 1 mm.[25] So, incision size is the main clinical factor in the amount of SIA after cataract surgery and therefore, in the improvement of visual outcome and high patient satisfaction.

Agarwal[26] has demonstrated an intervention called microphakonit (phako being done with a needle incision technology) that it is possible to remove cataract by phacoemulsification through a 0.9 mm microincision, using a 0.7 mm phaco tip. The problem now is the insertion of IOL and possibility of lens compression. Even with injector, it is still necessary to enlarge the incision. But Kaufmann et al. showed the negative consequences in terms of SIA, related to the enlargement of the incision for implantation of the IOL.[27] The result is also bad when authors try to introduce the lens through a tight microincision without enlargement. Moon SC et al. showed that excessive stretching may injure the cornea which does not have the capacity necessary to tolerate true elastic deformation.[28] The problem becomes serious when authors consider the multifocal implants or implants of high dioptric values (greater than or equal to 24 diopters), often of considerable thickness, whose insertion through the clear corneal microincision is almost impossible. The minimum width of the incision for these special implant must be 2.2 or 2.8 mm depending on the type of multifocal lenses, thus inducing astigmatism in a surgery which is intended to be refractive. How can surgeons overcome this problem?

Authors' TriMICS surgery technique begins as a classic BiMICS, but with two 1.0 mm incisions. The first two incisions are used only for cataract removal. Authors' procedure enjoys all the benefits of BiMICS but also its disadvantages, except that of the induction of surgical astigmatism. Authors' incisions are 1 mm length, therefore astigmatically neutral. How to solve the problem of inserting the IOL? Awaiting the development of new accurate material (IOL) that will help solve this issue, authors proceed to the injection of IOL through a sclerocorneal micro-tunnel.

The sclerocorneal incision through a tunnel is not new in cataract surgery. It was used in the past for extracapsular cataract extraction in order to reduce corneal astigmatism after cataract surgery. It was then a large and traumatic incision. With the advent of phacoemulsification, it decreased in size, but still big enough to induce some changes in corneal curvature.[29] The sclerocorneal micro-tunnel incision allows authors to reach their goal: the insertion of the IOL with injector without any impact on the corneal curvature. Other benefits of this technique are the good resistance to internal and external pressures and the lack of filtering bubble due to a good sealing.

Despite the advantage of keeping the corneal curvature intact, the sclerocorneal micro-tunnel incision has some drawbacks which are:

- A micro-bleeding at the site of the incision. This can be avoided by a good cauterization of the sclera before the incision and/or application of phenylephrine on the site before the incision
- Not suitable for topical anesthesia. Additional anesthesia is necessary: swab conjunctiva for about 30 seconds at the site of incision

With TriMICS, Authors believe that they have won not only the challenge to be neutral on shape and shift, but also to control exactly the astigmatism before and after the cataract surgery. Any grade or type of cataract can be operated by TriMICS. As MICS and astigmatically neutral cataract surgery, authors' technique is especially devoted for refractive cataract surgery and will be used for insertion of multifocal lenses, Toric lenses and even after corneal refractive surgery.

As with all surgeries, the TriMICS has some drawbacks:

- New instrumentation
- Special phaco tip
- Adapt the parameters of the phacoemulsification machine to new instruments
- Surge if surgeons don't use right parameters. Even with a hard cataract of grade 3–4 (LOCS III),[18] authors haven't any more surge
- Not all the machines are available for this technique
- Potential wound burn caused by thermal impact of the sleeveless phaco tip in a tight incision. The risk is almost zero. Indeed, the results of studies have shown that the energy necessary to cause a burn during biaxial phacoemulsification was much higher than the energy settings used clinically[9,30]

All of which (drawbacks) can be overcome after few weeks of training especially for ophthalmology surgeons who have already performed BiMICS.

As with all MICS, rupture of the posterior capsule is the most feared complication intraoperatively. Authors recorded no complications neither intra nor postsurgery. Even if their sample set of patients is small, authors can affirm that the occurrence of complications has become exceptional since the advent of new phacoemulsification machines that permit to realize phaco safely even when cases are difficult (cataract grade 3–4 (LOCS III).[18] There is also a risk of complications during the implantation of the implant. If the corneoscleral incision is not oblique enough, there can be an iris avulsion. Also for complications related to incision: a poorly made incision in the clear cornea causes a risk of forming descemetocele. The postsurgery complication to be feared is the increase of intraocular pressure due to the persistence of the viscoelastic material in the AC. This concern can be avoided by following the proper rinsing of the AC immediately at the end of the surgery.

Despite having to perform a third incision, the average total surgical time (time between the first incision and the insertion of the IOL) took 12 hours 30 minutes. This time is comparable to the corresponding times of standard coaxial, BiMICS and CoMICS (micro-coaxial cataract surgery).[31] Authors, effective phaco time (TPE) and phacotime (TPA) are also remarkable. Compared to those of literature, they are slightly short.[31-34] This is made possible due to authors' highly efficient of Stellaris device.

The first result of authors' pilot study suggest that the TriMICS technique does not induce any astigmatism and is therefore able to improve the predictability and precision of MICS according to authors' pre- and postsurgical keratometry and to their best corrected visual acuity results.

Conclusion

TriMICS seem to be a perfect match to not induce astigmatism surgery. Longer follow-up and more samples are need to confirm this surgery.

References

1. Kelman CD. Phacoemulsification and aspiration: A new technique of cataract extraction. Am J Ophthal. 1967;64:23.
2. Alio JL, Rodriguez-Prats JL, Vianello A, et al. Visual outcome of microincision cataract surgery with implantation of an Acri.Smart lens. J Cataract Refract Surg. 2005;31:1549-56.
3. Alio J, Rodriguez-Prats JL, Galal A, et al. Outcomes of microincision cataract surgery versus coaxial phacoemulsification. Ophthalmology. 2005;112(11):1997-2003.
4. Shearing S, Relyea R, Louiza A, et al. Routine phacoemulsification through a one-millimeter non-sutured incision. Cataract. 1985;2:6-11.
5. Agarwal A, Agarwal S, Agarwal AT. Phakonit and Laser Phakonit: lens surgery through a .9 mm incision. In Agarwal S, et al. Phacoemulsification, Laser Cataract Surgery and Foldable IOLs. 2nd edition. New Delhi: Jaypee Brothers Medical Publishers (P) Ltd.; 1998. pp. 204-16.
6. Agarwal A, Agarwal S, Narang P, et al. Phakonit: phacoemulsification through a 0.9 mm corneal incision. J Cataract Refract Surg. 2001;27(10):1548-52.
7. Alio JL, Rodriguez JL, Galal A. MICS: Microincisional Cataract Surgery. Eldorado, Panama: Highlights of Ophthalmology International 2004.
8. Tsuneoka H, Shiba T, Takahashi Y. Feasibility of ultrasound cataract surgery with a 1.4 mm incision. J Cataract Refract Surg. 2001;27(6):934-40.
9. Soscia W, Howard JG, Olson RJ. Bimanual phacoemulsification through 2 stab incisions. A wound-temperature study. J Cataract Refract Surg. 2002;28(6):1039-43.
10. Baykara M, Ercan I, Ozcetin H. Microincisional cataract surgery (MICS) with pulse and burst modes. Eur J Ophthalmol. 2006;16(6):804-8.
11. Paul T, Braga-Mele R. Bimanual microincisionnal phacoemulsification: the future of cataract surgery? Curr Opin Ophthalmol. 2005;16:2-7.
12. Crema AS, Walsh A, Yamane Y, et al. Comparative study of coaxial phacoemulsification and microincision cataract surgery. One-year follow-up. J Cataract Refract Surg. 2007;33(6):1014-8.
13. Dosso AA, Cottet L, Burgener ND, et al. Outcomes of coaxial microincision cataract surgery versus conventional coaxial cataract surgery. J Cataract Refract Surg. 2008;34(2):284-8.
14. Fine IH, Hoffman RS, Packer M. Optimizing refractive lens exchange with bimanual microincision phacoemulsification. J Cataract Refract Surg. 2004;30:550-4.
15. Weikert MP. Update on bimanual microincisional cataract surgery. Curr Opin Ophthalmol. 2006;17:62-7.
16. Cavallini GM, Campi L, Masini C, et al. Bimanual microphacoemulsification versus coaxial miniphacoemulsification: prospective study. J Cataract Refract Surg. 2007;33:387-92.
17. Fine IH, Packer M, Hoffman RS. Power modulations in new phacoemulsification technology: improved outcomes. J Cataract Refract Surg. 2004;30:1014-9.
18. Chylack LT Jr, Wolfe JK, Singer DM, et al. The lens opacities classification system III. The longitudinal study group. Arch Ophthalmol. 1993;111:831-6.
19. Omulecki W, Wilczynski M. Minimizing the incision in cataract surgery – a continuous challenge. Okulistyka. 2004;3(II):38-43.
20. Alió JL, Elkady B, Ortiz D. Corneal optical quality following sub 1.8 mm micro-incision cataract surgery vs. 2.2 mm mini-incision coaxial phacoemulsification. Middle East Afr J Ophthalmol. 2010;17(1):94-9.
21. Jiang Y, Le Q, Yang J, Lu Y. Changes in corneal astigmatism and high order aberrations after clear corneal tunnel phacoemulsification guided by corneal topography. J Refract Surg. 2006;22:S1083-S1088.
22. Olson RJ, Crandall AS. Prospective randomized comparison of phacoemulsification cataract surgery with a 3.2 mm vs. a 5.5 mm sutureless incision. Am J Ophthalmol. 1998;125:612-20.
23. Oshika T, Tsuboi S. Astigmatic and refractive stabilization after cataract surgery. Ophthalmic Surg. 1995;26:309-15.
24. Yao K, Tang X, Ye P. Corneal astigmatism, high order aberrations, and optical quality after cataract surgery: microincision versus small incision. J Refract Surg. 2006;22(9 Suppl):S1079-S1082.
25. Wilczynski M, Supady E, Piotr L, et al. Comparison of surgically induced astigmatism after coaxial phacoemulsification through 1.8 mm microincision and bimanual phacoemulsification through 1.7 mm microincision. J Cataract Refract Surg. 2009;35(9):1563-9.
26. Amar Agarwal, Athiya Agarwal, Sunita Agarwal. Microphakonit surgery perfomed with 0.7 mm tip. Ocular Surgery News Europe/Asia-Pacific. 2005.
27. Kaufmann C, Thiel MA, Esterman A, et al. Astigmatism change in biaxial microincisional cataract surgery with enlargement of one incision: a prospective controlled study. Clin Experiment Ophthalmol. 2009;37(3):254-61.
28. Moon SC, Mohamed T, Fine IH. Comparison of surgically induced astigmatisms after clear corneal incisions of different sizes. Korean J Ophthalmol. 2007;21(1):1-5.
29. He Y, Zhu S, Chen M, et al. Comparison of the Keratometric Corneal Astigmatic Power after Phacoemulsification: Clear Temporal Corneal Incision versus Superior Scleral Tunnel Incision. J Ophthalmol. 2009;2009:210621.
30. Soscia W, Howard JG, Olson RJ. Microphacoemulsification with White Star: a wound-temperature study. J Cataract Refract Surg. 2002;28:1044-6.
31. Izzet Can, Takmaz T, Yildiz Y, et al. Coaxial, microcoaxial, and biaxial microincision cataract surgery: prospective comparative study. J Cataract Refract Surg. 2010;36(5):740-6.
32. Kurz S, Krummenauer F, Gabriel P, et al. Biaxial microincision versus coaxial small incision clear cornea cataract surgery. Ophthalmology. 2006;113(10):1818-26.
33. Bovet J. Phaco chop for CoMICS (coaxial microincision cataract surgery). In: Ashok Garg, Jorge Alio, Robert J Weinstock, et al. (Eds). Mastering Phaco Chop Techniques. New Delhi: Jaypee Brothers Medical Publishers (P) Ltd.; 2009.
34. Bovet J. Phaco chop for BiMICS (bimanual microincision cataract surgery). In: Ashok Garg, Jorge Alio Robert J Weinstock, et al. (Eds). Mastering Phaco Chop Techniques. New Delhi: Jaypee Brothers Medical Publishers (P) Ltd., 2009.

Section 4

Personal Techniques for Particular Situations

16 Lens Salute Microphaco

Cyres K Mehta (India), Keiki R Mehta (India)

"All truth passes through three stages. First, it is ridiculed. Second, it is violently opposed. Third, it is accepted as being self-evident."

—Arthur Schopenhauer

Introduction

Cataract surgery has evolved over the past few decades with a progressive decrease in the size of the incision. Intracapsular surgery evolved into extracapsular cataract extraction after which with the advent of phacoemulsification through a tunnel, corneal or scleral, it was felt that the acme of cataract surgery had been reached. Microphacoemulsification, sleeveless bimanual phacoemulsification through a 1.2–1.4 mm clear corneal tunnel, has raised the bar further once again.

Microphaco, or bimanual phacoemulsification is not new. As far back as 1985, Dr Steven Shearing, MD, in Las Vegas USA propounded the separation of ultrasound/ aspiration and the irrigation handpiece.[1]

Soscia et al. have evaluated wound burn in two studies on cadaver eyes and found that wound burn is not generated when the phaco needle is naked (sleeveless), when an irrigating chopper (Olson irrigating chopper; Asico LLC, USA) is used and at worst only mild temperature elevation occurred at the tunnel. Wound burn only occurred when the fluid inflow was completely cut off at nearly 80% power, while using WhiteStar!

At the annual meeting of the Japanese Society of Cataract and Refractive Surgery in Kyoto in 1999, Crozafon reported using a 21 gauge sleeveless teflon (a poor thermal conductor) coated tip and the Optikon Pulsar unit.[2-4]

Also in 1999, Agarwal and coauthors presented phakonit through a 0.9 mm incision with constant dripping of cold balanced salt solution (BSS) over the phako needle. This is because authors felt that friction between the tip and the tunnel was the main factor for heat production and that pouring BSS on the incision site was required to disperse the heat buildup.

Donnenfeld et al. evaluated wound temperature using a micropulse system and showed only a minimal temperature elevation and comparable endothelial cell loss at three months as compared to conventional coaxial phaco.[4-7]

Tsuneoka and colleagues presented a study of 965 eyes in 2001 with no case of thermal burns using a Tsuneoka irrigating hook which later evolved into the Tsuneoka tip on the DUET system.[4-5]

These researchers emboldened authors to try out bimanual phaco through 1.2–1.4 mm incisions for themselves and the results were no different.

Fine, Olson, Mehta, Alio and others have expanded modified and refined this technique bringing it to its present level of refinement.[7-10]

Some of the names coined for this new technique are microphaco (Dr Randall Olson, USA) or Bimanual Phaco or Phakonit (coined by Dr Amar .Agarwal). Phakonit stands for *Phaco*emulsification with *N*eedle *I*ncision *T*echnology.[11-12]

The removal of the cooling irrigation sleeve and separation of infusion and emulsification/aspiration through two separate incisions is now a viable alternative to traditional coaxial phacoemulsification. Machines such as the AMO Signature, STAAR Sonic, Alcon Infiniti, Bausch & Lomb Stellaris and Dodick Nd:YAG Laser Photolysis systems offer the potential of offering relatively "cold" lens removal capabilities and the capacity for bimanual cataract surgery. Alio (Alicante, Spain) has described a technique using the Venturi pump system of the Alcon Accurus which maintains pressurized inflow and a surge-free system.[8-10]

Vejarano presented his technique of "safe chop" at the annual meeting of the Intraocular Implant & Refractive Society, India (IIRSI) in 2003, which showcases the importance of an irrigating chopper versus a non irrigating one. He sweeps the chopper in a counterclockwise manner after insinuating it in the space between the nucleus and the capsule. The irrigation exiting the chopper acts as a buffer zone between the nucleus and the capsule and a traditional Nagahara´s chop is employed which greatly simplifies chopping in hard cataracts.

Chiou and Bovet have used "cold phaco" technology and reported results with respect to corneal edema postoperatively, comparable with coaxial phaco.

The advantages in a smaller incision of 1.2–1.4 mm as compared to one of 2.8 mm is self-evident. It has been proved by topography and aberrometry (Zyoptics, Agarwal) to produce an astigmatically neutral incision. Secondly, the smaller the incision, the lesser is the chance of the entry of bacteria and fungi leading to endophthalmitis. Finally, the smaller the incision, the faster is the visual recovery of the patient.

Here authors have described their personal technique (Cyres K Mehta) that for them has made this surgery safe and reproducible.[13]

Surgical Technique

The two entry tunnels are made with diamond Meyco (Anton Meyer & Co Ltd., Switzerland) 613 knives, which create reproducibly a rectangular tunnel of 1 by 1.2 mm. Openings of consistent size are very important as a larger opening will lead to excessive leak and result in surge. However a very tight opening for the phaco needle, will result in no fluid exiting the eye on the sides of the needle and hence a greater likelihood of wound burn. The most stable incision is naturally one which is a little longer than it is wide, i.e. oversquare. However too long an incision can lead to trapping or oarlocking of the instrument in the tunnel, leading to lack of maneuverability. The tunnel must always be one gauge larger than the phaco tip in the interest of fluid egress from the sides which helps to cool the tip and prevent friction between tip and tunnel. Also the larger tunnel allows a little bit of additional maneuverability (Fig. 1).

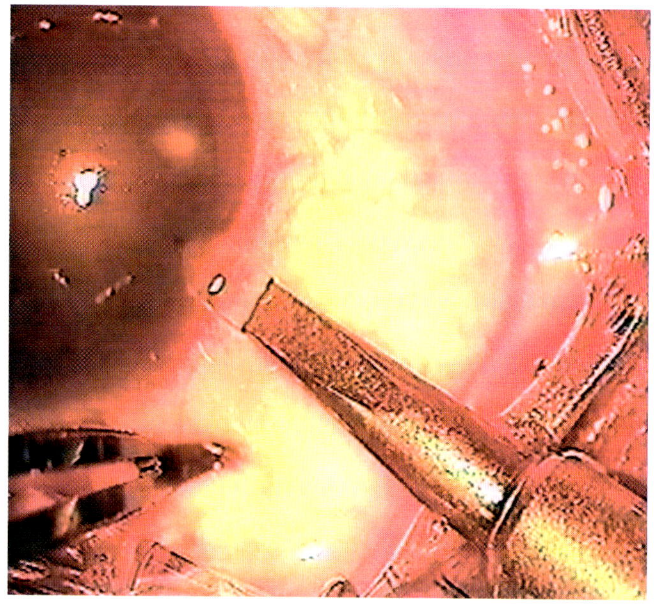

Fig. 1: Meyco 613 model; 1.2 mm diamond microport knife

Openings are best created at 2 o'clock and 10 o'clock so as to put the surgeons, hands at the angle of 90 degrees for efficient chopping maneuvers.

Inject viscoelastic and then introduce the Mehta microrhexis forceps (Indo-German Surgical Corporation, India). This is a reverse action forceps; it means that when surgeon compresses the lever, the forceps blades distract. Authors find this more accurate than a regular press and grasp forceps. A microrhexis forceps is a better alternative to a needle for a few reasons. A needle rhexis relies on the sharp tip of the needle to engage and pull the flap around a single pivot point, i.e. the minute opening created by the needle. Thus surgeon cannot tilt the needle or alter the line of pull as the tip will disengage from the flap. Also with a needle, a certain amount of flex is inherent compounding the problem. In hypermature cataracts, pediatric cataracts, eyes with high vitreous pressure when the rhexis runs out, pulling it in with a needle is difficult and sometimes not possible due to the line of pull and transmission of force required. A forceps however translates to a certain extent in authors' paracentesis opening (forceps is 1 mm wide and opening is 1.4 mm) can tilt and considerably vary its angle of pull. This makes rhexis a quick and reproducible affair. Unlike rhexis performed with a Utrata forceps in regular 2.8 mm phaco, surgeon will need more re-grasp, at least three to five as compared to two to three. However, as a happy consequence of a small opening, surgeons are spared having to refill the chamber with viscoelastic. A single filling usually suffices!

Authors prefer a rhexis 5 mm or larger for the lens salute procedure. Forceps of this kind are the evolution of Kershner's microrhexis forceps (Fig. 2).

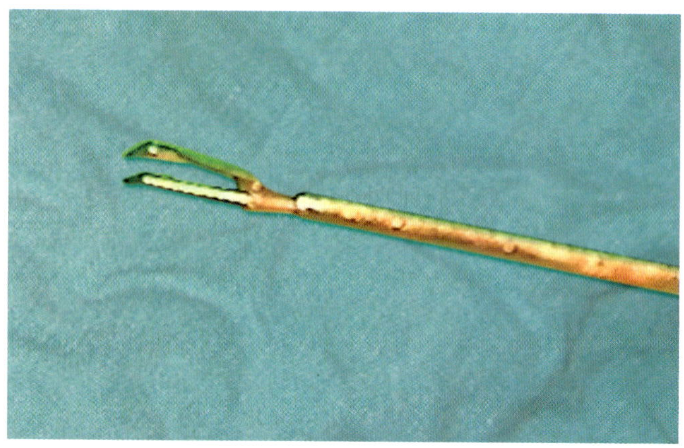

Fig. 2: Mehta microrhexis forceps–tips

Hydrodissection is carefully performed with a 24 gauge needle and BSS at two opposite poles. Before starting hydrodissection especially with high molecular weight (HMW) viscoelastics, remove viscoelastic from the anterior chamber with an aspiration cannula and low vacuum. Inject very small aliquots of fluid as the increased pressure in the anterior chamber can lead to an inadvertent blow out. This is because there is a limited exit pathway for fluid egress as compared to a 2.8 mm tunnel. Make sure surgeon can see the fluid wave move across to the opposite side of the lens. Once the nucleus elevates a little push it back down into the bag to "decompress" the lens. This has the effect of lysing all remaining cortico-capsular adhesions and prevents the creation of loculi of fluid below the lens which might blow out. Next through the right-hand opening slide the cannula all the way to the equator at 12 o'clock and progressively with low pressure inject fluid till the opposite pole of the lens tips up. This is the lens salute maneuver (Keiki R Mehta) which simplifies chopping in unstable anterior chambers (old generation of phaco machines) and hard nuclei while the general trend was still grooving and cracking. This technique depends on space creation below the nucleus for a chopper so that the nucleus is chopped through the densest part between the chopper and the tip. In lens salute and chop, the chopper and phaco tip approximate each other from opposite poles of the lens (Fig. 3).

The advantage of lens salute microphaco is that, unlike in a horizontal quick-chop with a sharp chopper primarily, there is no downward pressure on the posterior capsule at all. This is advantageous especially in cases with a zonular dehiscence, hard nuclei and cases where the rhexis has run away. Phacoemulsification in the iris plane or even a little

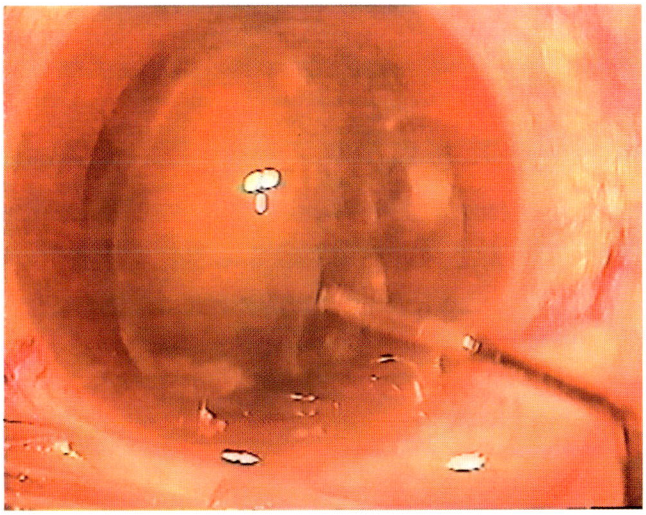

Fig. 3: Tipping up the nucleus in hydrodissection (lens salute position)

in the anterior chamber has its fair share of detractors and rightly so, as minimizing the quantum of ultrasound energy in the eye determines how fast the cornea will recover. Today even with hard cataracts, thanks to Dr Fine´s efforts at popularizing "power modulation", the amount of actual ultrasound time can be reduced to sub second levels. This allows a return to iris plane phaco as a safer quicker alternative to chopping in the bag. Secondly, all phaco in the iris plane is possible without any bevel up maneuvers and as Dr Fishkind has shown, the phaco energy radiates in a cone from the tip bevel. So bevel down means even less effective energy exposure for the endothelium. That´s why lens salute microphaco is a win-win situation. Clearer corneas at day 1 with less risk!

Once the lens has been tipped up, introduce the irrigating chopper, first always to blow up the anterior chamber and only then introduce the phacotip bevel down. Authors usually use 25% OziL power micropulses with burst mode on a 30 degree Kelman tip on the Infiniti system so authors can go between 1 to 2 micropulses per second all the way to continuous. These extremely short pulses allow the needle to cool between pulses.

The key to surge-less bimanual phacoemulsification is enough fluid inflow through the irrigating chopper. The amount of inflow must be greater than the outflow through the needle. One way to achieve this is to raise up the bottle, use a chopper of 18–20 gauge bore. Authors prefer the DUET system which uses a 20 gauge cannula open in the front with different interchangeable tips for adequate inflow. Do surgeons think their current chopper produces enough inflow? Let´s find out; raise up the bottle to the bottle height surgeons usually operate at and position the irrigating chopper at patient eye level. Open the irrigation and collect the inflow in a graduated measuring vessel. Over 1 minute most of surgeons will find a maximum of 25–30 cc of BSS in a minute with the average 21–22 gauge irrigating chopper made by most manufacturers. Surgeons need at least 40 cc/min to achieve a *relatively* surge-less situation during surgery. Inflow with the DUET (Microsurgical Technology, USA) is about 45 cc/min (bottle at 110 cm above eye level) *which increases to beyond 60 cc/min and more with the air pump*. Even with these high volumes, set their flow rate to less than half, it means 25 cc/min or less. This effectively eliminates surge. This DUET irrigating chopper is developed by Larry Laks of Microsurgical Technology and is a natural evolution of the Tsuneoka hook made by ASICO. As the flow is linear from the big single port, it does not have the restrictive turbulent flow of a side chopper with two side ports. The tip authors have used has been modified from the original

Nagahara (Cyres K Mehta) into a shorter tip with a ball at the end. In lens salute microphaco as authors are sometimes very close to the posterior capsule they prefer a rounded shorter tip to avoid mishaps (Fig. 4).

Using the Cruise Control (STAAR Surgical Company, USA) is another way out. It consists of a pencil length device connected to the aspiration line after the phaco handpiece, and basically acts as a flow restrictor while trapping nuclear debris in a plastic mesh. The flow restrictor is a simple constriction in the outflow pathway that by the laws of physics slows down outflow at occlusion break when the speed of outflow doubles and triples causing surge. Earlier, outflow restrictors had been tried but failed due to clogging by nuclear debris which is collected in this device by a side pathway thus leaving fluid passage though the narrow channel proceed unhindered.

In regular coaxial phaco the fluid currents move outwards from the needle and thus lead to particles being pushed away from the tip. In order to overcome this authors increase the vacuum levels even as high as 550 mm Hg in modern machines. However in bimanual phaco 350 mm Hg is more than adequate as having only one outflow and one inflow sets up a current that pushes the pieces towards the tip. The blast of fluid inflow can be used as a surgical tool as well to open up the bag, to push pieces around or to reposition nuclear material at the phaco tip. Remember to enter the eye with the irrigating chopper and to exit the eye with the irrigating chopper after surgeons have withdrawn the tip. First in last out, is a good rule to follow.

Open ended irrigating choppers are the way to go. Initially side opening choppers were popular but they have two disadvantages:

1. They do not let enough flow into the eye
2. Also during maneuvers if the irrigation ports accidentally exit the eye being situated as they are 2–3 mm away from the tip, the chamber will suddenly collapse.

Irrigation/Aspiration is performed with the DUET system with sand-blasted tips (Fig. 5A). The aspiration port is 0.3 mm. These tips fit in very snugly through the paracentesis openings as no leakage equals minimal surge when coupled with adequate inflow.

Lens injection is performed depending on which thin lens authors choose. Authors prefer the Acritec thin lens and have used the Thinoptx lens in the past as well (Figs 5B and C).

Such plate-haptic lenses have a well-documented propensity to supplant themselves against the posterior capsule. Will the ability of these thin lenses (basically plate-haptic lenses) to supplant themselves to the posterior capsule prevent migration of lens epithelial cells onto the posterior capsule? There is a question to study. The polymer they are made of causes a fibronectin pseudocapsule to form on the lens sticking it to the posterior capsule. Will this further diminish the chance of posterior capsular opacification? Only time will tell!

Another advantage of an acrylic polymer is that the fibronectin pseudocapsule isolates the lens from the ocular environment thus proving useful for uveitis patients. Acrylic lens for microphaco are gaining popularity worldwide (Figs 6A and B)

According to Arturo Pérez Arteaga from Mexico who uses Alcon´s Accurus system, the "vented gas infusion tubing" of the Accurus surgical system helps stabilize the anterior chamber during microincision cataract surgery.

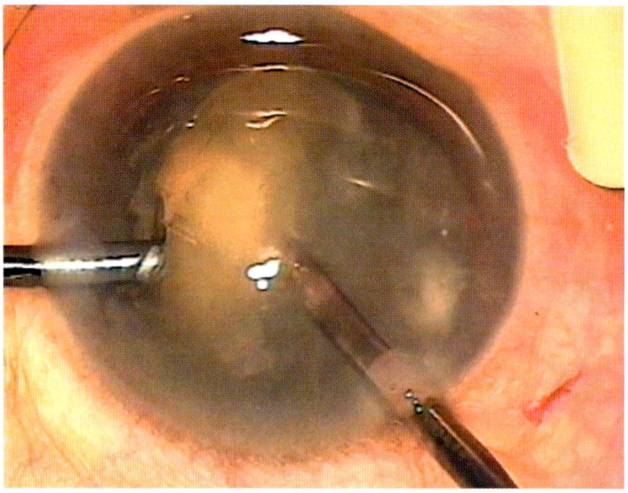

Fig. 4: Lens salute microphaco with the DUET

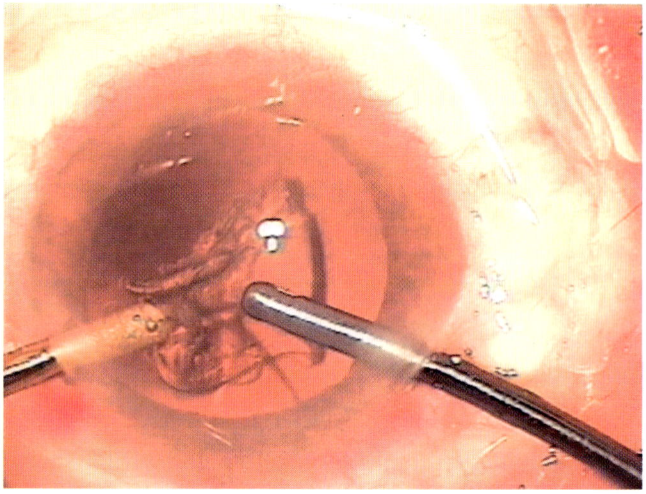

Fig. 5A: Irrigation aspiration with the DUET biaxial system

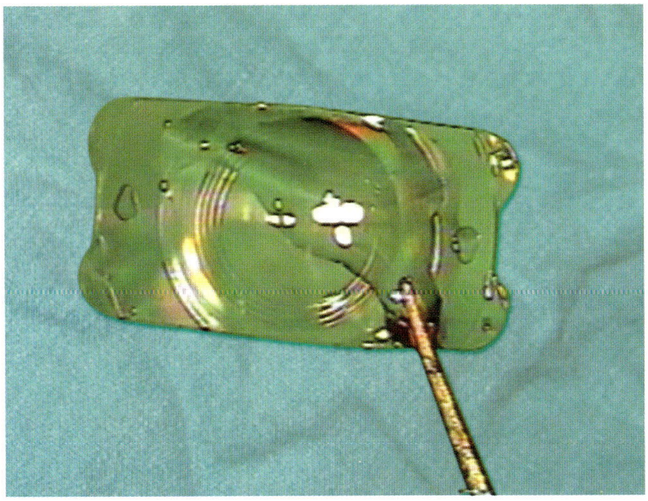

Fig. 5B: Thinoptx lens (notice rainbow colors)

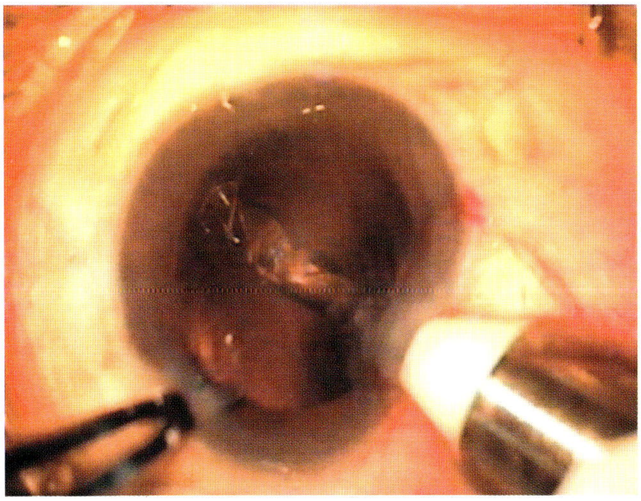

Fig. 5C: Thinoptx lens insertion

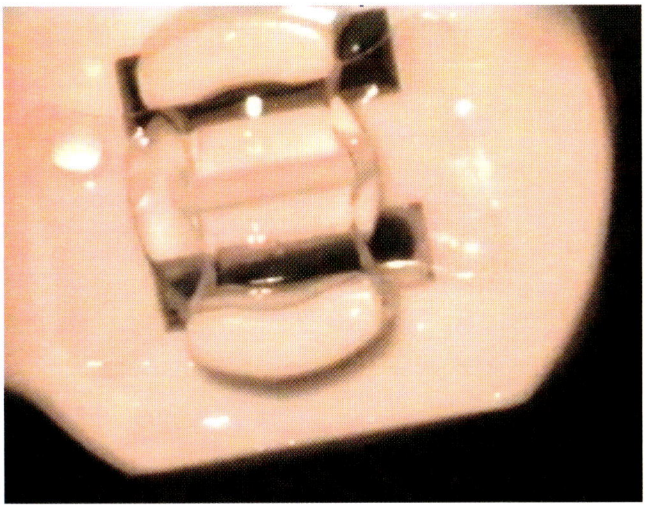

Fig. 6A: AcrysMart lens

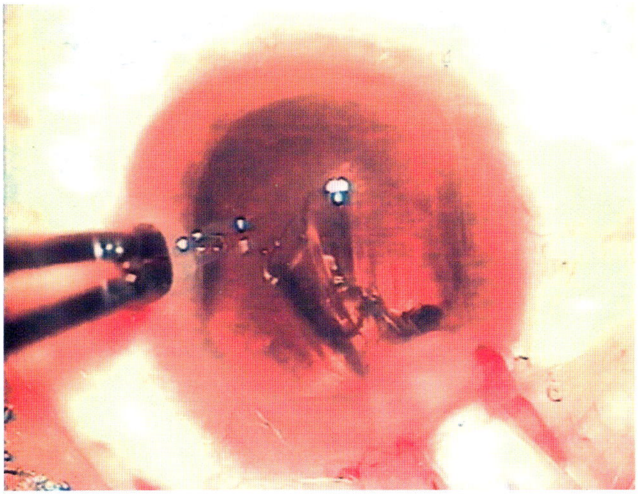

Fig. 6B: AcrySmart lens being injected

Authors use the ABS tip, and currently Kelman´s tip to perform microphaco safely with moderately high vacuum (200 mm Hg at venturi). Authors feel that this machine is the way forward because the Internal Forced Infusion and the venturi system.

"It is not the strongest of the species that survives, nor the most intelligent, but the one most responsive to change."

—Charles Darwin

References

1. Shearing SP, Relyea RL, Loaiza A, et al. Routine phacoemulsification through a one-millimeter non-sutured incision. Cataract. 1985;2(2):6-11.
2. Soscia W, Howard JG, Olson RJ. Microphacoemulsification with WhiteStar: a wound temperature study. J Cataract Refract Surg. 2002;28:1044-6.
3. Soscia W, Howard JG, Olson RJ. Bimanual Phacoemulsification through 2 stab incisions: a wound temperature study. J Cataract Refract Surg. 2002;28:1039-43.
4. Donnenfeld ED, Olson RJ, Solomon R, et al. Efficacy and wound temperature gradient of WhiteStar phacoemulsification through a 1.2 m incision. J Cataract Refract Surg. 2003;29:1097-100.
5. Tsuneoka H, Shiba T, Takahashi Y. Feasibility of ultrasound cataract surgery with a 1.4 mm incision. J Cataract Refract Surg. 2001;27:934-40.
6. Tsuneoka H, Shiba T, Takahashi Y. Ultrasound phacoemulsification using a 1.4 mm incision; clinical results. J Cataract Refract Surg. 2002;28:81-6.

7. Agarwal A, Agarwal S, Agarwal A. Phakonit and laser phakonit: Lens removal through a 0.9 mm incision. In: Agarwal A, Agarwal S, Sachdev MS, et al, (Eds). Phacoemulsification, Laser Cataract Surgery and Foldable IOLs. New Delhi: Jaypee Brothers Medical (P) Ltd.; 1999. pp. 204-16.
8. Fine IH, Packer M, Hoffman RS. New phacoemulsification technologies. J Cataract Refract Surg. 2002;28:1054-60.
9. Fine IH. The choo-choo chop and flip phacoemulsification technique. Oper Tech Cataract Refract Surg. 1998;1:61-5.
10. Fine IH, Hoffman RS, Packer M. The Staar Wave. Dev Ophthalmol. 2002;34:32-40.
11. Nishi O, Nishi K. Accommodation amplitude after lens refilling with injectable silicone by sealing the capsule with a plug in primates. Arch Ophthalmol. 1998;116:1358-61.
12. Agarwal A, Agarwal S, Agarwal A. Phakonit and laser phakonit: Lens removal through a 0.9 mm incision. In: Agarwal A, Agarwal S, Sachdev MS, et al. (Eds). Phacoemulsification, Laser Cataract Surgery and Foldable IOLs. New Delhi: Jaypee Brothers Medical Publishers (P) Ltd.; 1999. pp. 204-16.
13. Mehta C, Mehta K. Lens Salute Microphaco-A Tilt Above. J Intraocular Implant Refract Soc. 2004;1(2);5-10.

17 Micro-Biaxial Prechop Technique

Arturo Pérez-Arteaga (Mexico)

Introduction

During the reading of the book, you have seen many ways to perform cataract surgery using microbiaxial techniques with different nomenclature also.[1,6,10,11] At the prechopping field you have also read many ways to perform, either for coaxial or for biaxial techniques.[1-3] Most of the prechopping maneuvers need a particular instrumentation, a chopper (irrigating or not) and/or particular forceps; a lot of talent and money have been spent by doctors and industries in the creation and developing of choppers. In author's particular surgical practice, he has not been using any choppers for more than 8 years.[4] Author likes a lot to prechop with the same viscoelastic cannulas or with the irrigating cannula and the phaco tip; so, he has avoided the use of prechopping forceps, irrigating choppers or non-irrigating choppers. Author has to say that this was made possible because of the "Lens Salute" technique, described years ago by Keiki Mehta and very well explained in this textbook by his son, Cyres Mehta, in the chapter "Lens Salute Microphaco". These techniques to avoid choppers for cataract surgery (coaxial or biaxial) are the ones that author likes to share with you in this chapter.[5-8]

The objective of this chapter is to teach the technique regarding the performance of mechanical fragmentation of the cataract with two 25 G cannulas previous to start phacoemulsification, avoiding the use of prechop forceps, non-irrigating or irrigating choppers. This technique helps to decrease the possible damage to the capsular bag and the ciliary zonule, because it is performed at the iris plane.[4]

Instrumentation

It uses only the knives, the micro-capsulorhexis forceps, an irrigating cannula, a phaco tip, an aspirating cannula and two 25 G viscoelastic cannulas with their syringes for the entire lens extraction procedure.

The use of biaxial techniques is preferable, nevertheless is not mandatory; in all the cases that the surgeon has two incisions, exists the possibility to introduce two viscoelastic cannulas, making so the technique possible by complete; maybe the only one condition is that both incisions be separated by at least 120 degrees allowing this way the adequate transmission of forces. Maybe preferable to perform the technique under a biaxial approach because the incisions are smaller (700 micron in cases of micro-biaxial or microphakonit techniques)[9] and the advantage of a closed environment in the anterior chamber, avoiding the leakage, situation that improves the mechanical forces for nuclear fracture of the nucleus, and helps to protect the capsular bag and the endothelial cells. Nevertheless this technique is described here for biaxial and coaxial surgeons.

Surgical Technique

The main goal of this technique is to perform a mechanical fragmentation of the cataract outside the capsular bag, utilizing only the viscoelastic cannulas, avoiding the transmission of the mechanical forces to the capsular bag and zonule, but also far away from the endothelial cells of the cornea. It is a mechanical fracture of the nucleus at the iris plane in a bimanual fashion (Fig. 1).

The steps to perform this surgical technique are as follows:

1. A wide capsulorhexis is performed in order to facilitate the luxation of the nucleus outside the capsular bag (Fig. 2).
2. Vigorous hydrosurgery to facilitate the movement of the nucleus inside the capsular bag (Figs 3 and 4).
3. After the hydrodissection a rotation of the nucleus is performed developing a "hemi-luxation" of the nucleus, taking outside the capsular bag only one pole of the lens. This technique was described as "the lens salute technique" by Dr. Keiki Mehta from Mumbai

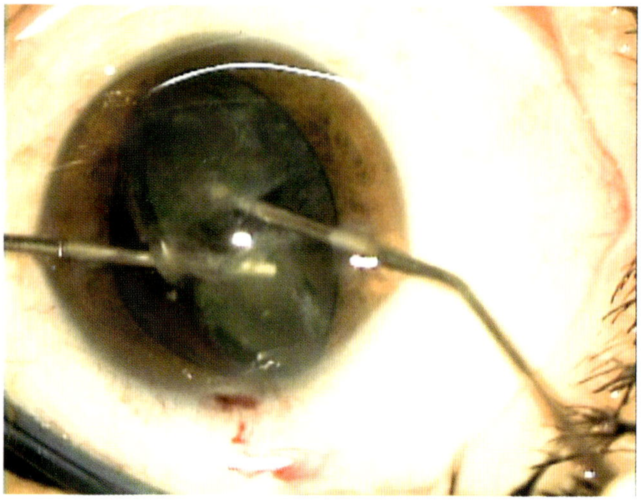

Fig. 1: Nucleus being fragmented at the iris plane with two 25 gauge cannulas

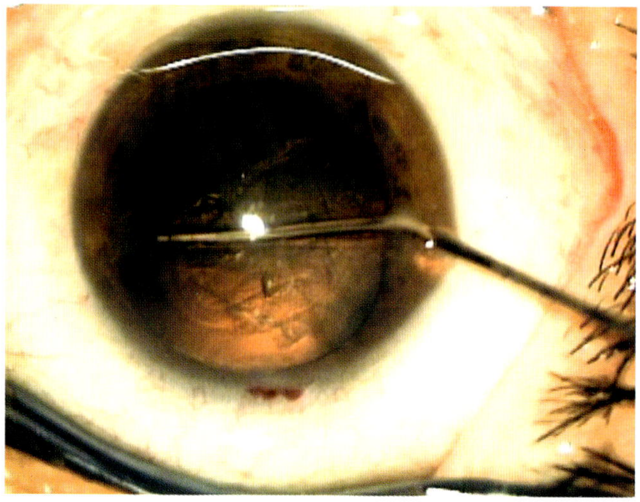

Fig. 2: Wide capsulorhexis

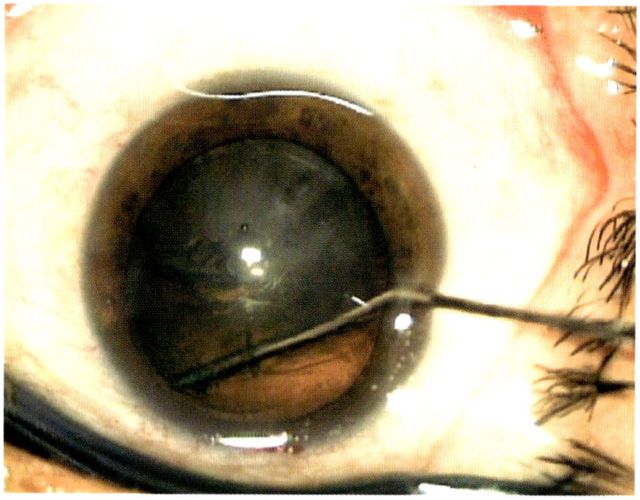

Fig. 3: Hydrodissection

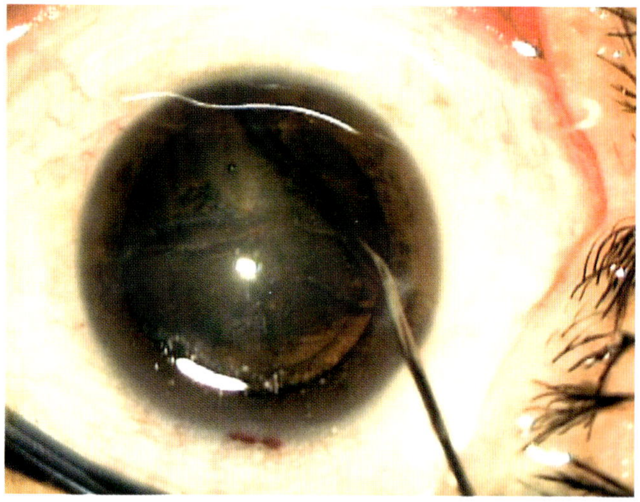

Fig. 4: Hydrodelamination

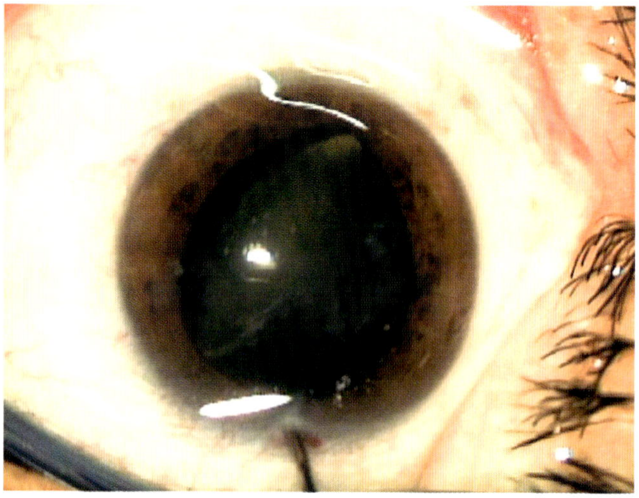

Fig. 5: Nucleus being placed in lens salute position

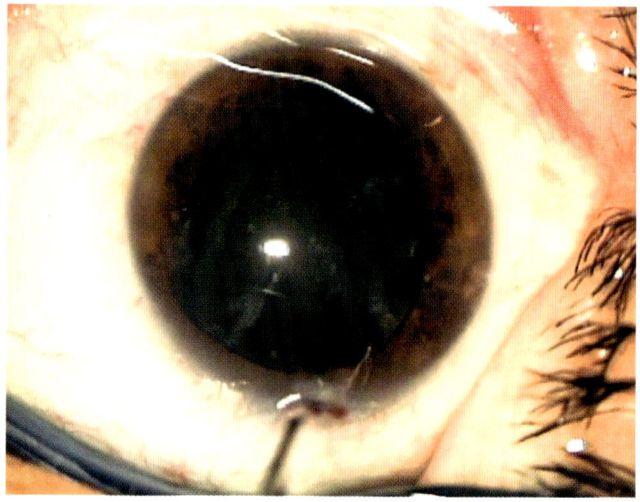

Fig. 6: Nucleus in lens salute position

India. The maneuver includes hydro-pressure, rotation and gentle mechanical pressure (Figs 5 and 6).

4. Once the nucleus is in lens salute position, the surgeon introduces the viscoelastic irrigating cannula through the non-dominant hand corneal incision and places viscoelastic between the rear part of the nucleus and the capsular bag, just to protect it from some eventual damage (Fig. 7).
5. Then, the surgeon introduces another viscoelastic cannula through the corneal incision for the dominant hand. It is helpful for the vector forces, if this incision is placed somewhere between 120 degree and 180 degree away from the non-dominant hand incision (at the opposite meridian). The surgeon introduces viscoelastic material between the nucleus and the corneal endothelium, with the objective to protect intraocular structures and finally place this cannula at the front of the lens in the central portion (Fig. 8).
6. Once the surgeon reaches this position, the work is to capture the nucleus between both instruments; our instruments are two viscoelastic (25 G) cannulas (Fig. 9).
7. The cannulas are introduced through the incisions with both hands. Beware to maintain the cannulas at

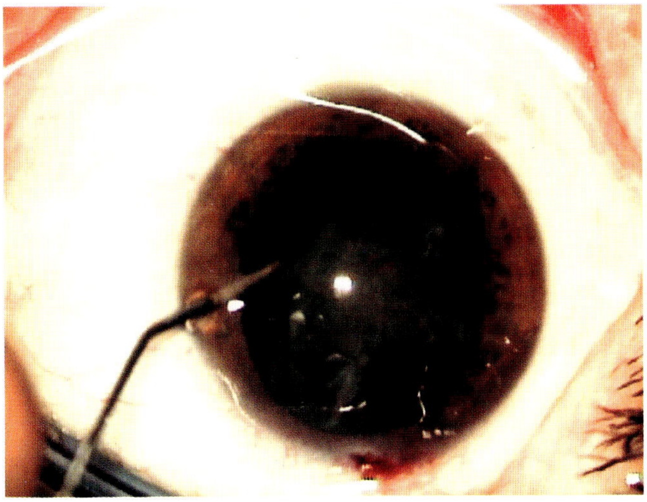

Fig. 7: Viscoelastic between the nucleus and the posterior capsule

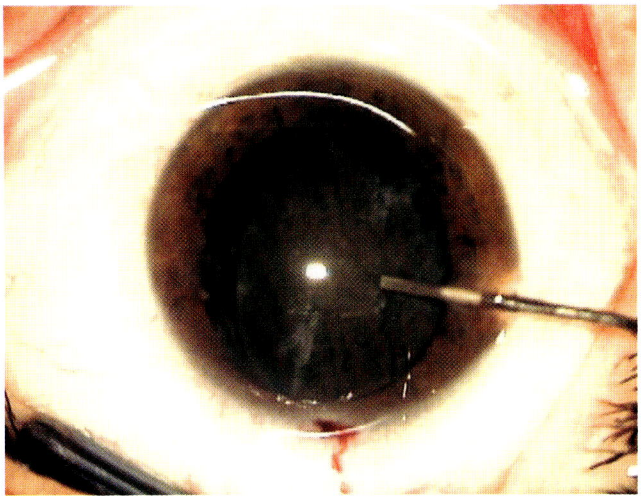

Fig. 8: Viscoelastic between the nucleus and the endothelial cells

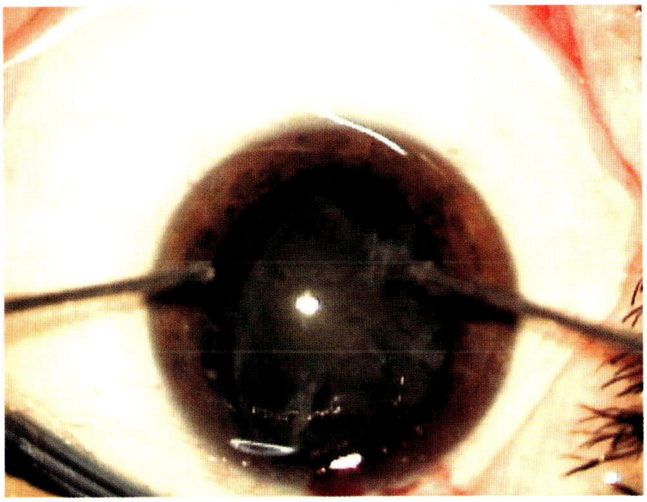

Fig. 9: Two 25 gauge cannulas and the nucleus at lens salute position

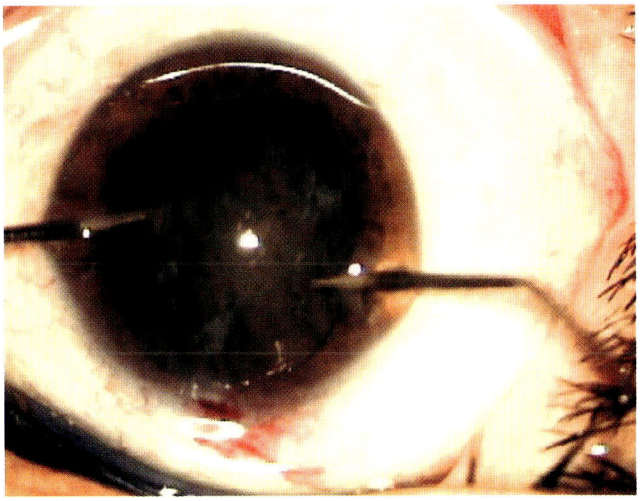

Fig. 10: Cannulas inside the eye

the iris plane, enough far away from the cornea and from the capsular bag (Fig. 10).

8. Then, with the anterior chamber wide open (full of viscoelastic) and with minimum leakage, in particular with microincisional techniques, the surgeon applies both cannulas at the nucleus margins holding this structure with both instruments (Fig. 11).
9. Then the surgeon applies gentle pressure between the two instruments with the nucleus in the middle trying to touch both instruments (Fig. 12).
10. Then a separation in the axis of the cannulas is enough force to separate the nuclear fragments (Fig. 13). This maneuver produces the first "crack" and then the nucleus is divided in two halves with a prechop technique, outside the capsular bag with the force of only two 25 G cannulas (Figs 1 and 14).
11. When possible, more nuclear fragmentations can be made in the same fashion; the surgeon is able to obtain 3, 4 or more nuclear pieces according to the applied forces and the advance of the learning curve. As in all the prechop techniques, as much as more pieces are obtained, less ultrasonic time and power will be needed (Figs 15A to E).
12. Once the prechop maneuvers are finished, multiple pieces are obtained (Fig. 16).
13. Then, the surgeon starts the phacoemulsification process, utilizing intermittent modulation modalities of ultrasonic power, and no more choppers are

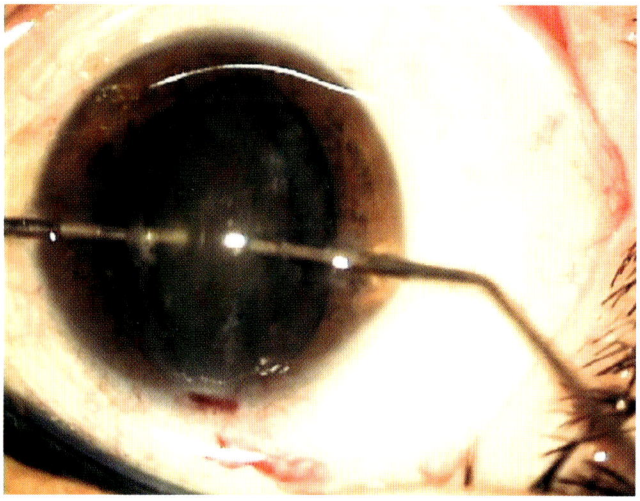

Fig. 11: Nucleus trapped between both cannulas. Notice the same axis between them

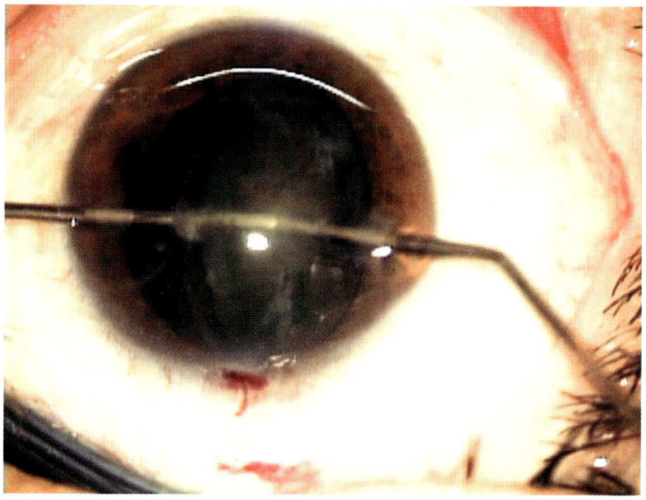

Fig. 12: Both cannulas are in contact

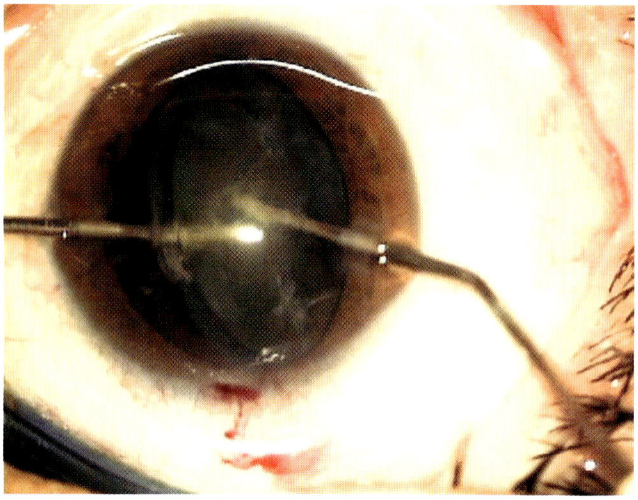

Fig. 13: Change in the axis of the cannulas

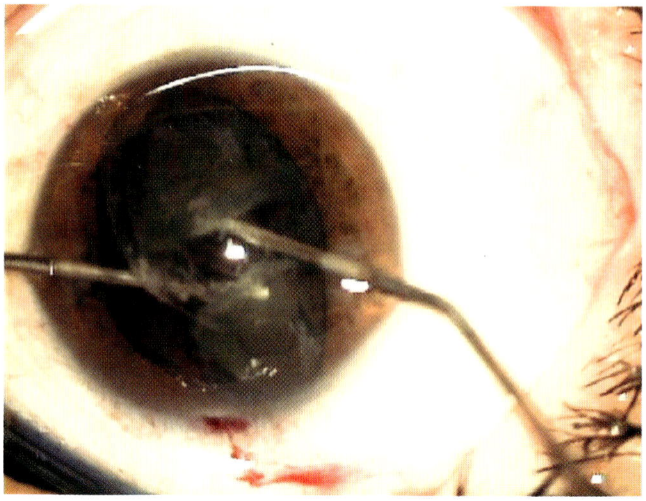

Fig. 14: Nucleus divided in two halves

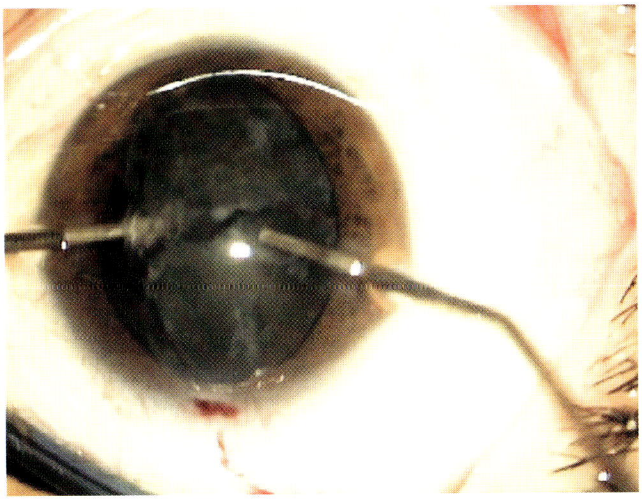

Fig. 15A: Cannulas placed at both sides of the nucleus

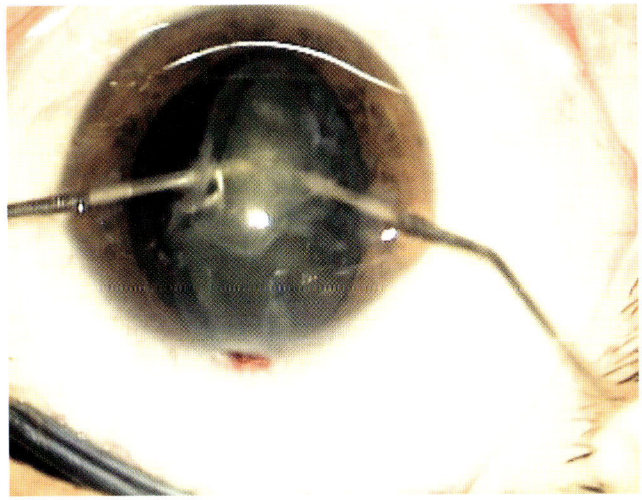

Fig. 15B: Creation of pressure between both cannulas

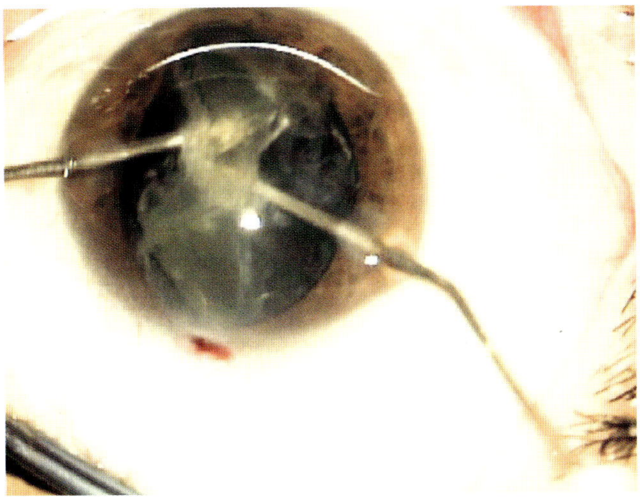

Fig. 15C: Separation of both cannulas creating a nuclear fragmentation

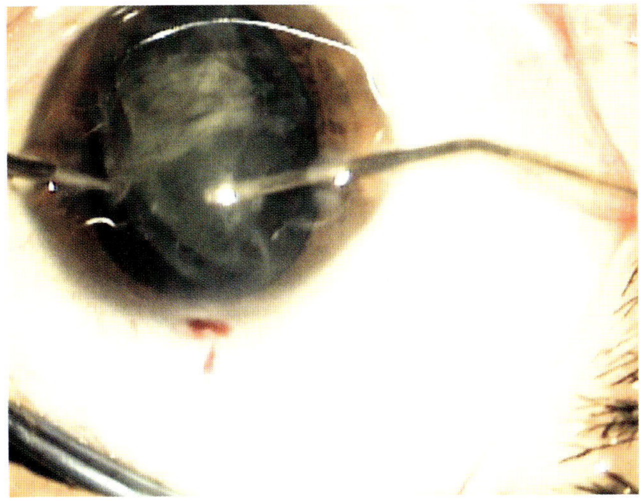

Fig. 15D: Nucleus divided in two pieces

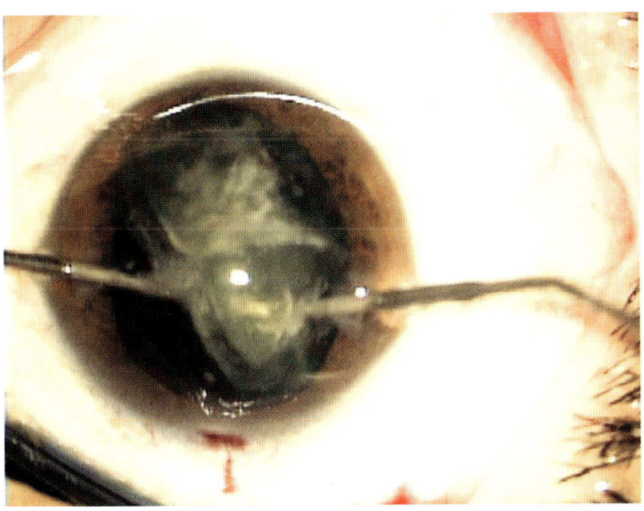

Fig. 15E: Multiple nuclear fragmentation

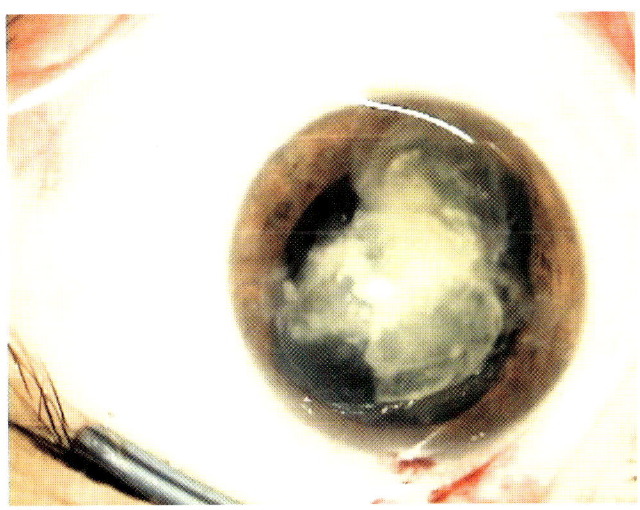

Fig. 16: Multiple nuclear pieces

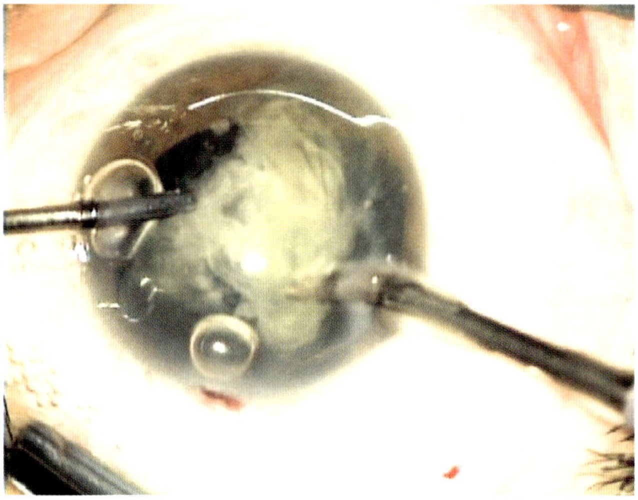

Fig. 17A: Starting phaco unburst or pulse mode

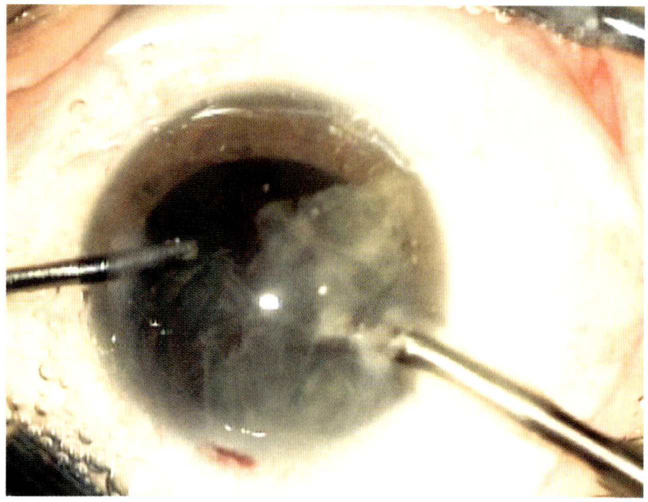

Fig. 17B: Notice that the phaco tip is not moving the fragmented pieces move to it by followability

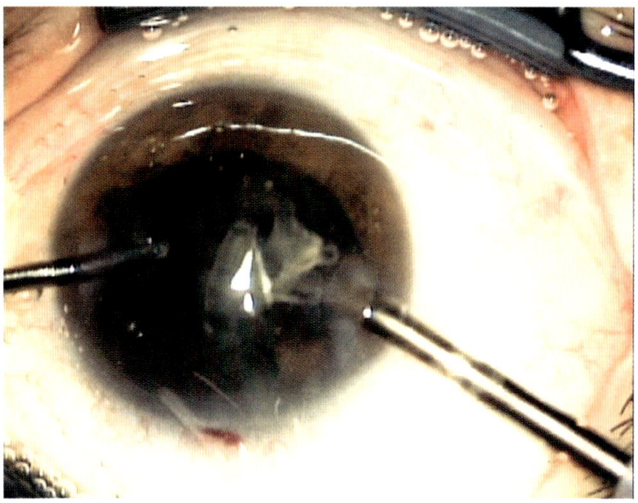

Fig. 17C: The epinucleus goes to the phaco tip by followability

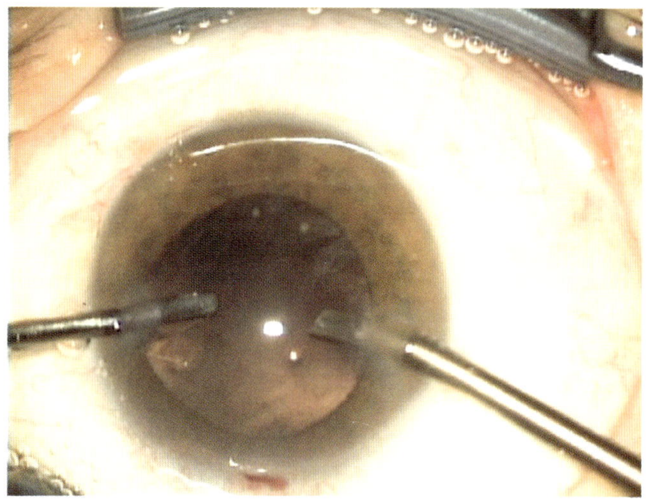

Fig. 17D: End of phaco notice the clear bag and the clean cornea

needed, just a second instrument (preferable an irrigating cannula) to serve for irrigation and as a help for the phacoemulsification (Figs 17A to D). Current phacoemulsification techniques are phacofragmentation techniques, followed by phacoaspiration assisted by ultrasound managed with intermittent power modulations.

14. At the end of the procedure, remember the advantage of the biaxial approach. While changing from phaco mode to I/A mode, and when finishing I/A and changing from I/A to fill the anterior chamber with viscoelastic, maintain always the nondominant hand with the irrigation on, and perform the changes only with the dominant hand. It will allow you to maintain a positive intraocular pressure during the changes of instrumentation, avoiding surge or flat anterior chamber. This is a realistic advantage of the biaxial approach impossible to be done under the coaxial approach (Fig. 18).

Variations to the Technique

In cases where the surgeon feels that the management of cannulas for prechopping can be difficult, the prechopping can be done with the irrigating cannula and the phaco tip (Figs 19A to D). The lens salute technique is again the basis for the well performance of the prechop. The surgeon places the nucleus at lens salute position; then introduces the irrigating cannula with the nondominant hand and the phaco needle with the dominant hand. With a small amount of vacuum and phaco power the phaco needle is embedded into the nucleus supporting it from the rear with

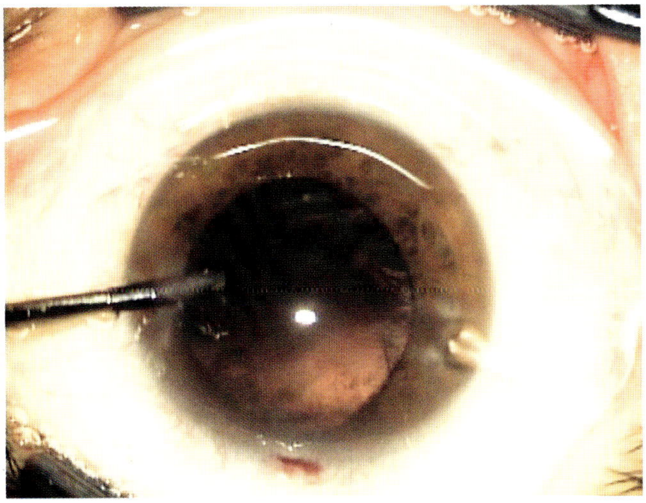

Fig. 18: Irrigating cannula maintained inside the eye to avoid negative intraocular lens

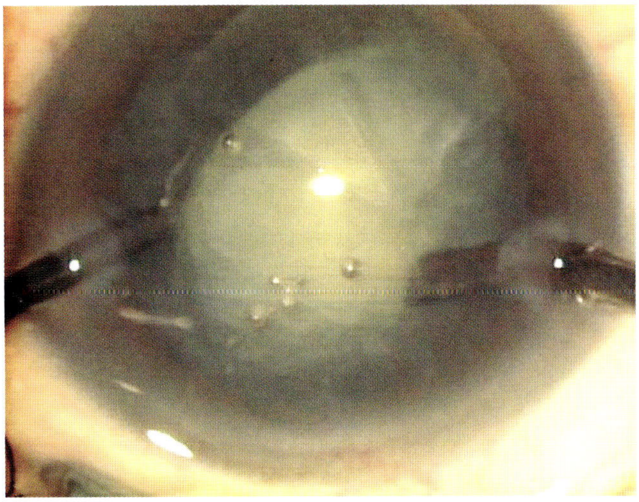

Fig. 19A: Phaco tip and irrigating cannula presented at both sides of the nucleus

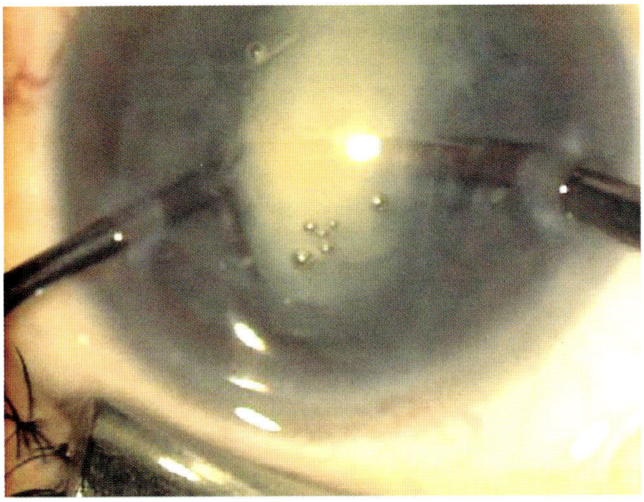

Fig. 19B: The nucleus is being captured between both instruments, with vacuum on

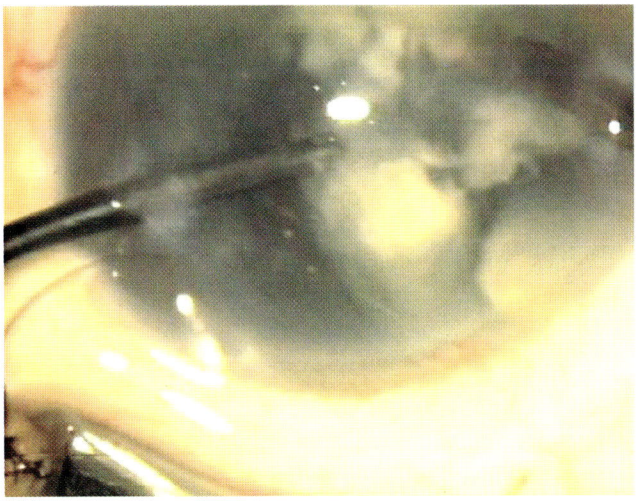

Fig. 19C: Nucleus has been fragmented in multiple pieces

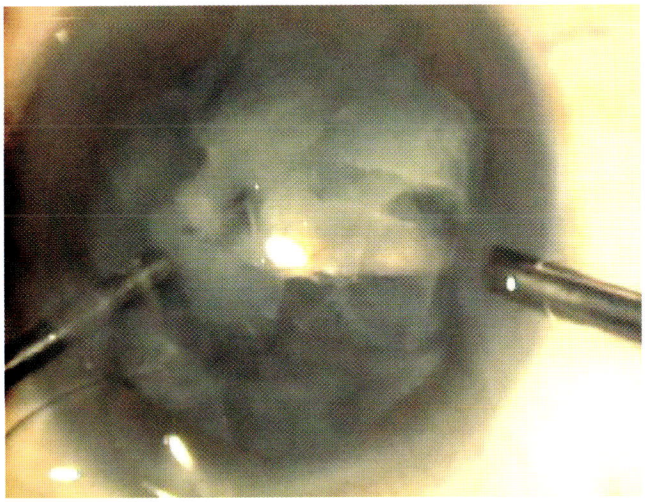

Fig. 19D: Starting to phaco multiple nuclear pieces

the irrigating cannula, avoiding this way the entrance again of the nucleus to the capsular bag with the pressure of the phaco needle. Deleting the phaco power but keeping the vacuum on, the nucleus is firmly held with the vacuum of the phaco handpiece, and in this moment the same movement of compression (described with the cannulas above) is performed, between the irrigating cannula and the phaco needle. The nucleus will fragment in two pieces easily with the irrigating cannula, avoiding this way the use of irrigating choppers. The key is to hold the nucleus with vacuum to avoid any undesired displacement. Once one fracture is done more fractures can be performed while performing phaco of the resulting pieces at the same time.

Another variation this technique is the "pull the nucleus technique", described in this textbook in the chapter of "Management of incomplete capsulorhexis". It also allows the performance of prechop with only use of an irrigating cannula and the phaco tip.

Conclusion

Author strongly believes that this technique is the latest and master evolution of the bimanual surgery. It combines the Bimanual Irrigation/Aspiration concepts, the art of the Phakonit, the latest evolution of microphakonit and the "state of the art" of the prechop concepts without any prechopper device, without irrigating chopper and with out stress over the zonule and posterior capsule. Future will tell...

The main advantages of this technique that author find are:

1. It keeps the anterior chamber wide open during the entire procedure (Fig. 18).
2. There is no stress over the zonule.
3. There is no need of a sharp instrument inside the eye.
4. There is no need to switch many instruments during the entire surgery; when the nuclear fragmentation has been done with the cannulas, there is only a switch to the phaco tip and the aspiration cannula.
5. There is less incision edema because there is not "inside and out" of many instruments.
6. Less time consuming; situation that can lead benefit for the patient.
7. There is less cost in the use of the viscoelastic cannulas for prechop in comparison to expensive prechopers (irrigating and no irrigating) or forceps.

References

1. Jorge Alió, José Luis Rodríguez-Prats, Ahmed Galal, et al. Outcomes of microincision cataract surgery versus coaxial phacoemulsification. Ophthalmology. 2005;112(11):1997-2003.
2. Roberto Pinelli, P Fazio. Dynamics of capsulorhexis. In: Ashok Garg (Ed). Mastering the Phacodynamics (Tools, Technology and Innovations).New Delhi: Jaypee Brothers Medical Publishers (P) Ltd.; 2007.
3. Sabine Kurz, Frank Krummenauer, Pia Gabriel, et al. Biaxial microincision versus coaxial small-incision clear cornea cataract surgery. Ophthalmology. 2006; 113(10):1818-26.
4. Arturo Pèrez-Arteaga. Biaxial pre-chop without choppers. In: Ashok Garg (Ed). Pre-chop Techniques. New Delhi: Jaypee Brothers Medical Publishers (P) Ltd.; 2008.
5. Kawai K, Suzuki T, Hayakawa K Tokai. The 23 gauge capsulorhexis forceps having a cystotome function. J Exp Clin Med. 2005;30(1):11-3.
6. Packer M, Hoffmann R, Fine H. Refractive lens surgery. Ophthalmol Clin North Am. 2006;19(1):77-88.
7. Arturo Pèrez-Arteaga. Prechop without pre-choppers and choppers conference by chop techniques symposium. World Ophthalmology Congress, Hong Kong, China, 2008.
8. Arturo Perez-Arteaga. Step by Step to Biaxial Lens Surgery. New Delhi: Jaypee Brothers Medical Publishers (P) Ltd.; 2008.
9. Agarwal A, Agarwal S, Agarwal A. Phakonit: lens removal through a 0.9 mm incision. (letter). J Cataract Refract Surg. 2001;27:1531-2.
10. Tsuneoka H, Takuya S, Takahashi Y. Feasibility of ultrasound cataract surgery with a 1.4 mm incision. J Cataract Refract Surg. 2001;27:934-40.
11. Aravind Haripriya, Srinivasan Aravind, Kavitha Vadi, et al. Bimanual microphaco for posterior polar cataracts. J Cataract Refract Surg. 2006;32(6):914-7.

18

Hypermature Cataract: Is It Impossible Management with Biaxial?

Luis Felipe Vejarano-Restrepo (Colombia)

Introduction

Any kind of cataract must be a challenge to every cataract surgeon, because there is no one exactly the same to another, even more the very hard and intumescent cataract, those always represent a real challenge in coaxial phaco even more in biaxial or through microincision.

In this chapter, author will try to explain the way how to deal with this very hard cataracts since the incision until the phacoemulsification passing through the rhexis, and the big differences between its management in intumescent and in the very hard with absorbed cortex also the hydrodissection, and not only that, also the big advantages in fluidics that gives the biaxial and micro-biaxial techniques over coaxial technique.

These kinds of cataracts are in the cataract classification as hypermatures but they are very different between both the management of each one since the capsulorhexis and the emulsification, surgeons have to deal in a different way.

As a review, author classified the cataracts related with maturity under the following heading.

Types of Cataracts

The following is a classification of the various types of cataracts:

Age-Related Cataract

1. **Immature senile cataract (IMSC):** Partially opaque lens, disc view hazy.
2. **Mature senile cataract (MSC):** Completely opaque lens, no disc view.
3. **Hypermature senile cataract (HMSC):** Liquefied cortical matter: Morgagnian cataract.

According to Maturity

1. **Immature:** Scattered opacities are separated by clear zones.
2. **Mature:** Cortex and nucleus become totally opaque.
3. **Intumescent:** The lens becomes swollen by absorbing water.
4. **Hypermature cataract:** Mature cataract, which has become smaller and has a wrinkled capsule as a result of leakage of H_2O out of lens.
5. **Morgagnian cataract:** Hypermature cataract in which total liquefaction of cortex allows the nucleus to sink inferiorly.

Classified by Location of Opacity within Lens Structure

Anterior Cataract

1. Anterior cortical cataract
2. Anterior polar cataract
3. Anterior subcapsular cataract

Nuclear Cataract

Grading correlates with hardness and difficulty of surgical removal

1. Grey
2. Yellow
3. Amber
4. Brown/Black

Posterior Cataract

1. Posterior cortical cataract
2. Posterior polar cataract (importance lies in higher risk of complication—posterior capsular tears during surgery)
3. Posterior subcapsular cataract (PSC)

Management through Biaxial Technique

The biaxial (less than 1.5 mm) or micro-biaxial (less than 1 mm) technique that separates the two functions in the phacoemulsification technique (irrigation/manipulation from the aspiration/emulsification) not only has the big advantage of the incision size in this kind of challenge cataract but also has more than one advantage beginning with the capsulorhexis avoiding the evacuation of the ophthalmic viscoelastic device (OVD), diminishing the risk of the anterior capsular tear, better and safer manipulation of the capsule and also provide an easy hydrodissection because the use of less liquid in the bag to get a free nucleus; also depending on the fluidics, the stability of the anterior chamber during the emulsification is perfect, guaranteeing less risk of posterior capsule rupture, endothelial cells and uveal trauma giving to the patient a better postoperative period and faster recovery of his visual acuity.

Incision

In regard with the side port incision, it must be as watertight as possible when the instrument (irrigating chopper) is in position, but without compromising its maneuverability, and this is a very important issue, since in biaxial this is the instrument that makes most of the movements necessary to emulsify the nucleus. For this reason, author uses a trapezoidal shape side port incision, which internally maintains very good watertightness and externally has more room for a wider arch of movement of the instrument, if surgeons feel the instrument gets stuck at the incision, it is a good idea to apply a small amount of viscoelastic on the chopper to make its movement easier.

Author has found that performing a trapezoidal 0.9/1.3 mm (inner/outer size) incision, let him to use the Vejarano's Irrigating Chopper® (AC7340; Accutome, Malvern, USA) (Fig. 1), which for biaxial has 20 gauge (approximately 0.9 mm diameter), with almost no leakage and very good maneuverability. To achieve a good architecture, author uses a 0.9/1.3 mm diamond knife (Accutome, Malvern, USA) (Fig. 2) to perform this incision, but an alternative is to use 20 gauge vitreoretinal blades (Fig. 3) or 1.2/1.4 mm steel blades (MicroSurgical Technology, Redmond, USA) (Fig. 4). When performing the main incision, author uses 1.2 mm diamond lancet or the same 0.9/1.3 mm diamond knife to avoid additional expenses (both Accutome, Malvern, USA), using a 20 gauge phaco microtip, author thinks that it is not indispensable that the main incision has a trapezoidal shape because in biaxial the phaco needle does not move considerably, just back and forth, to look for the pieces and back to the center to emulsify them, even more could bring near to the internal lip of the incision to unoccluded the tip facilitating the emulsification and avoiding the excessive movements of the second instrument preventing additional damage or deformation of the side port incision.

The incision width is not determined arbitrarily but is contingent upon the needle diameter. A common misconception is that a 0.9 diameter instrument will fit in a 0.9 mm incision. This will cause excessive stretching of the incision, and may tear it, compromising its watertightness and due to the too tight contact between the tissue and the phaco tip, will increase the risk of thermal damage because the fluid going out helps to cool the needle's shaft. On the other hand, a too big incision will increase the leakage and will compromise the anterior chamber stability. According to the gauges of the irrigating instrument and the phaco

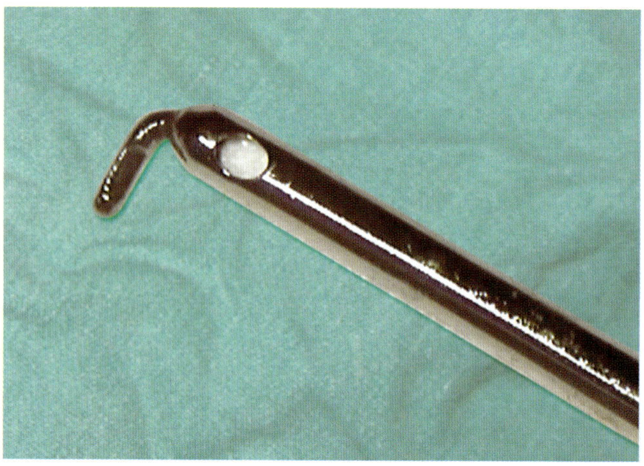

Fig. 1: Vejarano's Irrigating Chopper 20 gauge with oval lateral holes

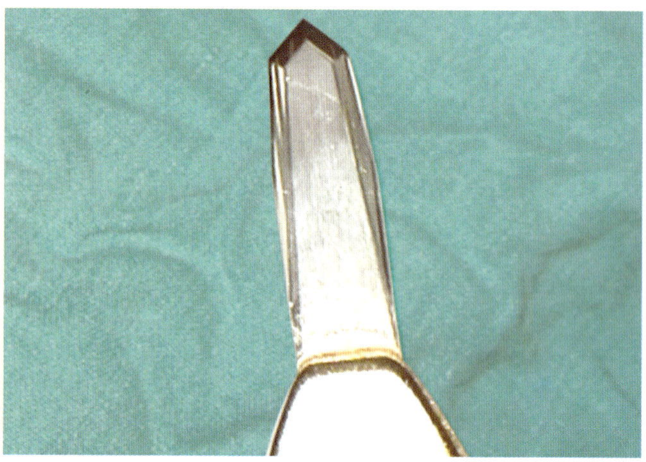

Fig. 2: Diamond blade for side port incision

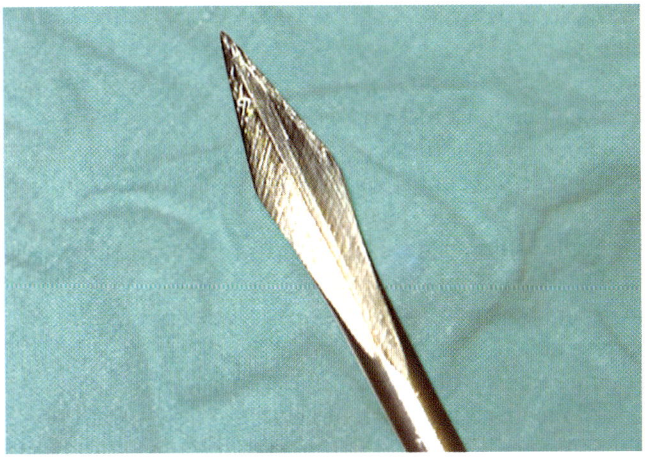

Fig. 3: MVR blade 20 gauge

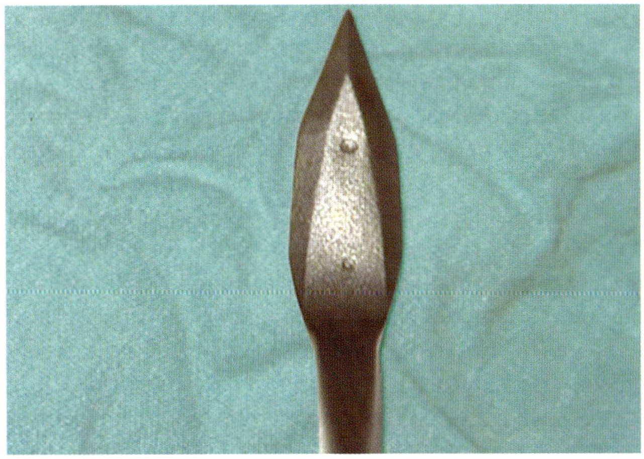

Fig. 4: Trapezoidal metal blade

needle that surgeons use, they can determine the proper size of their incisions. Surgeons calculate the circumference length of the instrument using the formula [2 ($\pi \times r$)], where "r" means radius of the instrument in mm. Then, since each lip of the incision covers a half, not the whole length of the instrument's circumference is needed (and the incision length corresponds to one incision's lip length), so surgeons have to divide the result by two (in order to find out how long is half of the circumference of the instrument and therefore the incision length). Moreover, the cornea has elastic properties and so surgeons have to take in account the tissue compliance that empirically, according with the true incision length measured in author's procedures, author has calculated in 20%. Thus, the final formula to decide upon the right length of the incision is:

[2 (π r) /2] – 20%. This may be simplified as: $\pi \times r \times 0.8$.

For instance, for a 0.9 mm tip (approximately 20 gauge) the incision length should be:

$\pi \times r \times 0.8 = \pi \times 0.45$ mm $\times 0.8 \approx 1.1$ mm.

For a 1.1 mm tip (approximately 19 gauge), the incision length should be:

$\pi \times r \times 0.8 = \pi \times 0.55$ mm $\times 0.8 \approx 1.3$ mm

(Table 1).

TABLE 1 Incision size depending on the phaco needle gauge and its outer diameter[1-4]

Gauge	Milimeters	Incision
18	1.22	1.53 mm
19	1.02	1.28 mm
20	0.91	1.14 mm
21	0.81	1.01 mm
	0.71	0.89 mm

Capsulorhexis

For author, this step is one of the most important in the whole procedure; depending on the type of cataract based on the anterior classification (at the beginning of the chapter), author has a different kind of hard cataracts, there are some, with some kind of red reflex and this could confuse him with a standard nuclear cataract, but those also have a very hard nucleus, surgeons have to be aware of that to avoid complications.

So even in those with some red reflex is better to assure a complete continuous capsulorhexis staining the anterior capsule, to get better control and visualization, avoiding any zonular stress because in any of these cataracts the zonula mostly is weak.

Now depending on if the cataract is intumescent or just hard with absorbed cortex, the capsulorhexis management is different.

Intumescent Cataracts

As author pointed out before, where the lens becomes swollen by absorbing water, the whole capsular bag is tense because of the liquid inside of it, so exist a big chance that when surgeons puncture the anterior capsule and release the tension inside, the tear goes out to the periphery; to avoid this, there are many tips: one of those is taking a Pentacam preoperatively with dilated pupil and measure the anterior chamber and nuclear thickness[5] and depending on that surgeons will be sure if it is a real intumescent cataract or just milky.

Knowing whether it is a real intumescent cataract, first of all surgeons have to fill the anterior chamber with the dye of their preference; author always uses trypan blue, but diluting the commercially available 0.1% solution to a 0.05% solution, with very good results in contrast and visualization because of its cost, and it's very easy to obtain; also it stains perfectly the anterior capsule even diluted, after that, leave it for at least 30 seconds and remove it all with viscoelastic, the best kind of visco device in this case because of its rheological properties is the cohesive one, because of the small incision is almost impossible to come out from the anterior chamber through the incision and also it maintains the anterior capsule flat enough to try to avoid any unexpected tear.

Now, the next step is to make a puncture in the anterior capsule and release the tension inside, there are many tricks of this as well; first, surgeons can do it with a needle engage in a syringe and immediately inside the bag, aspirate the milky substance through the needle or switch to a cannula to aspirate it (Fig. 5); after this, surgeons can do either take out the needle or cannula and introduce the microutrata forceps (MicroSurgical Technology, Redmond, USA) and make the rhexis or depending on the amount of the milky substance that surgeons removed and the size of the nucleus; surgeons can fill the bag with viscoelastic to separate both capsules and give some shape to the bag improving their maneuvers to make the rhexis (Fig. 6). Another maneuver is also make a small central tear with one of the tips of the microutrata (Fig. 7A) (MicroSurgical Technology, Redmond, USA) and immediately lift up

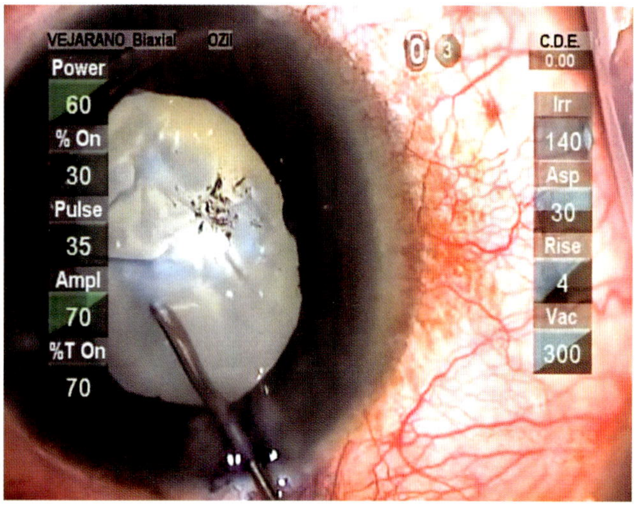

Fig. 5: Needle puncture of the anterior capsule to release the tension inside the capsular bag

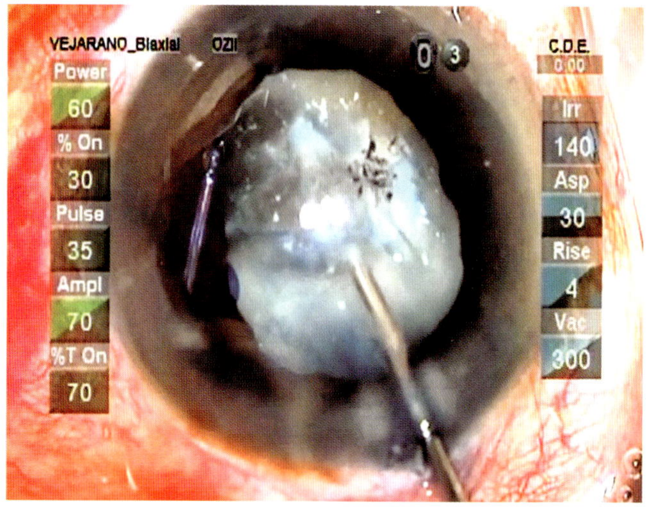

Fig. 6: Filling the capsular bag with viscoelastic after aspiration of the milky substance

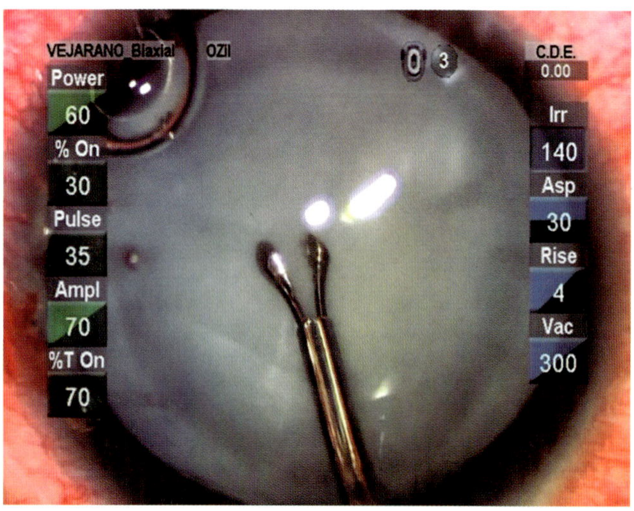

Fig. 7A: Begin the tear directly with the tip of the microutrata and lift the flap to initiate the rhexis

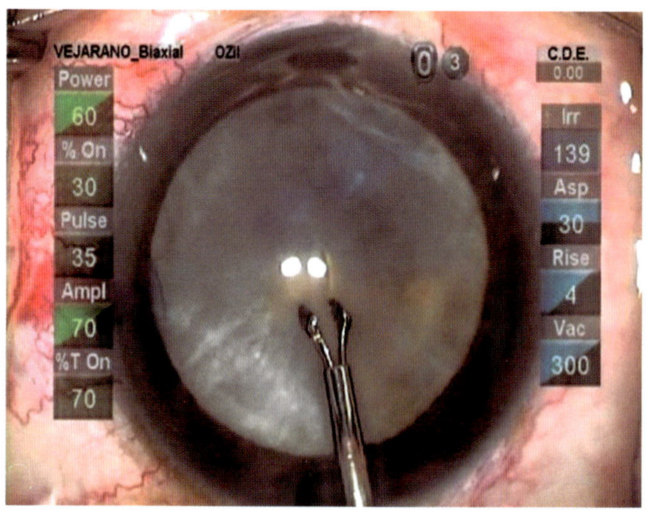

Fig. 7B: Begin the tear directly with the tip of the microutrata and lift the flap to initiate the rhexis

a flap of the anterior capsule and begin the rhexis tear, releasing tension and leaving to the liquid comes out of the bag making some pressure over the posterior lip of the incision forcing to take out some viscoelastic mixed with the cataract substance, then refill the anterior chamber with clear viscoelastic and continue the rhexis.

Other maneuver is introducing the phaco needle bevel down aspirate the anterior capsule just at the center and release a short burst of ultrasound to open the anterior capsule in a circular shape and immediately aspirate some material that also diminishes the tension and facilitate the rhexis after this.

Hard Cataract with Reabsorbed Cortex

All of these cataracts don't have almost any cortex material but instead of the intumescent cataracts, there are zonular traction and stress because of the fibrosis or retraction of the anterior capsule; so after stain and flattening the capsule, surgeons can make with one of the microutrata tips (MicroSurgical Technology, Redmond, USA) a central tear (Fig. 7B) and start the rhexis in slow manner avoiding any zonular tension. If there are some fibrosis underneath of the anterior capsule, surgeons have to try to go peripherally of this avoiding to go through it (Fig. 8) but if it is impossible to avoid, surgeons must to make it in a very slow motion avoiding any sudden force that can direct the tear toward the periphery. In some cases, the fibrosis covers almost the whole anterior capsule preventing a normal rhexis with the microutrata, then surgeons have to use a microscissors (MicroSurgical Technology, Redmond, USA) to cut the fibrosis and continue the rhexis; nevertheless there are some cataracts with severe fibrosis and the whole rhexis needs to be performed with microscissors (MicroSurgical Technology, Redmond, USA) using both incisions (lateral and main) to achieve complete continuous capsulorhexis (Figs 9A and B).

When surgeons finally can start the rhexis, surgeons have to always lift it up and fold it over to have a real control of the tear, take it as many times as surgeons need it; also the size of the rhexis is very important in these cases, even the best size is 5.5–6.0 mm to avoid posterior capsule opacification by preventing the contact of both capsules with anterior capsule over the optic zone of the intraocular lens (IOL), here surgeons need a bigger size of

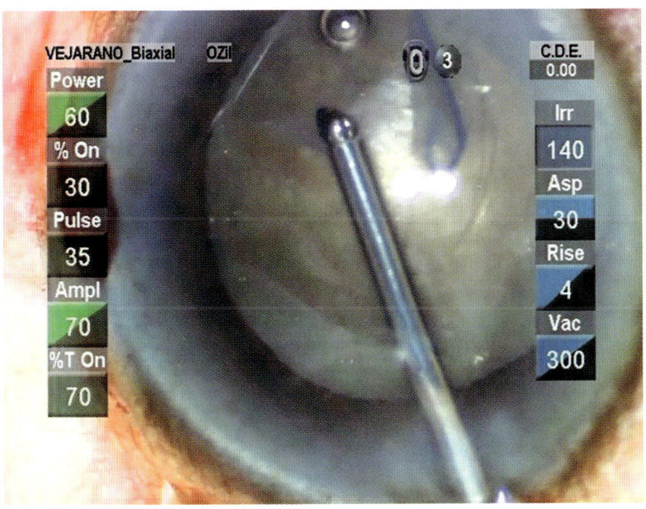

Fig. 8: Avoid the subcapsular fibrosis making the rhexis more peripheral

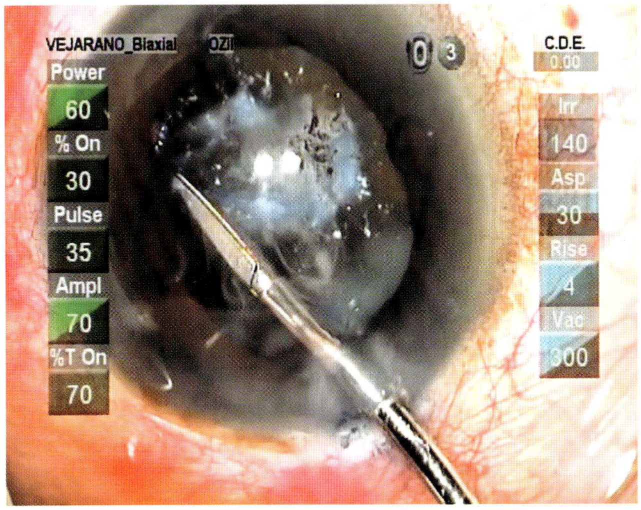

Fig. 9A: Rhexis with microscissors because the severe fibrosis of the anterior capsule using the main incision

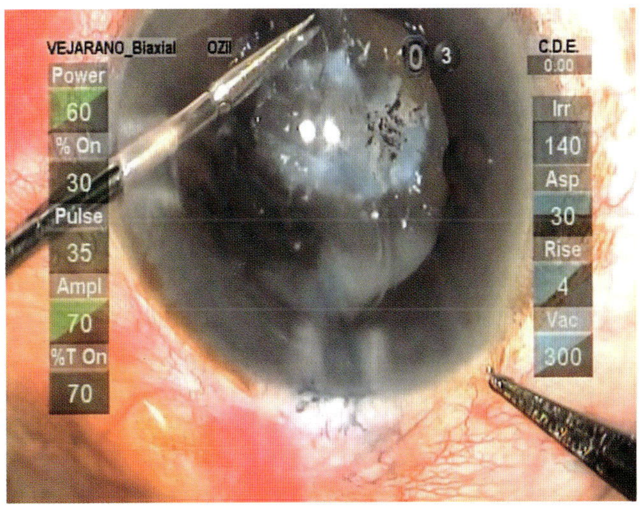

Fig. 9B: Rhexis with microscissors because the severe fibrosis of the anterior capsule using the side port incision

the rhexis because this facilitates the removal of the pieces of the nucleus that are very large, rigid and sticky from the bag preventing any zonular traction, tension and forces against the zonular fibers avoiding zonular dialysis; like any other rhexis surgeons have to finish it from outside to inside.

Hydrodissection

This is another surgical step with very high importance; more in this kind of cataracts surgeons always have to be sure that the nucleus is free from the adherences of the bag principally from the equator joints and also from the posterior capsule plaque.

Unlike the coaxial phaco, here the incision is very small and tight, so to prevent any sudden rise of the intraocular pressure that can cause backward distension of the zonula, inject balanced salt solution (BSS) into the bag before. Surgeons must extract some amount of viscoelastic from the anterior chamber. Always use a blunt cannula. Begin with an anhydric dissection, which means that lift the anterior capsule in its edge separating the anterior surface of the nucleus with the posterior surface of the anterior capsule. In hard cataracts with reabsorbed cortex where the union between both is very tight, it helps to create some space that allows to introduce the cannula and liquid; because in the intumescent cataracts, when surgeons aspirate the hydrate cortex most of the times the nucleus is already loose and it isn't necessary to make hydrodissection.

Release a stream of BSS in a controlled and continuous fashion, because it is impossible to see the wave underneath the nucleus; surgeons have to be aware when the nucleus goes up and goes forward against the edges of the rhexis, in this precise moment stop to inject BSS and push back the nucleus 180° away from the injection side to avoid bag hypertension that can cause an explosion of the posterior capsule and nucleus drop by the blockade the way out of the BSS (capsular block syndrome) and also the push back of the nucleus allows to emerge the fluid, retained underneath of the hard cataract, releasing the nucleus from equator adherences facilitating its rotation.

Surgeons always have to be sure that the nucleus is free of all its joints with the capsule, rotating it with careful bimanually with two hooks under viscoelastic substance (Sinskey, Lester or Kuglen) or with a curve blunt cannula irrigating permanently to avoid zonular stress because, as author told before, in almost of the cases it is weak.

Phacoemulsification

When performing biaxial or micro-biaxial microincision phacoemulsification surgery, knowledge and management of fluidics are crucial.[1,2,6,7] The issue of destabilization of the anterior chamber during the procedure, mentioned by several authors,[8,9] like Tsuneoka,[10] is due basically to the fact that more fluid is going out of the eye than the amount that is entering onto the anterior chamber in a given moment. Although smaller-incision surgery promotes a more tightly closed and stable anterior chamber, the equilibrium between inflow and outflow rates is critical. This has been one of the biggest problems for surgeons initiating biaxial or micro-biaxial, since the irrigation rate in this technique is usually less than in standard coaxial phacoemulsification (Table 2). The factors that influence the fluid balance in biaxial or micro-biaxial microincision phacoemulsification are several:

- The infusion rate of the irrigating instruments. This is determined by the fluidic resistance of the irrigating line and instruments (determined by the inner diameter of tubing and instruments—chopper—and the irrigating port size), and the pressure of the fluid (bottle height or amount of positive pressure applied to the bottle by any active system)

The flow of the fluid may be calculated using the Poiseuille's equation (Table 3):

$$F = \Delta P \, \pi \, r^4 / 8 \, \eta \, L$$

where, F: flow; ΔP: pressure gradient; π: 3,1416; r^4: radius of the tube at fourth power; η: viscosity of fluid; L: length of the tube. So inflow is related directly to the

TABLE 2 Comparative inflow between coaxial and most of the irrigating choppers in the market

Irrig. Chopper	Gravity 2 Extenders	IOP 100 mm Hg	AVGFI 120 mm Hg
Coaxial	114 cc/min	142 cc/min	131 cc/min
Tsuneoka	74 cc/min	88 cc/min	75 cc/min
Olsoni-II	73 cc/min	81 cc/min	77 cc/min
Nagahara	74 cc/min	84 cc/min	75 cc/min
Braga-Mele	60 cc/min	68 cc/min	61 cc/min
Vejarano Hor.	57 cc/min	66 cc/min	60 cc/min
Vejarano Inf	44 cc/min	55 cc/min	45 cc/min
Vejarano 22 Ga.	44 cc/min	55 cc/min	54 cc/min
Irrig. 20 Ga.	53 cc/min	67 cc/min	64 cc/min
Irrig. 22 Ga.	46 cc/min	58 cc/min	53 cc/min

TABLE 3 Relative flow depends on the phaco needle diameter based on Poiseuille's law (courtesy: Uday Devgan, MD)

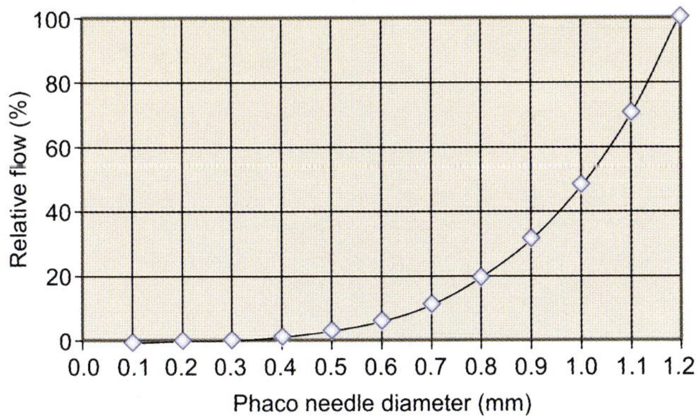

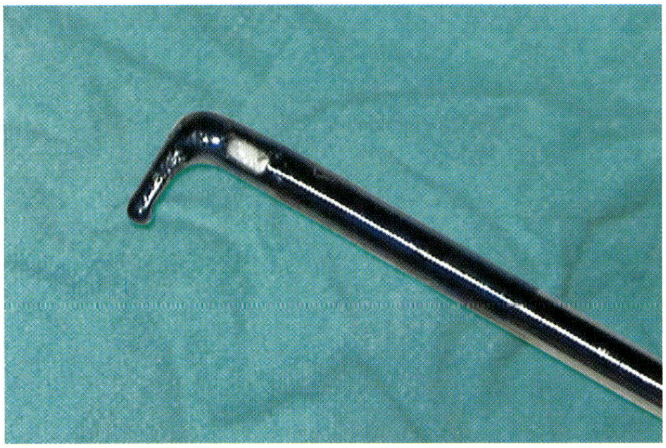

Fig. 10: Vejarano's Irrigating Chopper 22 gauge with rectangular lateral holes

radius of the tube or instrument's hollow shaft and the pressure gradient of the fluid (determined by gravity according to bottle height, or amount of positive pressure applied to the bottle by any active system), and inversely related to the length of the tube and the viscosity of fluid. In clinical settings, usually the first two factors may be modified easily and on the other hand the last two usually are rather constant.

- The amount of leakage through the incisions, determined by the relation between the outer diameter of the instruments (Phaco needle and irrigating chopper) and the incisions architecture (shape, size and presence of an inner valve)
- The amount of fluid aspirated through the phaco needle, determined by the resistance of the aspirating line (determined by the inner diameter of tubing, needle and tubing compliance) and the level of vacuum in venturi pumps and the level of flow and vacuum in peristaltic pumps

This may be calculated again using the Poiseuille's equation (Table 3) and directly related with inner diameter of tubing and needle (which determines the resistance), and the pressure gradient inside the tubing (determined by the level of vacuum in venturi pumps and the level of flow and vacuum in peristaltic pumps).

It is necessary to maintain equilibrium between those factors, in order to achieve a stable anterior chamber, without jeopardizing the intraocular tissues (iris, endothelium, posterior capsule).

To reach that goal the surgeon must take in account several issues: infusion rate of the irrigating instruments, amount of leakage through the incisions, and amount of fluid aspirated through the phaco needle.

In biaxial or micro-biaxial, surgeons have to try to forget the high vacuum levels that surgeons are used to, because the inflow that surgeons can get through any irrigating chopper never will be like the one that surgeons can obtain through the coaxial irrigation in standard phacoemulsification (Table 2), but it is very similar with the new micro-coaxial phacoemulsification with the new ultrasleeve, the inflow in biaxial with the Vejarano's Irrigating chopper 20 gauge (AC7340; Accutome, Malvern, USA) (Fig. 1) is the 49% of the coaxial and 84% of the micro-coaxial, the inflow in micro-biaxial with the Vejarano's Irrigating Chopper 22 gauge (MicroSurgical Technology, Redmond, USA) (Fig. 10) is the 41% of the coaxial and 70% of the micro-coaxial, and the micro-coaxial is the 58% of the standard coaxial phaco (Table 4) so surgeons must change and adapt their parameters depending of the irrigating chopper that surgeons are going to use (depends on its own inflow), for example if it has frontal irrigation, surgeons have to reduce their parameters in average to 65%, if it has inferior irrigation to 58% and if it has lateral irrigation to 50% (based on the data of the Table 2 comparing with a coaxial inflow).

TABLE 4 Comparative inflow depending on the phaco tip, sleeve and incision size in coaxial and micro-coaxial phacoemulsification (courtesy: Armando Crema, MD)

Irrig/min	*% Irrig*	*Tip*	*Incision*
136 ml	100%	1.1 flared	2.75 mm
106 ml	78%	1.1 flared Mini/Tape	2.75 mm
95 ml	69%	1.1 flared	2 to 2.2 mm
79 ml	58%	Tapered or Mini-flared	2 to 2.2 mm

Also surgeons have to modulate their aspiration flow avoiding surpassing levels above 25–30 cc/min, and use the fluidic control software of their phaco machine with bimodal or linear aspiration. This reduces the rise time and makes more controllable the events inside of the anterior chamber.[11-13] Since the goal of the surgery is not solely to maintain the anterior chamber space, but to permit the emulsification of the nucleus. It is necessary to use levels of vacuum which allow surgeon achieve a good enough purchase of the nucleus and its fragments, and perform an effective chopping procedure. In peristaltic machines, it is necessary to use standard flow levels between 25 cc/min and 30 cc/min and vacuum levels of 250–300 mm Hg, and in venturi machines a level of vacuum of 120–160 mm Hg.

Remember the Poiseuille's equation, so with a smaller diameter of the needle, the flow will be less (Table 3) and the vacuum needs to be higher to be comparable with bigger needle diameter in holding power.

In biaxial technique, although any emulsification technique can be used like divide and conquer, nucleus disassembly or nucleus fracture, because of the bare tip and less maneuverability for the small incisions; those techniques, which are through microincision, aren't the most recommended in hypermature cataracts because the tight incisions make the whole maneuvers more difficult to emulsify this kind of nucleus.

For those reasons, it is better in these hypermature cataracts to use chopping techniques, the one that surgeons used to but the author manages and recommends the using of technique that author himself developed since 1998 and is called Vejarano's Safe Chop.

To perform the emulsification of the nucleus author uses his Safe Chop technique.[14-24] Author will provide a brief description of the technique in the following paragraphs.

After aspirating the anterior cortex and epinucleus, the phaco tip, bevel down is placed in the proximal portion of the nucleus and pulsed or preferably burst ultrasound

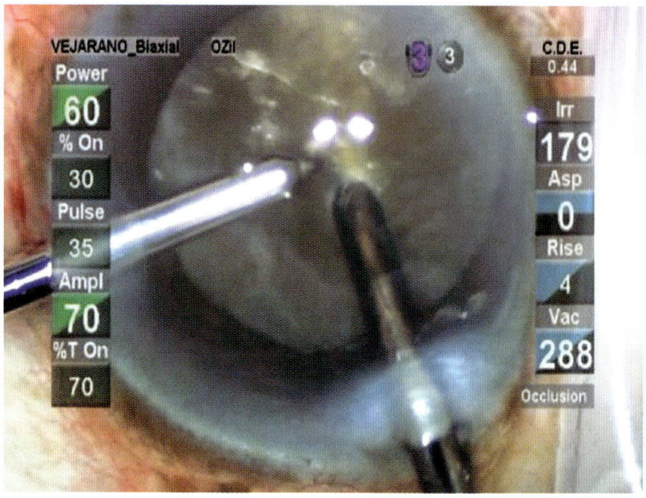

Fig. 11: Impaling the nucleus with the phaco tip bevel down, before the chopping maneuver

energy is applied, so that it penetrates deep in the nuclear core (Fig. 11).

When the tip is buried into the nucleus, the foot pedal is switched to position two. In this moment the irrigating chopper is lightly rotated horizontally (tilted), so that the longest length of the tip is not presented toward the space between the continuous curvilinear capsulorhexis (CCC) edge and the lens material (space that in brunescent and very hard cataracts is very small, even absent). The tilted chopper is slid beneath of the anterior capsule, 180° apart of the side port incision (Figs 12A to C), maneuver that is much easier to perform, than trying to slide it under the anterior capsule, just in front of the phaco tip. Afterward, when reaching the equator of the nucleus, the chopper is rotated vertically and moved inside the bag, to the position in front of the phaco tip (Figs 13A to C), and the chopping maneuver takes place. In hard cataracts, author holds the nucleus between the two instruments for a moment, and applies a small amount of additional pulsed ultrasound

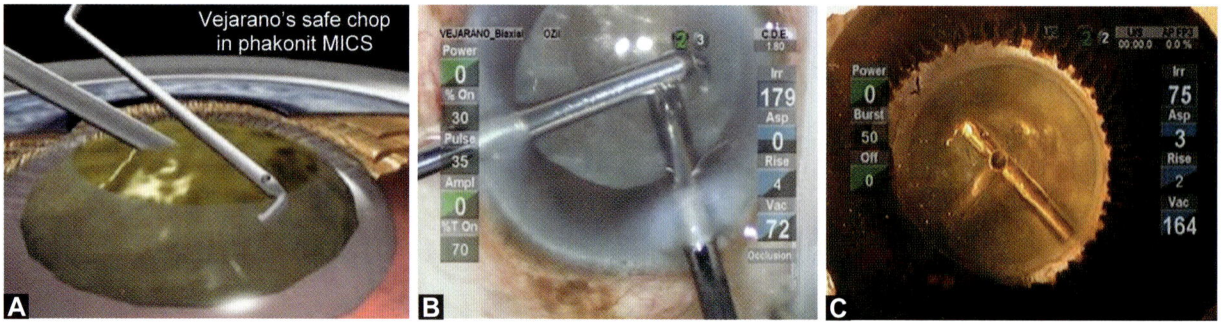

Figs 12A to C: Irrigating chopper tilted sliding underneath anterior capsule avoiding its damage, going to equator capsular bag previous to its rotation; (A) 3D animation, (B) Surgeon view, (C) Miyake view

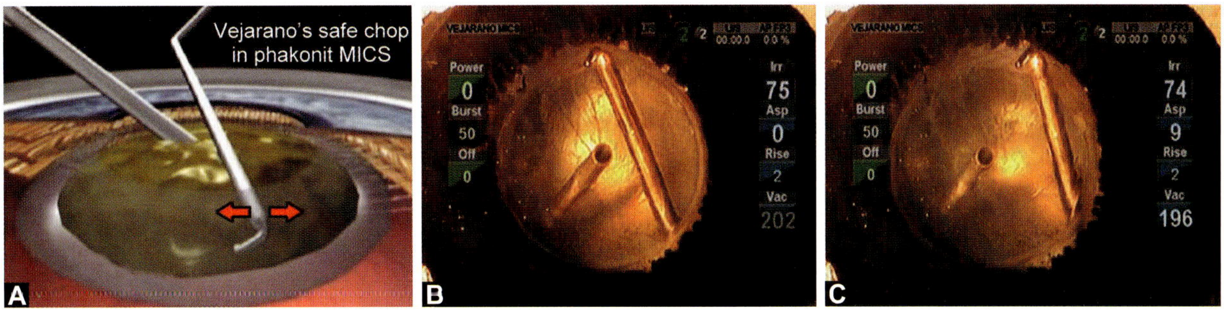

Figs 13A to C: Irrigating chopper underneath anterior capsule inside the capsular bag rotating until inferior part of the nucleus; (A) 3D animation, (B) and (C) Miyake view

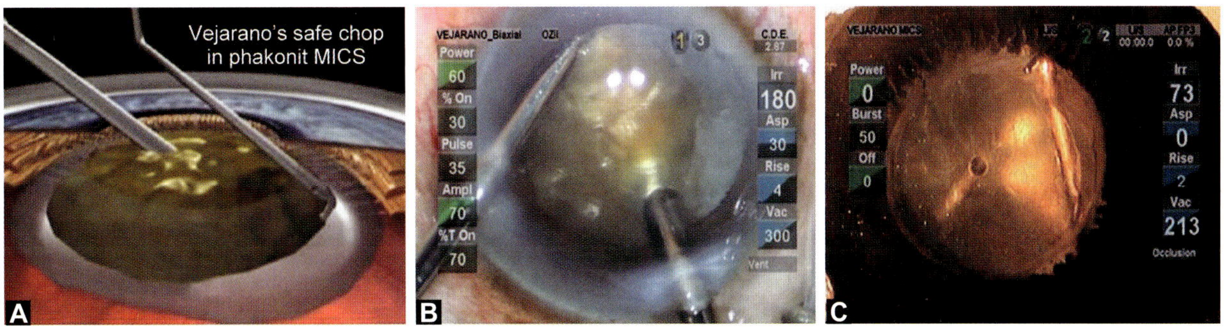

Figs 14A to C: Irrigating chopper is in position to make the chopping maneuver at inferior equator of the nucleus; (A) 3D animation, (B) surgeon view, (C) Miyake view

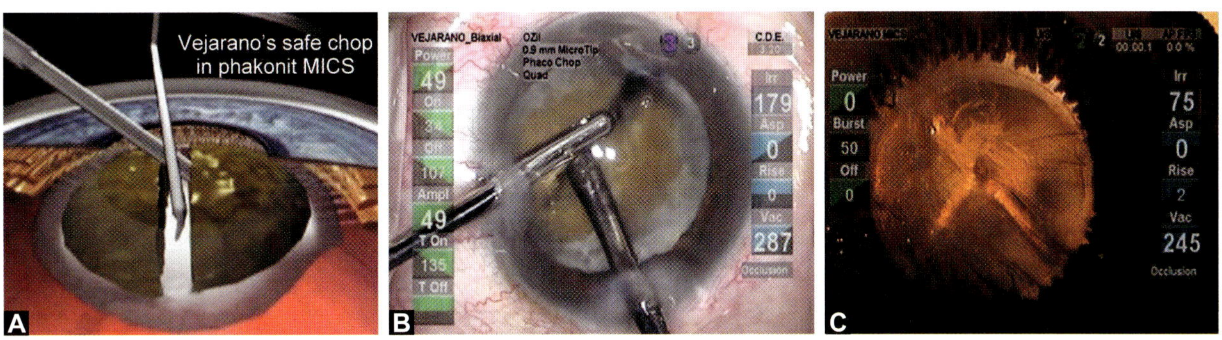

Figs 15A to C: Irrigating chopper is introduced along the fracture line avoiding any damage of the anterior capsule and giving it the safe position inside the capsular bag to rotate it again; (A) 3D animation, (B) surgeon view, (C) Miyake view

energy, so that the tip penetrates deeper in the nuclear material improving the holding power (Figs 14A to C). This allows us to gain improved control of the whole nucleus during the chopping process, since it doesn't become easily dislodged, as long as the high vacuum and the deep position of the tip maintain a tight occlusion seal around the tip. One very important advantage of this technique is that with this very good purchase of the nucleus, especially in hard cataracts, the chopping process is more effective, and helps us to separate the leather like very hard posterior layers of those cataracts, that often represent a challenge to the surgeon.

After dividing the nucleus in halves, author rotates it 45° to try to get the first piece of the heminucleus. The technique to avoid damaging the CCC while chopping the nuclear fragments, is to insert the irrigation chopper now vertically and always along the fracture lines of the nucleus (Figs 15A to C), where there is more room for the chopper, and move it to reach its chopping position again only when it is already at the lens' equator, inside the capsular bag, in this way making this step completely safe (where the name of the technique comes) and repeat it as many times as necessary to remove the first piece (Figs 16A to C).

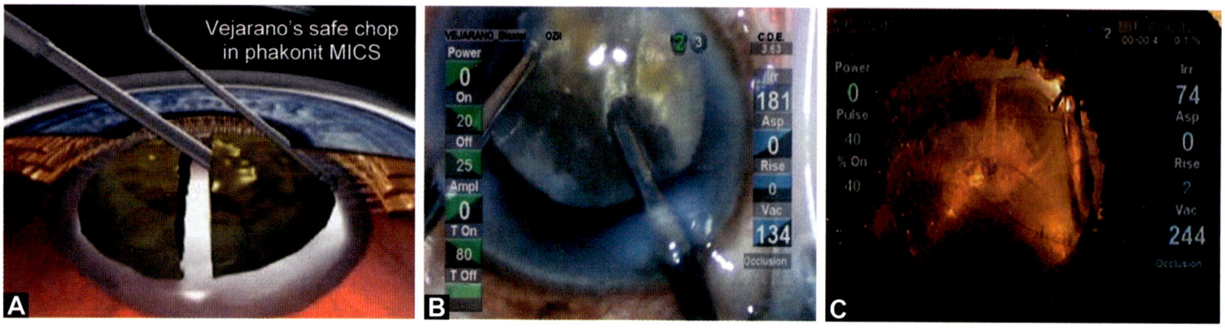

Figs 16A to C: The safe maneuver is repeated as many times as is necessary, rotating the irrigating chopper close to the equator until inferior nucleus and making the chop to obtain nuclear pieces to emulsify them at the center; (A) 3D animation, (B) surgeon view, (C) Miyake view

The features of the fluidic and design of the Vejarano's irrigating chopper (AC7340; Accutome, Malvern, USA and MicroSurgical Technology, Redmond, USA), with lateral oval irrigating ports and olive at the end of the tip makes easier the step of sliding the chopper's tip inside the bag, since it inflates the bag (Fig. 13A) and also protects the posterior capsule of any damage.

The subsequent fragments are managed in the same way; when several nuclear fragments have been emulsified, the amount of remaining nuclear material is less and author will have more room in the center, so it is not usually necessary to go beneath the anterior CCC in order to chop them.

The epinucleus when exists is aspirated using a flip technique, and protecting the posterior capsule with the irrigation chopper used like a barrier, since its tip has an olive to avoid damaging tissues, and also its flow will move away the capsule.

Bimanual irrigation/aspiration of cortical remnants, using bimanual handpieces and, if necessary, posterior capsule polishing are done.

The use of capsular tension rings (CTR) depends if the nucleus is subluxated because of the capsular retraction or if surgeons feel that the zonular support is very weak.

The decision of the IOL is still a point of discussion, also if surgeons have to enlarge the main incision (this is the way how author does) or if surgeons make a new one between their two incisions only to introduce the IOL that means a third incision.

Conclusion

Author had been doing biaxial since October 2002 and micro-biaxial since November 2005 and his entire cataract surgery switch to microincision in December 2005 so author stopped to make coaxial since then, this means that any kind of cataract could be extract by phacoemulsification through microincision with biaxial or micro-biaxial technique.

Those techniques are very reliable and safe if surgeons understand the fluidics even more than the power modulation, because only with pulse mode is possible to achieve the technique and there isn't a single case reported with corneal burn with biaxial, surgeons don't need obligatory a power modulation software in their machine but of course that is better; if surgeons control the fluidic, surgeons will avoid the instability of the anterior chamber giving less endothelial and uveal trauma, there won't be turbulence and the followability and holding power remains identical, then, surgeons can make any kind of cataract with any technique of their preference, always following the advice of the experts who make a lot of this cataracts. Never forget that the hypermature cataracts are different to any of regular cataracts; surgeons don't have red reflex, the anterior capsule is very thin and fragile with great chance of producing a peripheral tear, always make a big capsulorhexis to supply enough room to remove the pieces from the bag to the iris plane to emulsify them, the most of the zonular support are weak, the hardness and the adherence of its fibers are bigger and the energy delivered could be higher therefore the surgical time.

Even with those difficulties is possible to make them giving to the patient the whole benefits of this technique, like:

- Smaller incisions: Less invasive approach
- Really anastigmatic incisions: Doesn't matter the position temporal or superior, author induces only 0.06 D
- Really watertight incisions
- Less possibility of iris extrusion even in intraocular floppy iris syndrome (IFIS)
- Higher resistance to postoperative trauma

- Minimum uveal trauma because of minimal turbulence
- Less amount of endothelial cell lost because of minimal turbulence and low ultrasound emission
- Faster corneal stability and visual recovery
- Deep anterior chamber along the whole surgery
- Less BSS consumption in each case, author spends only 60–80 cc in regular cases and 120 cc in hypermature cataracts
- Less fluctuation and mobilization of vitreous because the stability of the anterior chamber during the whole procedure, so it's better in refractive lens exchange (high myopes and hyperopes) and patients with previous retinal tears or retinal surgery
- Avoid the high intraocular pressure depending on the high inflow in coaxial, then is better in glaucoma patients and also keep the safety range of retinal irrigation, that is 3 minutes at 70 mm Hg, after this surgeons could cause retinal damage; with biaxial technique surgeons can obtain between 20 mm Hg and 30 mm Hg during the surgery but in coaxial surgeons can arise until 60 mm Hg or more, so the risk for retinal and optic nerve damage is higher
- Better maintenance of the anterior chamber with viscoelastic during the rhexis, when introduces a CTR and management of small pupils
- Surgeons can make the rhexis from both incisions
- Surgeons can switch the hands in phaco
- It is possible to perform this technique with any machine
- Hyperpulses is not a mandatory necessity
- Easiest removal of subincisional cortex
- The irrigation is a third instrument
- The main incision helps to mobilize fragments
- Theoretical less incidence of endophtalmitis
- Indicated in cases of previous penetrating keratoplasty (PKP), radial keratotomy (RK) or Seton devices
- Better control in uveal effusion
- Better management of complications
- In any case, mainly in complicated
- Better to teach in right and left handed Residents or Fellows

There are good softwares and new machines that help with the learning curve.

Take Home Pearl

First of all, never sub-estimate the hypermature cataracts, they always are more difficult and challenge than a regular ones; about the incision, always make it with precalibrated knives to obtain more anterior chamber stability avoiding leakage; in rhexis always help surgeons with staining the capsule even it has some red reflex. This gives surgeons more control and safety, don't forget that their major goal in intumescent cataracts is to decrease the intracapsular pressure to avoid peripheral tears and to avoid any subcapsular fibrosis and peripheral traction in hard ones without cortex; the hydrodissection is mandatory with mobilization of the nucleus in hard ones and in the intumescent sometimes it isn't necessary but always be sure that the nucleus is free before to begin the phacoemulsification, finally in phaco, use their favorite technique but author prefers to recommend always chop in these cataracts.

Comment

Author hopes that with this chapter and the whole book, more and more surgeons take the challenge to give the next step in the future cataract surgery and don't fall in the false believe that microincision is not good enough because the perfect IOL is not developed now and surgeons need to enlarge the incision, remember at the beginning of the phacoemulsification when only exist the rigid IOLs author enlarged the incisions but with the benefits of the phaco against of the extracapsular, so as surgeons read before, the IOL is not an advantage of the technique, the biggest advantage is the calm intraocular environment during the whole procedure that increases the visual prognosis to the patient.

References

1. Vejarano L Felipe, Alejandro T. Fluidics in bimanual phaco. In: Agarwal A, (Ed). Bimanual Phaco: Mastering the Phakonit/MICS Technique. Thorofare: Slack Inc.; 2004.
2. Vejarano L Felipe, Alberto V, Alejandro T. Fluidics in phakonit. In: Garg A, (Ed). Mastering the Art of Bimanual Microincision Phaco (Phaconit/MICS). New Delhi: Jaypee Brothers Medical Publishers; 2005.
3. Arturo Perez-A. Accurus forced infusion good for MICS Ocular Surgery News U.S. Edition, June 1, 2003.
4. Tablas_Utiles. Available from http://www.inoxidable.com/tablas_utiles.htm [Access on January 2012].
5. Ocular Surgery News. Latin America Edition. 2006;1-3.
6. Vejarano L Felipe, Alberto V, Alejandro T. Fluidics in phakonit and microphakonit. In: Garg A, (Ed). Mastering the Phacodynamics (Tools, Technology and Innovations). New Delhi: Jaypee Brothers Medical Publishers; 2007.
7. Vejarano L Felipe, Alberto V, Alejandro T, et al. Fluidics in biaxial lens surgery. In: Arturo Perez-Arteaga (Ed). Step by Step Biaxial Lens Surgery. New Delhi: Jaypee Brothers Medical Publishers; 2008.
8. Blumenthal M, Assia E. Using an anterior chamber maintainer to control intraocular pressure during phacoemulsification. J Cataract Refract Surg. 1994;20:93-6.

9. Agarwal A, Agarwal S, Agarwal A. Antichamber collapse. J Cataract Refract Surg. 2002;28:1085.
10. Tsuneoka H, Shiba T, Takahashi Y. Ultrasonic phacoemulsification using a 1.4 mm incision: clinical results. J Cataract Refract Surg. 2002;28:81-6.
11. Vejarano L Felipe, Alejandro T. Facoemulsificación: Equipos y Sistemas. In: Virgilio Centurion, (Ed). El libro del cristalino de las Américas. São Paulo: Editorial Santos; 2006.
12. Vejarano L Felipe, Julian OM, Alejandro T. Phacoemulsification: equipments and systems. In: Garg A, (Ed). Mastering the Techniques of Advanced Phaco Surgery. New Delhi: Jaypee Brothers Medical Publishers; 2008.
13. Vejarano L Felipe, Julian OM, Alejandro T, Jerome B. Phacoemulsification machines and systems for biaxial lens surgery. In: Arturo Perez-Arteaga (Ed). Step by Step Biaxial Lens Surgery. New Delhi: Jaypee Brothers Medical Publishers; 2008.
14. Vejarano L Felipe, Alejandro T, Alberto V, et al. The safer and most effective techniques in cataract surgery. Highlights of Ophthalmology. 2004;32(2):10-6.
15. Vejarano L Felipe. Preliminary results on phakonit, the new era for phaco surgery. Ophthalmology Times.
16. Vejarano L Felipe, Alejandro T. Vejarano safe chop makes transition to chopping easier. Ocular Surgery News. 2005;23(5):10-1.
17. Vejarano L Felipe, Alejandro T. Vejarano safe chop, makes transition to Chopping easier. Ocular Surgery News Europe/Asia-Pacific Edition. 2005;16(5):19-22.
18. Vejarano L Felipe, Alejandro T. Vejarano's safe chop technique: a safer chopping. Techniques in Ophthalmology. 2005;3(3):109-15.
19. Vejarano L Felipe, Alberto V. Safe chopping in bimanual phaco. In: Agarwal A, (Ed) Bimanual Phaco: Mastering the Phakonit/MICS Techniqal. Thorofare: Slack Inc., 2004.
20. Vejarano L Felipe, Alberto V, Alejandro T. Implantation techniques in microphaco: Vejarano's safe chop in phakonit. In Garg A, (Ed). Mastering the Art of Bimanual Microincision Phaco (Phaconit/MICS. New Delhi: Jaypee Brothers Medical Publishers 2005.
21. Vejarano L Felipe, Alejandro T, Vejarano Alberto. Safe chop: a safer technique in phaco chop. In: Boyd S, Dodick J. Highlights Collection, vol. I, New Outcomes in Cataract Surgery. Panamá: Highlights of Ophthalmology; 2005.
22. Vejarano L Felipe, Alejandro T. Using safe horizontal chopping to prevent ruptures. In: Agarwal A, (Ed). Phaco Nightmares. Thorofare: Slack Inc.; 2006.
23. Vejarano L Felipe, Alejandro T. Phakonit and Microphakonit. In: Virgilio Centurion (Ed). El libro del cristalino de las Américas. São Paulo: Editorial Santos; 2006.
24. Perez-Arteaga Arturo, Vejarano L Felipe, Alejandro T, Jerome B. Biaxial cataract surgery: personal techniques. In: Arturo Perez-Arteaga, (Ed). Step by Step Biaxial Lens Surgery. New Delhi: Jaypee Brothers Medical Publishers;.2008.

19

Biaxial Microincision Phacoemulsification for Difficult and Challenging Cases[1]

I Howard Fine (USA), Jorge L Alió (Spain),
Richard S Hoffman (USA), Mark Packer (USA)

Core Messages

The advantages of biaxial microincision phacoemulsification have been elaborated in a variety of papers within the literature.[2-10] Author and colleagues believe that the technique has distinct fluidic advantages.

- By separating inflow from aspiration and phaco, all of the fluid is coming in through one side of the eye and exiting through the opposite side of the eye
- There are never competing currents at the phaco tip
- It is easier to achieve a nearly closed system
- Author and colleagues can address certain cases that would be less advantageous, or even impossible, with the use of a coaxial phaco tip

High Myopia

In highly myopic eyes, author and colleagues are able to achieve a situation in which they can maintain the anterior chamber in a completely stable configuration, never trampolining the vitreous face, by keeping the irrigating handpiece in the eye throughout the case. Chopping can take place in the usual manner, and with the completion of chopping, mobilization of segments and the epinucleus, author and colleagues can keep the irrigating chopper in the eye, remove the phaco needle, infuse viscoelastic, remove residual cortex, and then infuse viscoelastic for the implantation of the intraocular lens (IOL) without ever shallowing the anterior chamber. Author and colleagues believe that there may, eventually, be a documented decreased incidence of retinal detachment in high myopia as a result of non-trampolining of the vitreous face during phaco, and the implantation of IOLs that fill the capsule, such as dual-optic IOLs or IOLs that arch posteriorly, as does the Crystalens.

Posterior Polar Cataract (Fig. 1)

In the situation of posterior polar cataracts, 35% have defective posterior capsules[11,12] and almost all of them have weakened capsules, so it is very important to not over-pressurize the eye and perhaps force nuclear material through the defective posterior capsule. By the same token, it is important to not shallow the chamber and have the nucleus come forward, and possibly open the defect in the posterior capsule. These cases are advantageously done with biaxial microincision phacoemulsification, because of the anterior chamber stability.[13]

Author and colleagues do hydrodelineation, without hydrodissection, and then carefully chop the endonucleus into pie-shaped segments and evacuate them from the eye. Once the endonucleus is removed, author and colleagues viscodissect (Viscoat®, Alcon Laboratories, Fort Worth, Texas) the epinucleus up from its position against the

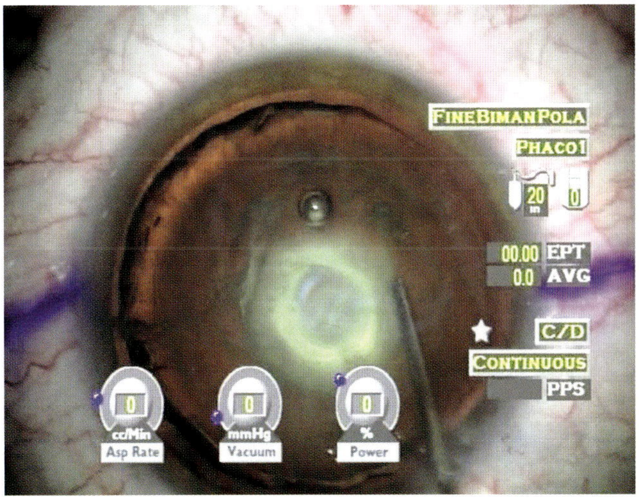

Fig. 1: Hydrodelineation of a posterior polar cataract

cortex without removing the irrigating chopper. In this way, author and colleagues have a layer of cortex and viscoelastic under the epinucleus when they evacuate it, so should the capsule open, it is less likely that they will spill lens material into the vitreous. Once the epinucleus is gone, they leave the irrigation system in the eye, remove the phaco needle, and add Viscoat®. Author and colleagues viscodissect the cortex up into the plain of the capsulorhexis, in the same way and remove it while having a thick layer of viscoelastic on top of the fragile posterior capsule. They never polish the posterior segment of the capsule prior to the IOL implantation, but would rely on YAG laser if there were visually significant opacities within the visual axis, postoperatively.

Posterior Subluxed Cataracts (Fig. 2)

For posterior subluxed cataracts, which are hinged to a small zone of attached zonules, author and colleagues will go through a pars plana incision and prolapse the lens, in its capsule, up into the anterior chamber and then add viscoelastic (Viscoat®) under the lens. They will then phaco the lens with biaxial microincision instrumentation utilizing an irrigating cannula in the left hand and a phaco needle in the right, keeping the irrigation on top of the viscoelastic, but below the cataract. They don't try to disassemble these cataracts, but phaco them from the outside in. In general, with the irrigation under the nuclear material, author and colleagues have a system in which there is fluid circulating in a circuitous pattern on top of the viscoelastic, and chips that are liberated from the mass of the nucleus tend to circulate entirely within the anterior segment and not get deposited into the vitreous. After removal of the cataract, they do a partial anterior vitrectomy and implant, through a 2.5 mm incision, a foldable intraocular lens, with the haptics under the iris and the optic on top. This allows the haptics to indent the undersurface of the iris and be easily identifiable. Author and colleagues then suture the haptics to the iris and nudge the optic beneath the pupillary margin. They have had great success with this technique.

Mature Cataract with Zonular Dialysis (Fig. 3)

In cases in which there is a dialysis of the zonular apparatus during phacoemulsification, as in a case of unrecognized pseudoexfoliation in the presence of a dense cataract, author and colleagues can hold the nucleus with the phaco tip, remove the irrigating chopper, place viscoelastic under the lens, and then put the irrigating handpiece, without a chopper, under the lens and again phaco the lens entirely within the plain of the capsulorhexis. Nuclear material can be mobilized from the posterior chamber with an unsleeved phaco tip because there is no irrigation going along with the phaco tip, as in coaxial phaco, which would force the nuclear material into the vitreous cavity. This is not possible with a coaxial phaco tip. In these cases they also see chips that circulate in the fluid above the viscoelastic, which is sitting on top of the vitreous, but they do not see chips that move posteriorly. Once this has been completed, they will do a biaxial microincision partial anterior vitrectomy, or a pars plana 25 gauge transcleral microincision vitrectomy, and implant an anterior chamber lens, or a posterior chamber lens, and suture it to the iris.

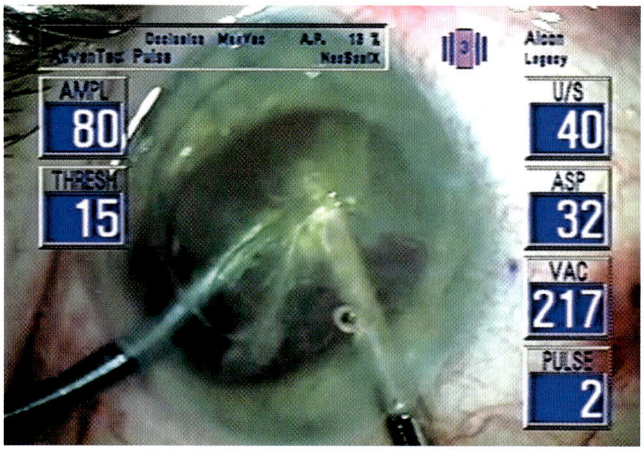

Fig. 2: Phacoemulsification of a subluxed cataract in the anterior chamber

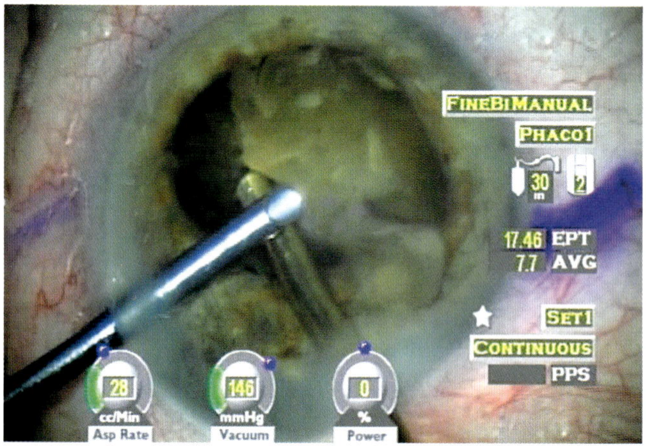

Fig. 3: Bringing nuclear material out of the posterior chamber with an unsleeved phaco tip in the presence of zonular dialysis

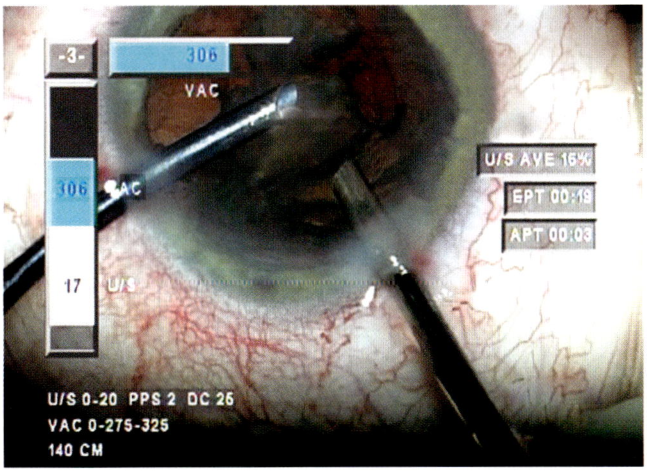

Fig. 4: Completing phacoemulsification in the presence of a punctured posterior capsule

Punctured Posterior Capsule (Fig. 4)

In the case where the capsule is punctured during the course of phacoemulsification, author and colleagues can continue the irrigation high in the anterior chamber and go back into the endolenticular space with the unsleeved phaco tip, and complete the phacoemulsification without further enlarging the puncture in the posterior capsule. Without removing the irrigator, author and colleagues then remove the cortex, and then instill more viscoelastic. They then implant the lens into the capsular bag or into the ciliary sulcus. Residual viscoelastic should be removed with a vitrector to avoid the possibility of bringing vitreous to the wound. This procedure would be impossible with a coaxial phaco tip because a continuously changing fluid wave from the phaco sleeve would enlarge, or extend, the capsular tear out to the periphery of the capsule, with loss of lens material into the vitreous.

Posterior Capsule Rupture (Figs 5 and 6)

In an extensive posterior capsule rupture, author and colleagues can bring the entire endonucleus up into the anterior chamber by holding it with the phaco tip. Very little fluid leaks out of the incision when they remove the irrigator, place Viscoat® under the nucleus, and replace the irrigator under the lens. They then proceed with phacoemulsification in the plain of the capsulorhexis or in the anterior chamber, with the irrigator beneath the nucleus as they carousel, or phaco, it from the outside in. They can then proceed with cortical clean-up in a similar manner, or first perform a partial anterior vitrectomy, either through

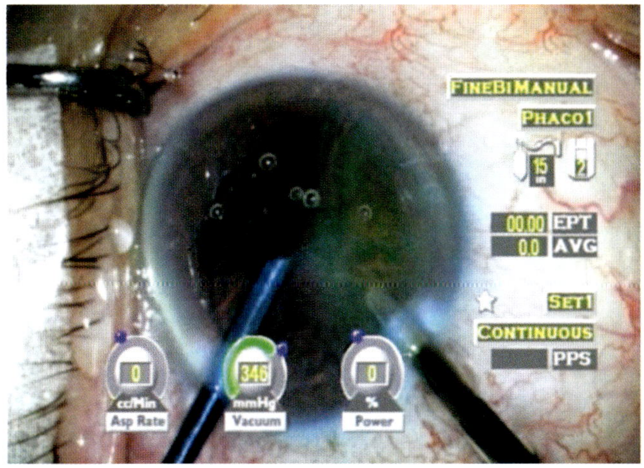

Fig. 5: Holding the Nucleus with an unsleeved phaco tip prior to removing the chopper and adding viscoelastic under the nucleus in the presence of a large posterior capsule rupture

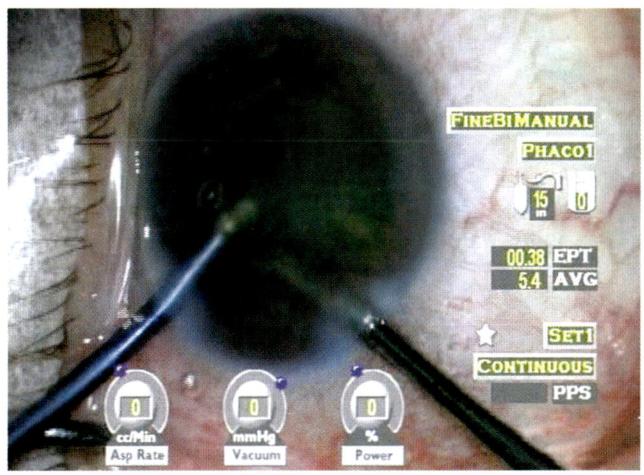

Fig. 6: Irrigating below the cataract in the presence of a capsule rupture.

the pars plana, or through side-port incisions biaxially. Once all residual cortex has been removed, they implant a posterior chamber lens into the ciliary sulcus.

Pseudoexfoliation (Fig. 7)

In post-filtration surgery, in the presence of pseudo-exfoliation, author and colleagues like to use an endocapsular tension ring that they can introduce through a side-port with an injector, following gentle cortical cleaving hydrodissection. The injector doesn't enter the incision; it is just held against the incision, and the forces on the capsule as the endocapsular tension ring is being inserted are contained by the use of a Lester hook in the

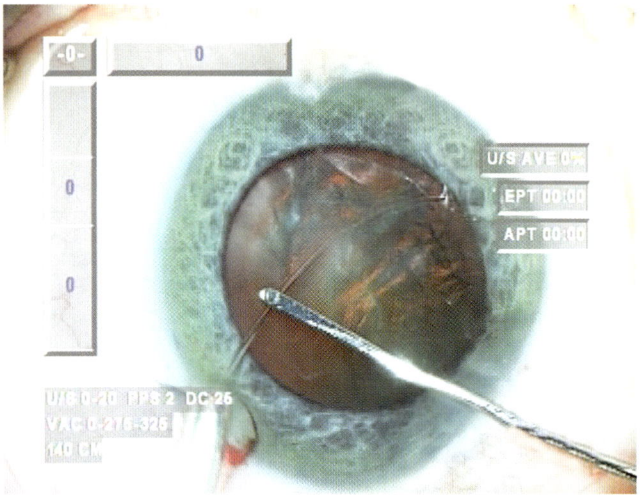

Fig. 7: Injection of a capsule tension ring through a microincision controlled by a Lester hook in the right hand

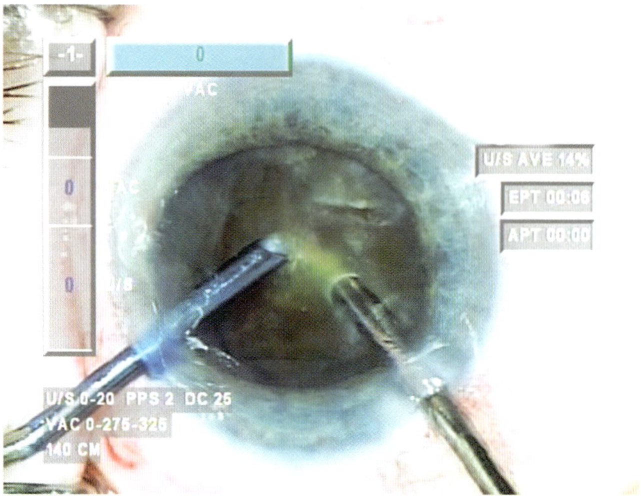

Fig. 8: Chopping a rock hard nucleus

opposite hand (Fig. 7). Author and colleagues then proceed with biaxial microincision horizontal chopping of the lens so as to not add any downward force on the lens which might stress the residual zonules. Cortical clean-up is facilitated in the presence of an endocapsular tension ring, by performing gentle cortical cleaving hydrodissection prior to the implantation of the ring. The lens is then implanted into the capsular bag through an incision between the two side-port incisions, which is our routine method for IOL implantation in the presence of two 1.1mm phacoemulsification incisions.

Rock-Hard Nuclei (Fig. 8)

Author and colleagues can phacoemulsify rock-hard nuclei with the same facility and ease with which they do softer nuclei with biaxial microincision phacoemulsification, and they usually end up with average phaco powers under 10% with effective phaco times under ten seconds, in spite of the density of these nuclei. This is an enormous advantage in terms of corneal, endothelial protection because of the great stability of the anterior chamber. Author and colleagues prefer a 30° phacoemulsification tip used with the bevel down. This allows the achievement of vacuum once the tip touches the endonucleus. A bevel-up tip must go deeply into the nucleus before occlusion and vacuum are achieved. With a bevel-down tip, they are also sending all of the energy toward the nucleus and none toward the corneal endothelium or trabecular meshwork. Finally, one can mobilize pie-shaped segments from the level of the capsulorhexis up, rather than having to go deeply into the endolenticular space to achieve occlusion to mobilize these segments, as author and colleagues would have to with a bevel-up configuration.

Switching Hands (Fig. 9)

In cases of zonular dialysis, another advantage of biaxial microincision phacoemulsification is that surgeon can use the phaco tip with either hand. After inserting an endocapsular tension ring through one of the microincisions, author and colleagues would hydroexpress the lens into the plain of the capsulorhexis and then utilize the phaco tip in either the right, or left, hand, depending on the location of

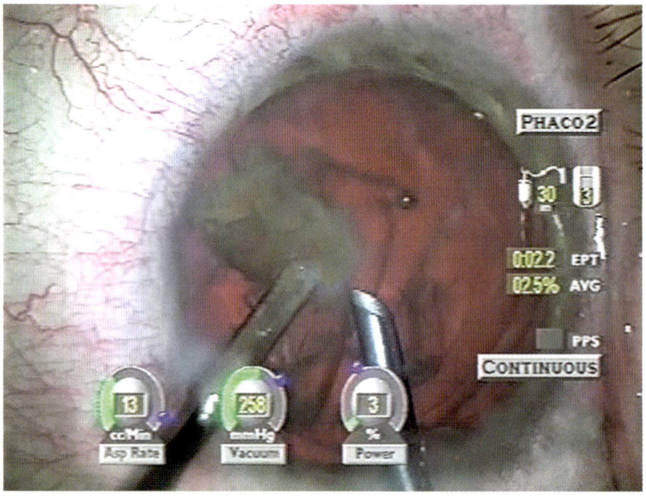

Fig. 9: Phacoemulsification in the left hand in the presence of zonular dialysis (surgeon's perspective)

the zonular dialysis. For dialyses that are on the operating surgeon's right side, author and colleagues would use the phaco tip in the right hand, drawing material in the anterior chamber toward the area of weakened zonules, rather than away from it, which would stress the intact zonules. For dialyses that are on the left-hand side, author and colleagues can use the phaco tip in our left hand and the irrigating chopper in the right to remove the nucleus, thereby closing the zonular dialysis with the activation of flow and vacuum toward the left side.

Microcornea or Microphthalmos (Fig. 10)

For very small eyes, the use of biaxial phacoemulsification is an enormous advantage because the smaller size of the instruments avoids creasing of the cornea, which compromises visualization of intraocular structures. A coaxial tip, which is much larger in size, would indent the cornea as it was manipulated and partially obscure the visualization of the intraocular structures. This has turned out to be especially advantageous in cases with a microcornea or a microphthalmic eye in the presence of an unusually large lens.

Large Iridodialysis and Zonular Defects (Fig. 11)

In cases where there are large iris defects and missing zonules, author and colleagues will straddle that area with our microchopper and phaco tip, fractionate the anterior chamber with Healon 5 to keep the vitreous back and proceed in the usual manner. This has been very efficacious and has not resulted in bringing vitreous out of the posterior segment. This is exemplified in the case of a woman who had 100° of ciliary body and iris, except for the pupillary margin, excised in management of a choroidal/ciliary body malignant melanoma, resulting additionally in fragile and atrophic sclera and conjunctiva at the tumor site.

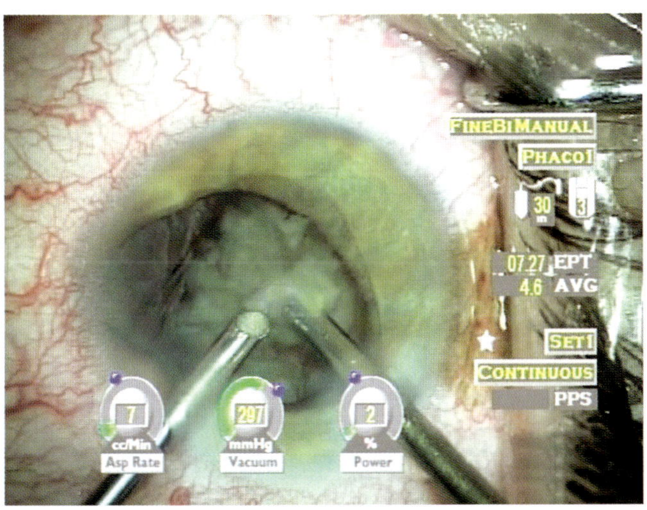

Fig. 10: Micro instruments phacoing a large dense nucleus in an eye with micro cornea and iris coloboma

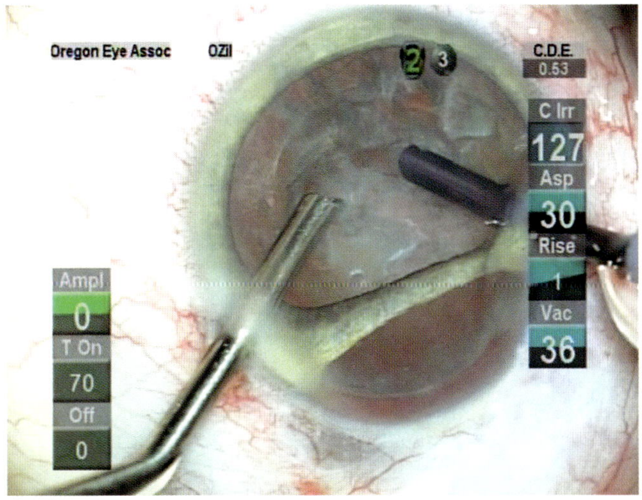

Fig. 11: Initial chop of the cataract post 100° ciliary body excision for malignant melanoma

In this case, author and colleagues were able to perform biaxial microincision phacoemulsification through two microincisions on each side of the 100° of atrophic sclera and conjunctiva, and missing ciliary body and iris. The advantage here is that with the vitreous face open to the anterior chamber, they wanted to be drawing material toward the area of missing zonules, after having sequestered the vitreous in that area with Healon 5 (Advanced Medical Optics, Santa Ana, California). Phacoemulsification performed through an incision in other locations would bring vitreous to the phaco tip and provide a much more challenging situation. The IOL was implanted nasally over the intact zonules to force the lens to push against the capsular fornix in the area of missing zonules, rather than to pull away from the area of missing zonules if it had been implanted in the temporal periphery.

Intraoperative Floppy Iris Syndrome (Figs 12 to 16)

Author and colleagues find biaxial microincision phacoemulsification enormously useful in cases of intraoperative floppy iris syndrome (IFIS). If they have

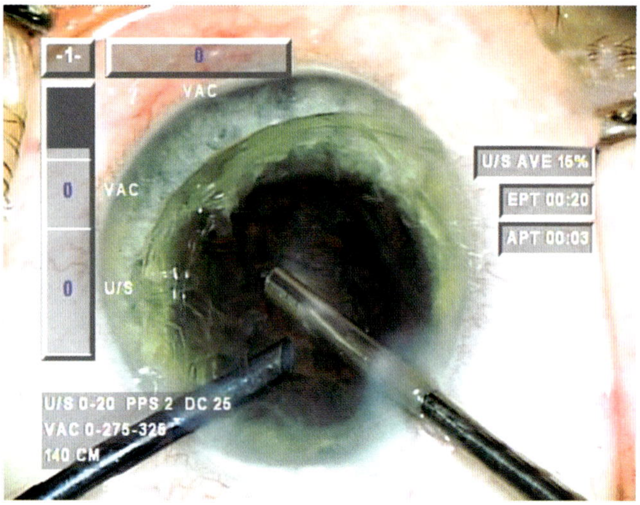

Fig. 12: Epinucleus holding the iris back after carouseling the endonucleus in the presence of intraoperative floppy iris syndrome (IFIS)

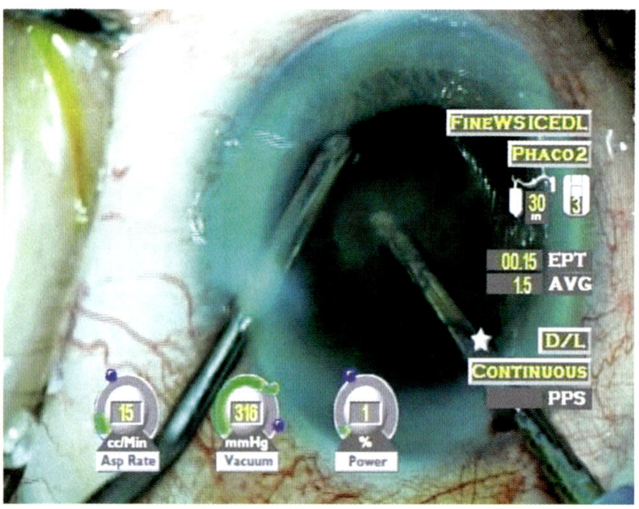

Fig. 13: Endonuclear disassembly in the anterior chamber with the irrigator tamponading the iris

adequate dilation in the presence of a floppy iris, they will perform gentle cortical cleaving hydrodelineation and hydrodissection, and then hydroexpress the lens into the plain of the iris. They will then carousel the endonucleus in the plain of the capsulorhexis with the irrigating cannula held high in the anterior chamber. Holding the irrigator high in the anterior chamber allows for a tamponading of the iris by the fluid which then disallows floppiness, or billowing, of the iris. After removing the endonucleus in the plain of the capsulorhexis, they see a fully intact epinuclear shell, which had been sitting on top of the iris, helping to hold it back. This is an extremely advantageous technique for nuclei of less hard densities that can be carouselled and phacoed in the anterior chamber without threatening the corneal endothelium.

For harder cataracts, and in the presence of pupils that will not dilate well, they will dilate the pupil with Healon 5, do a rather large capsulorhexis and then do one endolenticular chop. They then keep the irrigating chopper high in the anterior chamber and with the unsleeved phaco tip, bring nuclear material up to the chopper held high in the anterior chamber for further disassembly. This allows, once again, a tamponading of the iris and prevention of billowing or floppiness. They try to keep the phaco needle occluded and in foot position two or three, but with a clearance of occlusion, they go to foot position one in order to minimize evacuation of Healon 5, which is holding the pupil open.

After the endonucleus is removed in this way, they remove the epinucleus. Since it is harder to keep the tip occluded with epinuclear trimming and flipping, there tends to be evacuation of Healon 5 and a reduction of the size of the pupil, although because of the irrigator held high in the anterior chamber, it does not billow. Author and colleagues then have to re-instill Healon 5 to expand the bag and redilate the pupil prior to cortical clean-up. Then, once again, holding the irrigator high in the anterior chamber, they keep the aspirating microincision handpiece occluded by going circumferentially around the capsulorhexis, with the port facing the capsule fornix, removing the cortical material from only the fornix of the capsule, letting it sit as a cluster in the central portion of the capsule. After all of the cortex has been mobilized from the capsular fornix, author and colleagues remove the residual cortex from the eye. In this way, they are able to keep Healon 5 in the eye and disallow miosis of the pupil until the case is complete.

In some cases, the pupil is intractably small and won't respond to Healon 5 expansion. In these cases, author and colleagues may use a pupil expander ring (Morcher Pupil Expander Ring, Type 5S, FCI Ophthalmics, Marshfield Hills, MA; or a Malyugin Ring, Catalog # MAL-0001, MicroSurgical Technology, Redmond, WA). These are implanted through a 2.5 mm clear corneal incision to enlarge the pupil (Fig. 14), after which biaxial phacoemulsification is then performed through the two side-port incisions and the larger incision remains sealed during the operation because of its self-sealing construction and architecture. The pupil expander rings are advantageous because the pupil can be moved away from the incisions just by pushing on the ring.

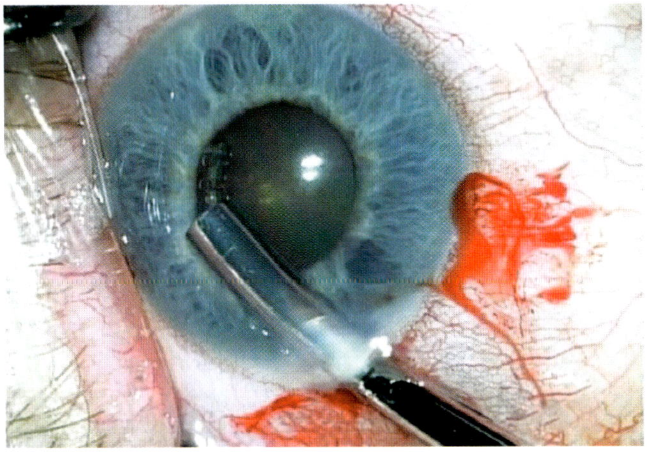

Fig. 14: A Morcher Pupil Expander Ring (Type 5S, FCI Ophthalmics, Marshfield Hills, MA) is injected through a 2.5 mm clear corneal incision

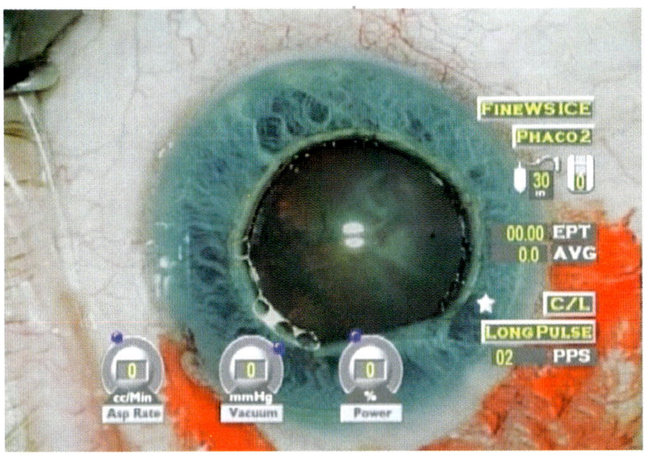

Fig. 15: The Morcher Pupil Expander Ring in place

With the ring in place (Fig. 15), author and colleagues have found in some cases that they were unable to adequately perform hydrodissection or hydrodelineation. If they cannot perform our hydrosteps because of the tendency for the pupil to extrude, they will use a bevel-down phaco tip to bowl out the center of the cataract, and then do inside-out hydrodelineation, as described by Abhay Vasavada.[14] They then chop the residual endonucleus in the usual fashion, and then remove the epinucleus as well.

In some cases, they may perform subincisional cortical removal by using a coaxial irrigation handpiece in the 2.5 mm incision to hold the iris back, while going to a distal location through a microincision with a 0.2 mm port aspirator to remove the subincisional cortex (Fig. 16). This has been very efficacious.

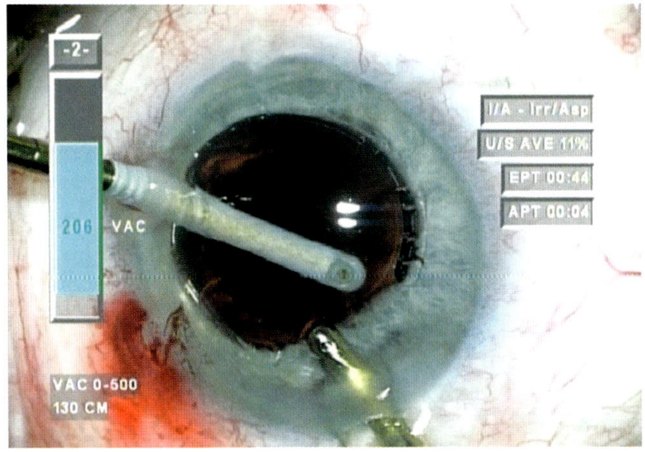

Fig. 16: The use of a coaxial irrigation handpiece with a micro aspirator to remove subincisional cortex

Every Small Pupil must be Viewed as a Potential Intraoperative Floppy Iris Syndrome

They believe that every small pupil must be viewed as a potential floppy iris case because there have now been identified multiple other drugs and neutraceuticals that have anti-alpha-1A properties and therefore which create an intraoperative floppy iris syndrome. They no longer stretch small pupils because if they become IFIS cases they have exacerbated the floppiness by disrupting the only portion of the iris (the pupil) which retains structural integrity. The only exceptions to that are pupils that are bound down by inflammatory pupillary membranes, or that have a long history of exposure to miotic drops, and a clear absence of medications that might produce a floppy iris.

Iris Bombé (Figs 17 to 20)

For pupils that are completely bound down by a pupillary membrane, they will use biaxial phacoemulsification. Commencing with a small iridotomy peripherally, close to one of the microincisions (Fig. 17), Viscoat® is used to elevate the iris and its cannula to sweep the pupillary membrane from the anterior lens capsule. Author and colleagues then stretch the pupillary membrane in one direction and the iris just distal to the pupillary membrane in the opposite direction in the same meridian (Fig. 18). This results in a lysing of the pupillary membrane for several clock hours from the pupil itself, and allows us to go back, and using tangential forces with a microincision

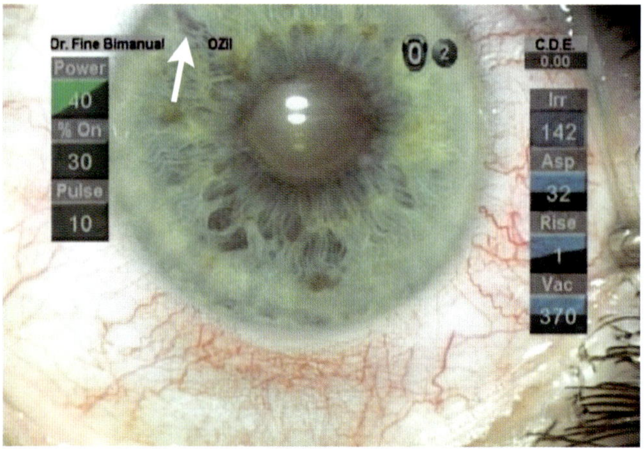

Fig. 17: Preoperative image of an eye with a bound down pupillary membrane. Arrow indicates small, peripheral iridotomy.

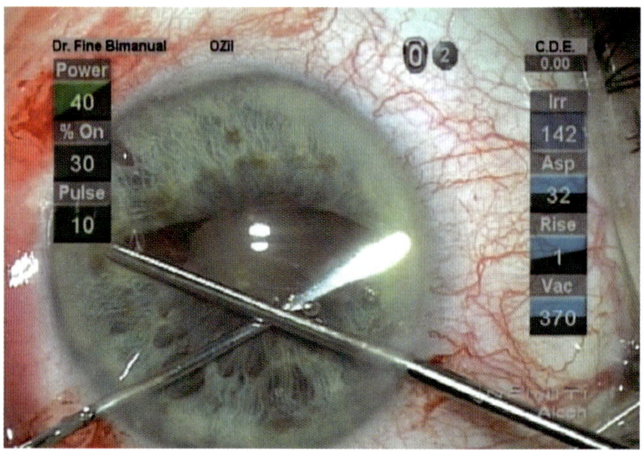

Fig. 18: Stretching the pupillary membrane in one direction and the iris just distal to the pupillary membrane in the opposite direction in the same meridian

capsulorhexis forceps, strip the pupillary membrane from the pupil (Figs 19 and 20). Following this, Healon 5 allows for maximum dilation of the pupil and they proceed in the usual manner.

Very Shallow Anterior Chambers (Fig. 21)

For very shallow anterior chambers biaxial phacoemulsification is also a great advantage because the instruments are indeed smaller and fit more readily in the eye; however, if the anterior chambers are too shallow (Fig. 21) they perform a 25 gauge transcleral pars plana vitrectomy, before proceeding with biaxial phacoemulsification. It is very important in using these microvitrectors to use a finger of the non-dominant hand to maintain tactile contact with

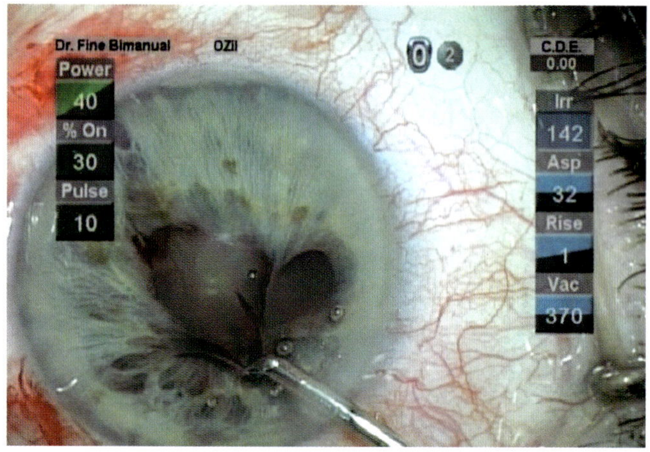

Fig. 19: Stripping the pupillary membrane

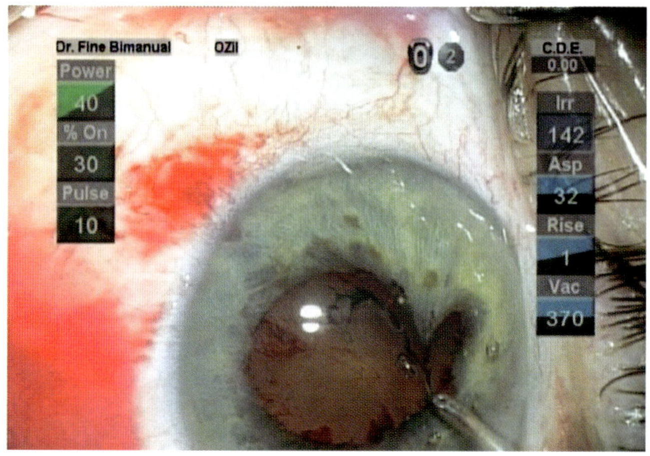

Fig. 20: Releasing the last adhesion of the pupillary membrane

the eye, so that one doesn't over-soften the eye. These vitrectors are capable of between 1,200 and 1,500 cuts per minute. In spite of their small gauge, unless care is taken, one can overly soften the eye, retroplacing the lens and creating new difficulties and challenges.

Refractive Lens Exchange (Figs 22 to 25)

Author and colleagues can do refractive lens exchange very easily, and safely, with biaxial microincision phacoemulsification. Author and colleagues do cortical cleaving hydrodissection and no hydrodelineation. They then hydroexpress the lens into the plain of the capsulorhexis, and carousel it, without any phacoemulsification energy for soft lenses, usually encountered in refractive lens exchange (Figs 22 and 23). They do an entirely fluidic-

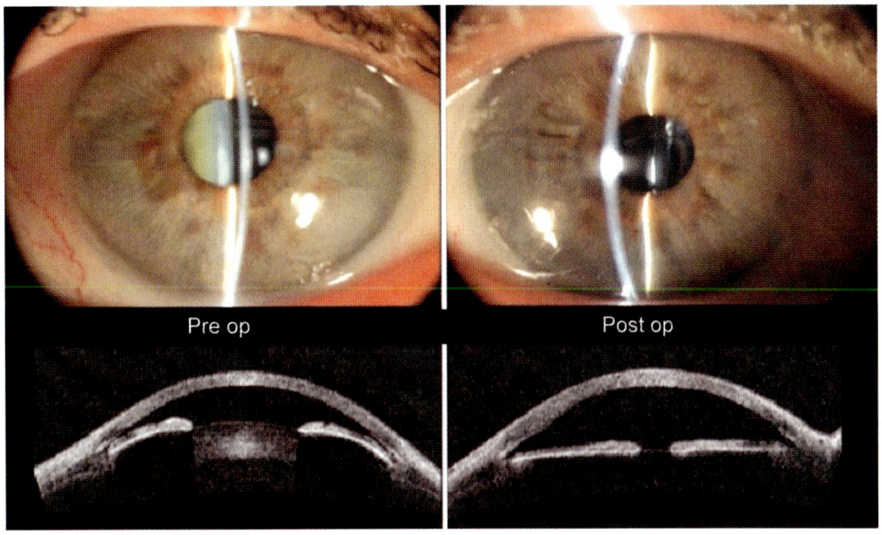

Fig. 21: Preoperative slit-lamp and optical coherence tomography (OCT) images of a very shallow anterior chamber. The post-operative images demonstrate the increase in anterior chamber depth due to the 25 gauge transcleral pars plana vitrectomy

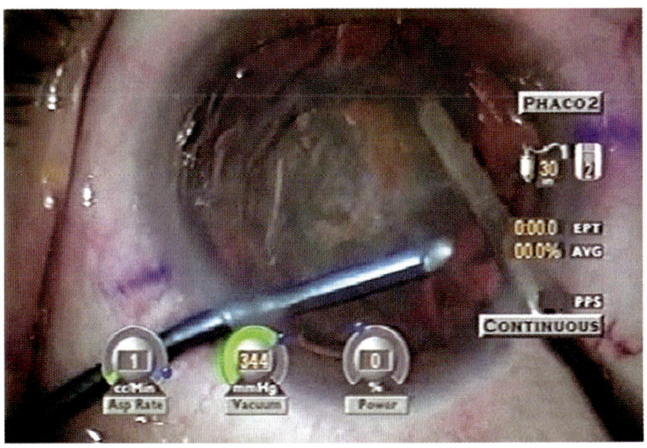

Fig. 22: Carouselling the nucleus in refractive lens exchange without using any phacoemulsification energy

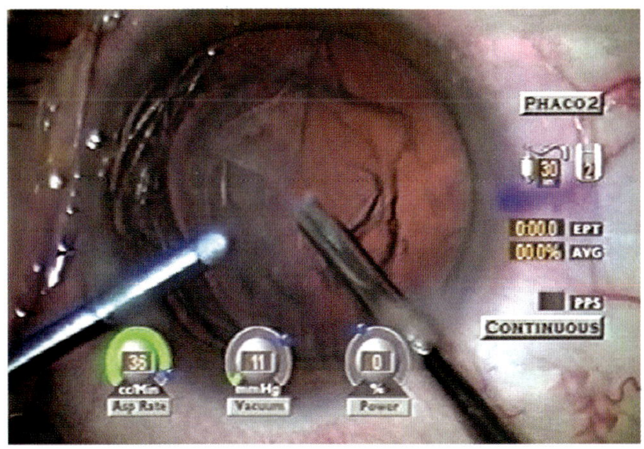

Fig. 23: Endonucleus removal complete with only cortex remaining. No phacoemulsification energy was used to remove the endonucleus

based extraction and then, because of cortical cleaving hydrodissection, they are able to evacuate the cortex by just tilting the phaco tip back into the posterior chamber where it jumps into the phaco tip as a single piece (Figs 24 and 25).

Refractive Lens Exchange in Post Radial Keratotomy (Fig. 26)

In cases where previous radial keratotomy (RK) has been performed, they can do biaxial microincision clear lens or cataract removal by going between two previously placed radials, making it much less likely that they will rupture the radial incisions during the course of the lens extraction. They then make an incision between our two microincisions for implantation of the IOL, but in the presence of previous RK, they make it through the posterior limbus for implantation of the IOL.

Intraocular Cautery (Fig. 27)

They have found that they can, with biaxial microincision instruments, do intraocular cautery by using an irrigating cannula in one of the microincisions and a microincision bipolar cautery in the other. Pinching the irrigation tubing allows bleeding to take place, clearly identifying the point

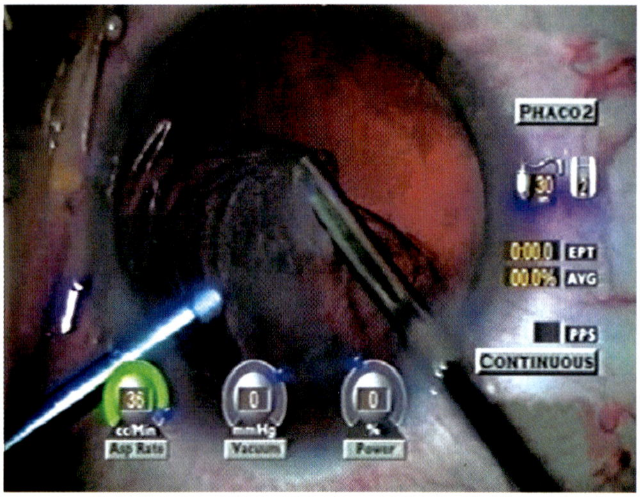

Fig. 24: Removing cortex in refractive lens exchange by tilting the phaco tip back into the posterior chamber.

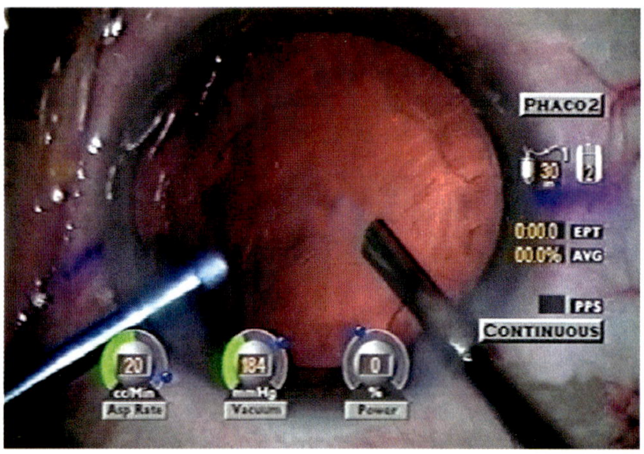

Fig. 25: Cortex completely removed

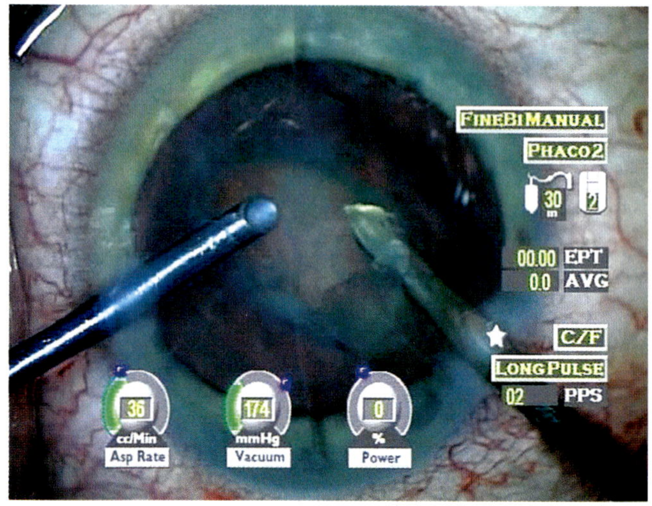

Fig. 26: Bimanual microincision phacoemulsification of a cataract between radial keratotomy incisions

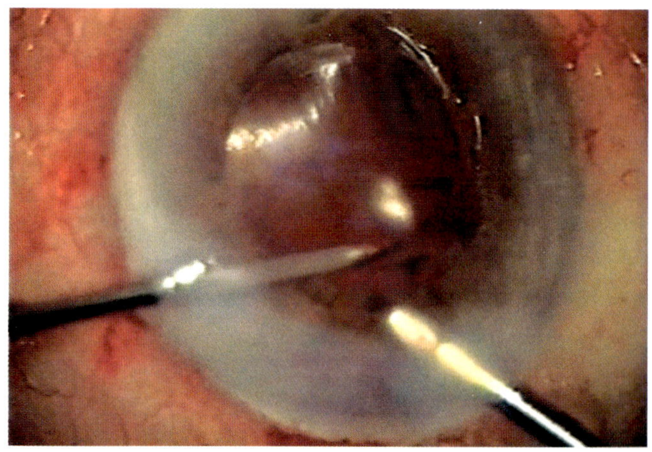

Fig. 27: Bipolar intraocular microcauterization with easy identification of the bleeding point by pinching the infusion tubing

source because the eye softens and the bleeding points start to ooze. They cauterize them precisely with the bipolar cautery, and therefore, minimize trauma to intraocular structures by avoiding more cautery than is necessary.[15]

Biaxial Microincision Instruments (Figs 28 and 29)

There are a number of other instruments that have been developed for use through 1.1 mm microincisions. Iris reconstruction is very much easier utilizing intraocular forceps that stabilize the iris for suturing. New intraocular needle holders are also usable through a 1.0 mm incision. In this way, very fragile and atrophic irides can be sutured without putting excessive stress on the iris tissue. The knots are tied with a Siepser external tying mechanism,[16] and the knots are cut with an intraocular microincision scissors, which is also admissible through a 1.0 mm incision.

For late reopening of capsular bags to recenter IOLs, author and colleagues can enlarge a capsulorhexis in the late postoperative period by nicking the rhexis with a microincision intraocular scissors, and then tearing a larger opening with a microincision capsulorhexis forceps. Viscodissection of the lens,[17] within the capsular bag, can be accomplished through microincisions which also allow for repositioning of IOLs without the need to make larger incisions to manipulate them intraocularly. There are currently additional microincision instruments under

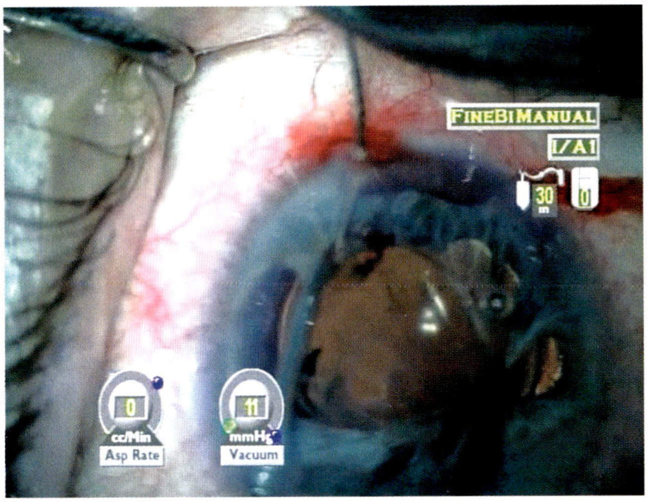

Fig. 28: Suturing of atrophic iris using microincision intraocular forceps

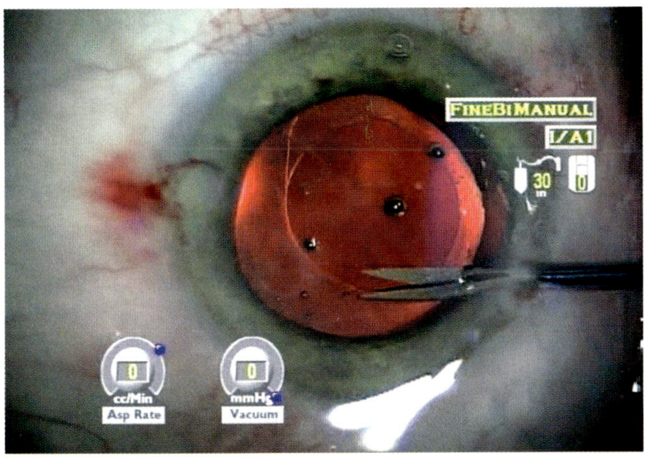

Fig. 29: Nicking the capsulorhexis with microincision scissors prior to enlarging the capsulorhexis

a state of development, including microincision Colibri forceps, microincision iris graspers, and microincision intraocular lens holders and cutters.

Take Home Pearls

Author and colleagues believe biaxial microincision phacoemulsification is a technique that has a very short learning curve, is highly atraumatic, and is unquestionably the technique of the future. For those who are willing to go through the short learning curve now, it represents the best and safest technique at present for the management of certain difficult and challenging cases.

- The separation of infusion from aspiration and ultrasound energy allows us to use the incoming fluid wave as a unique instrument to hold back floppy irides.
- Author and colleagues can sequester the anterior segment from the posterior segment in cases of ruptured capsules and zonular dialyses.
- Is especially useful in situations in which the smaller instrumentation of biaxial phacoemulsification are required, such as in high hyperopia, small eyes, and crowded anterior chambers.
- Has unique advantages in high myopia and posterior polar cataracts.
- New instrumentation facilitates
  - repositioning decentered lenses in fibrosed capsules;
  - control of bleeding pre-, intra- and post-operatively;
  - intraocular suturing, especially following iris trauma.

References

1. Fine IH, Alio JL, Hoffman R, et al. Biaxial microincision phacoemulsification for difficult and challenging cases. In: Jorge L Alió, Fine IH (Eds). Minimizing Incisions and Maximizing Outcomes in Cataract Surgery. New York: Springer Science+Business Media; 2010. pp. 163-74.
2. Girard LJ. Ultrasonic fragmentation for cataract extraction and cataract complications. Adv Ophthalmol. 1978;37: 127-35.
3. Shearing SP, Relyea RL, Loaiza A, et al. Routine phacoemulsification through a one-millimeter non-sutured incision. Cataract. 1985; 2:6-10.
4. Hara T, Hara T. Endocapsular phacoemulsification and aspiration (ECPEA) – recent surgical technique and clinical results. Ophthalmic Surgery. 1989;20(7):469-75.
5. Tsuneoka H, Shiba T, Takahashi Y. Feasibility of ultrasound cataract surgery with a 1.4 mm incision. J Cataract Refract Surg. 2001;27:934-40.
6. Agarwal A, Agarwal A, Agarwal S, et al. Phakonit: phacoemulsification through a 0.9 mm corneal incision. J Cataract Refract Surg. 2001;27(10):1548-52.
7. Tsuneoka H, Shiba T, Takahashi Y. Ultrasonic phacoemulsification using a 1.4 mm incision: Clinical results. J Cataract Refract Surg. 2002;28:81-6.
8. Tsuneoka H, Hayama A, Takahama M. Ultra small-incision bimanual phacoemulsification and AcrySof SA30AL implantation through a 2.2 mm incision. J Cataract Refract Surg. 2003;29(6):1070-6.
9. Fine IH, Packer M, Hoffman RS. Power modulations in new technology: Improved outcomes. J Cataract Refract Surg. 2004;30:1014-9.

10. Fine IH, Hoffman RS, Packer M. Optimizing refractive lens exchange with bimanual microincision phacoemulsification. J Cataract Refract Surg. 2004;30:550-4.
11. Osher RH, Yu BC-Y, Koch DD. Posterior polar cataracts: a predisposition to intraoperative posterior capsule rupture. J Cataract Refract Surg. 1990;16:157-62.
12. Vasavada AR, Sing R. Phacoemulsification in posterior polar developmental cataracts. In: Lu LW, Fine IH. Phacoemulsification in Difficult and Challenging Cases. New York: Thieme; 1999. pp. 121-8.
13. Aravind H, Aravind S, Vadi K, Natchair G. Bimanual microphaco for posterior polar cataracts. J Cataract Refract Surg. 2006; 32(6):914-7.
14. Vasavada AR, Raj SM. Inside-out delineation. J Cataract Refract Surg. 2004;30(6):1167-9.
15. Fine IH, Hoffman RS, Packer M. Bimanual bipolar diathermy for recurrent hyphema following anterior segment intraocular surgery. J Cataract Refract Surg. 2004;30(9):2017-20.
16. Seipser SB. The closed chamber slipping suture technique for iris repair. Ann Ophththal. 1994;26(3):71-2.
17. Fine IH, Hoffman RS. Late reopening of fibrosed capsular bags to reposition decentered intraocular lenses. J Cataract Refract Surg. 1997;23:990-4.

20 Complications in Phaco; How to Deal with Them

Luis Felipe Vejarano-Restrepo (Colombia)

Problems Constructing the Incision

Complications may arise from a faulty constructed incision. If the tunnel is too long (longer than 2.00 mm) passing the phaco tip through it and turning the tip downward to perform the procedure creates undue striae and makes visualization difficult. Surgeons can get oarlocked as they try to manipulate the phaco needle. Moreover, the increased wound distortion will pose the risk of incisional burn, as author will discuss later.

The tunnel can be too short (shorter than 1.4 mm) with a premature entry into the anterior chamber. The anterior chamber will tend to shallow, which can itself cause problems. Moreover, it is easier that iris prolapse occurs. To avoid this situation angle somewhat anteriorly the blade when making the tunnel.

Using dull blades (it is no matter if they are made of diamond or sapphire) may cause the incision roof to tear when surgeons direct the tip of the blade downward to the anterior chamber. If surgeons feel that they will need to apply too much pressure in order to make the blade enter into the anterior chamber, stop and change it. It is better to use a sharp metal blade than a dull diamond blade.

Sometimes during the clear cornea incision construction irregular cut at the corners (dog-ears) may be formed. Usually they do not pose additional problems, but a way to avoid them is to make initially a groove of around 250 microns before entering the blade to construct the tunnel. If surgeons are planning to wide the incision to insert a rigid polymethylmethacrylate (PMMA) they will have to suture it, and this technique allows a better apposition of the wound edges.[1] If the incision is so poor that it really can't be fixed, abandon it. Hydrate it or suture it and move to a new location and make a fresh incision.

Incisional Burns

The technique of lens extraction by phacoemulsification has revolutionized cataract surgery. However, the production of ultrasound energy is associated with heat generation that can result in ocular tissue damage. Incisional burns are a risk whenever surgeons use an ultrasound tip.[2-3] The cause of an incisional burn is heat transfer from the needle to the tissue surrounding it; the degree of injury is directly related to the total amount of heat absorbed.

Higher phaco power and a longer duration of phaco time (especially when using continuous mode) tend to increase the needle temperature Therefore, the judicious use of phaco energy at lower power settings, the use of pulsed or burst modes, and the new options of turning off the energy during a period of time through the cycle of pulses, [WhiteStar´s cool phaco (AMO Sovereign) or Infiniti´s duty cycle and Legacy´s Everest software (Alcon)] or using hybrid phaco technology [NeoSoniX (Infiniti & Legacy; Alcon) and Staar Sonic Wave System] will also help reduce the risks for corneal burns. A critical issue is the presence of an effective cooling of the needle and the tissue during the ultrasound energy delivery, which is achieved by the flow of irrigation fluid inside the barrel of the phaco needle (aspiration flow rate) and, more important, outside the needle (irrigation through the silicone sleeve) and outside the sleeve (fluid leaking through the incision). In standard phacoemulsification the wound size is big enough to allow the passage of the tip and the sleeve, but the outflow through the incision is very little (to avoid an unstable anterior chamber). Since the flexible irrigation sleeve fills the wound, it reduces even more the flow around the sleeve, particularly in a tight wound. In this setting a complete occlusion of aspiration and therefore complete blockage of irrigation may result in a wound burn.

When the incision is too tight, the irrigation sleeve is compressed against the phaco needle and against the tissue around it, and so there will be contact between the tip and the sleeve and there will not be cooling fluid separating the needle from the corneal tunnel (a similar situation may occur when the phaco needle is pressed against the wound due to an excessively steep approach). It has been shown that the position of the needle in the incision is a very important factor in temperature increase. Experimentally using three different tips, when in the primary position, the temperature remained under 36°C, but when the tips were in the roofing position, a marked temperature increase (51.4°C) was observed with the standard tip; with the MicroTip, a temperature increase occurred but was lower than with the standard tip; with the Mackool tip, the temperature remained stable. The temperature around the incision site increased with all tips when they were moved toward the corner of the incision, which resulted in direct contact with the silicone sleeve. This change was most obvious with the standard tip (temperature 51.5° C), and a wound burn was observed. With the MicroTip, the temperature increase was moderate (44.2°C), and the wound burn area was smaller. With the Mackool tip, the temperature increased the least (42.1°C).[4] This direct relation between the position of the phaco tip and thermal injury, was also shown by Tsuneoka in an experimental study in porcine eyes, and indicates that it is advisable to keep the tip in a central primary position, avoiding roofing or flanking it too much (to limit the temperature buildup due to friction between the tip and the sleeve, that will be transmitted to the adjacent tissue). For the same reason, it is important to make the incision not too tight.[5] Some strategies have been used to design safer phaco needles. The Mackool phaco tip (Alcon) has a rigid polyamide outer sleeve designed to decrease heat buildup and transfer, whereas The MicroFlow® tip (Bausch & Lomb, Claremont, Calif., USA) designed by Barrett has a series of longitudinal grooves that ensures infusion even if the sleeve is compressed.[6] Measures that serve to cause the least wound distortion and so the least needle/sleeve/tissue compression, include: temporal approach, avoiding an excessively long corneal tunnel, and minimizing excess lifting or depression of the handpiece. One option in cases of deep set eyes is the angulated tip such as the Kelman.

Although the theoretical risk of incisional burns is also present when using sleeveless microincisional phacoemulsification, no one case has been reported. Moreover experimentally, it has been shown that ultrasound phacoemulsification produced almost no temperature elevation at the incision site as long as the infusion liquid was adequately circulated around the ultrasound tip, even when the tip was in contact with the 1.4 mm incision corner.[6] In other experiment using cool phaco with a bare 19 gauge aspiration needle in human cadaver eyes, a wound burn could not be produced at the highest energy settings unless all flow into the eye and all aspiration were occluded. These settings are well beyond clinically applicable conditions.[7] In 305 eyes reported by Agarwal and 637 eyes reported by Tsuneoka, no one had clinically significant burns.[8,9] At equilibrium, additional irrigation fluid will not enter the eye unless fluid or other materials, such as viscoelastic or the lens material, leave the eye. In an experimental study both the cohesive and dispersive viscoelastic agents were associated with a delay from the onset of phaco power to the onset of irrigation flow, and this lack of irrigation and aspiration resulted in the greatest thermal rise and caused wound damage.[10] For these reasons, it is very important that just after entering the phaco needle to the anterior chamber full of viscoelastic, to aspirate for a while to ensure irrigation and aspiration flow, before the onset of phacoemulsification power.

It is important to watch for the production of a "milky" material while emulsifying the nucleus, which suggests poor irrigation and aspiration and, therefore, poor cooling. This is a warning sign indicating that a thermal injury may ensue if ultrasound is not stopped and the problem is not solved.

Generally, the burn associated with phacoemulsification involves primarily the roof of the incision. It has a spectrum from a slight graying or whitening of the corneal tissue, which rarely has any lasting consequence, to collagen shrinking and extensive whitening of the anterior lip of the wound resulting in gaping that may lead difficulties with wound closure and different amounts of astigmatism.

Shallow Anterior Chamber

Some eyes have anatomically a shallow anterior chamber. In these cases, it is very important to use viscoelastics to deepen the anterior chamber, but in eyes with extremely crowded anterior segments it could be difficult, and if too much viscoelastic is injected, the intraocular pressure (IOP) will overly increase and may cause iris prolapse. Chang has described that an automated pars plana vitreous tap is useful to expand the anterior segment when extremely shallow anterior chambers do not deepen sufficiently with viscoelastic injection alone.[11]

When occurring during the procedure shallowing is due to either extraocular or intraocular causes. To determine the origin, touch the eye gently and feel the IOP. If the eye is soft, the problem is external. It may be a tight lid speculum or tight drapes, or there may be problems in the incision (leakage) that will need sutures. If the IOP is high, either it may be a fluid misdirection syndrome. The cause of the misdirection is the presence of zonular dialysis that allows fluid to flow around the equator into the vitreous. Check with the anesthesiologist if there is no cardiovascular contraindications, and use mannitol (0.75–1 gm/kg) intravenously to dehydrate the vitreous. It will take

10–15 minutes to lower the IOP. If it does not work, other option is to perform a sclerotomy to try to drain misdirected liquid from vitreous cavity. Lower the bottle and decrease flow rates to achieve a lower flow-type emulsification to diminish the risk of fluid going back through the zonules and rehydrating the vitreous. If the IOP remains high after these measurements, it could be the result of a suprachoroidal effusion/hemorrhage. Use indirect ophthalmoscope to confirm the diagnosis. Fortunately with small incision cataract surgery, it is improbable that an effusion turns into an expulsive hemorrhage, but to tamponade it surgeons need to close the eye, placing sutures. Never enlarge the incision trying to finish the case. The procedure must be finished in a second stage.

Lens-Iris Diaphragm Retropulsion Syndrome: Excessive Anterior Chamber Deepening

Lens-iris diaphragm retropulsion syndrome (LIDRS) is characterized by anterior chamber deepening, pupil dilation and concave shape of the iris. The excessively deep chamber makes the surgery technically more challenging and painful for the patient under topical anesthesia. Cionni and Osher theorize that it is caused by a reverse pupillary block, and so must be solved equalizing the fluid pressure between the anterior chamber and the posterior chamber. They indicate that it can be managed simply separating the iris from the anterior capsule rim with the phaco needle, the irrigation/aspiration (I/A) tip or any other second instrument. The iris immediately returns to a more physiologic position with correction of the chamber depth.[12]

Detached Descemet Membrane

This uncommon complication may occur during a manipulation of the wound including injection of viscoelastic, implantation of an intraocular lens (IOL), passing of instruments into the eye or enlargement of the incision. When using dull blades, they instead of sharply incising Descemet's membrane, may catch it and push it ahead of them.

When small it is usually asymptomatic, but when it is severe enough will cause corneal edema. A large Descemet detachment may appear to be a retrocorneal membrane; however, this is contiguous with the normal Descemet detachment and endothelium in the periphery. The differential diagnosis includes a residual fragment of anterior capsule.

The clue to avoid this complication is a careful placement of instruments inside the eye. Try to avoid pressing forcefully the phaco tip. A newly designed irrigation sleeve (Microsmooth® Alcon) with a more slippery material, may diminish the friction when entering through the wound. Before injecting anything (viscoelastics, balanced salt solution, air) the surgeon must be sure that the tip of the cannula is in the anterior chamber, well beyond the incision, and not dissecting the Descemet. If, upon placing an instrument within the eye, the surgeon feels unusual resistance, the instrument should be retracted and wound size or visualization should be improved before the instrument is again placed into the anterior chamber. If surgeons have caught a piece of the membrane, the careful placement and removal of instruments becomes critical for the remainder of the procedure. For an intraoperatively diagnosed detachment, involving not more than one-fourth of the corneal area, the surgeon may make a stab incision in a location away from the wound, and inject air or a viscoelastic into the eye to force the membrane back to its original position. An injection of air at the end of the procedure may help to keep the Descemet reattached, by compressing it to the cornea. However for large detachments, encompassing one-third or more of the corneal surface area, the best option is repositioning it surgically. A patient with this condition usually presents on the first postoperative day with a significant amount of corneal edema that does not resolve.

The Descemet membrane can be reattached to the cornea using 10-0 monofilament sutures passed through the cornea, according with the classic technique described by Vastine.[13] The surgeon may make a new paracentesis site at the limbus, to get a good approach to a site in the anterior chamber where to inject air or a viscoelastic to push the detached Descemet membrane into its proper position; then places the sutures starting posterior to the limbus, passing anteriorly into the anterior chamber, through Descemet and into the cornea stroma.

Other alternative is the injection of sulfur hexafluoride gas[14] which may be used at the time of surgery or afterward if surgeons notice a detachment postoperatively. The risk is the IOP increase, so it is mandatory to monitor it. A very good description of the procedure has been done by Dr Fishkind.[15] A new technique for intracameral gas injection that can be performed by one person at the slit lamp microscope or in a minor operating room with minimal equipment has been described.[16]

Capsulorhexis Related Complications

The anterior continuous curvilinear capsulorhexis (CCC) should be capable of preserving the integrity of the capsular bag against the asymmetric forces that occur during phacoemulsification and IOL implantation.

In regard with surgeon's control, a larger diameter capsulorhexis is more challenging because the anterior capsular contour more dramatically slopes away from the instrument as it moves toward the periphery. Because of this, a smaller rhexis should be attempted if difficulty with visualization or control is encountered. If necessary, surgeons may enlarge it in a second maneuver. Always remember that when in the periphery, the capsulorhexis tear can encounter a zonular attachment that can work as a straight edge, sending the tear out to the capsular fornix and possibly around and through the posterior capsule. Once an errant tear begins to extend radially it becomes much harder to control.

Because pediatric anterior capsules are very elastic, these capsulorhexis are among the most difficult to achieve, since after pulling the leading edge the resulting tear is overly rapid and tends to advance away from, rather than toward, the grasping instrument. A recent study showed that the new viscoadaptative agent Healon 5 (sodium hyaluronate, 2.3%) appears to lead to a higher CCC completion rate in children.[17]

It is crucial to keep the anterior chamber pressurized, so that the anterior face of the lens is flattened. The most common cause of anterior capsule convexity is intraoperative anterior chamber shallowing due to egress of fluid or viscoelastic through the wound due to an excessive instrument pressure on the posterior incision lip, or an over-sized incision or a tight lid speculum, which may cause vector forces in the anterior segment such that the lens pushes forward and the capsulorhexis tends to tear outward. Interrupting the rhexis to refill the anterior chamber with viscoelastic and solving the problem (sutures in the wound, repositioning the lid speculum) is important in this situation. A shallow anterior chamber may also be the natural result of a small globe. Moreover in cases of white hypermature cataracts, if there is liquefied cortex, the resulting intralenticular fluid pressure may also encourage peripheral extension of the capsular tear, and in this setting it is even more important to keep the anterior capsule flattened. Cohesive viscoelastics perform better in flattening the anterior capsule surface than dispersive viscoelastics, but dispersives are more retentive. Using both of them with the Arshinoff's soft shell technique is a good option[18].

The farther the capsule forceps is from the tearing point, the more difficult it is to direct the tear. If this starts to happen, the flap must be regrasped closer to the leading edge of the tear. Regrasp frequently, at least at every three clock hour of circumference, to optimize control of the base of the flap. It is very important in order to guide the flap and to monitor the direction of the tear as it develops. Delayed recognition of a peripherally escaping tear may preclude any chance to redirect it in time. Surgeons are not in a rush; a couple of minutes inverted in performing carefully the capsulorhexis are well worthwhile.

In white and brunescent cataracts capsule may be very thin and friable, and due to the presence of a poor red reflex or even absence of it, it is difficult to distinguish the capsule from the cortex and to follow the leading edge. Other causes of poor visualization are decreased corneal clarity, small pupils, anterior cortical opacity (spokes), and vitreous opacities such as asteroid hyalosis or hemorrhage. Currently the best way to maximize visualization, and so improve control, is using an anterior capsule staining method. Trypan blue 0.05–0.1%, gentian violet 0.001%, indocyanine green (ICG) 0.5%, fluorescein 2%, and the patient's autologous blood may be used, but it has been shown that trypan blue, ICG and gentian violet are more effective in staining the capsule.[19-21] Although author used gentian violet 0.01% in more than 500 cases, author had one case of corneal edema probably related with the dye (wrong dilution?), and now author prefers for safety reasons to use trypan blue 0.05%.

There are several techniques to use this dye. In one the anterior chamber is filled with air and several drops of dye from a 1 mL syringe are placed through a 30 gauge cannula directly onto the anterior capsule surface. The air is then exchanged for viscoelastic and the capsulotomy is performed in the usual manner. Due to the good tolerance and very good staining capabilities of trypan blue 0.05%, surgeons may obviate the initial air, injecting the dye directly into the anterior chamber, just after performing the side port incision. It will dilute in the aqueous humor, but by the time that surgeons replace it with viscoelastic, around ten seconds later, the capsule is already stained. Other option is to use the Arshinoff's ultimate soft-shell technique, having the anterior chamber partially filled with Healon 5 and advancing the injecting cannula along the lens surface almost past its center.[22] Author has injected trypan blue over the lens surface, below other viscoelastics (methylcellulose 2%, Viscoat®) and it also works rather well, but the viscoelastics becomes stained in some degree, limiting visualization. Avoid injecting it forcefully in the periphery, since it may diffuse to the vitreous through weak zonules. Some surgeons inject the dye in the subcapsular space through a capsule puncture, but doing this into these frequently overly hydrated lenses might result in an uncontrolled capsular rip. Supracapsular dye application is sufficient, and avoids this potential complication.

Without a red reflex the anterior capsule edge cannot be visualized during sculpting or chopping and, especially in chopping techniques, there is the risk of tearing it with the instrument. Dye staining of the anterior capsule is also helpful in this sense, since the surgeon will be able to see the edge. The Vejarano´s safe chop, discussed in other section of this book, is a very good option to avoid damaging the anterior capsule edge during the phacoemulsification.

When a peripherally escaping tear occurs, the best way to rescue it is to refill the anterior chamber, fold the flap over the anterior capsule for better visualization, regrasp it close to the leading edge of the tear, and pull centripetally, rather firmly. If the tear redirects to the central area, follow the rhexis in the standard manner. If the tear extends more peripherally, stop, and initiate tear from the other direction attempting to connect the CCC from the other side. Sometimes surgeons will end up with a single radial tear in the capsulorhexis (tear drop shape). In this case surgeons must remember during the procedure that this area is weakened, and that the full extent of the radial tear is concealed by the iris, so surgeons cannot exert pressure on that area. A chopping technique would be preferable. Others advice using a cystotome to offset the forces transmitted to this weakened area makes numerous relaxing incisions in the capsulorhexis for 90°;[23] making a second radial tear 180° away or converting to a can-opener capsulotomy. Author thinks that usually these maneuvers are not necessary.

Other techniques have been described in this situations, like pushing the nucleus with a second blunt-tipped instrument through the side port incision, to make the anterior capsule more concave.[23]Gentle hydrodissection is important to minimize capsular stress with rotation. Place the needle or cannula for hydrodissection opposite, rather than in the region of the potentially torn capsule. Phaco chop can reduce capsular stress compared with sculpting techniques. Other alternative may be elevating the nucleus out of the capsular bag to the plane of the anterior chamber, where it can be emulsified.

Avoid pushing the optic toward the tear during IOL inserting maneuvers. If the position of the tear will cause that the leading haptic presses the weakened area, one can instead initially place the leading IOL haptic in the angle, and dial IOL into position by always decentering the optic away from the capsulorhexis tear.

Surge Control

When occluding the phaco tip, the nuclear fragment will cause the aspiration line´s vacuum to build up. In the moment that the occlusion is broken, and the fragments are rapidly aspirated, the fluid in the anterior chamber (which has reached a high pressure while the occlusion lasted) tends to rush into the aspiration line through the phaco tip, and the phenomena of surge may occur.

This situation is even more critical in phakonit/MICS cases, since the irrigation rate is always lower than in standard phacoemulsification. Surge control may be managed using several approaches and strategies that will be discussed below.

Some machines have additional features designed to diminish the possibility of surge. The AMO Prestige (Allergan, Irvine, California, USA) decreases its pump speed as the actual vacuum approaches the maximum vacuum preset.[24] Deflection of a flow-sensitive diaphragm on the aspiration side is translated into voltage, which decreases the pump speed when 50% of the targeted vacuum has been reached.[25] The Sovereign (Allergan, Irvine, California, USA) merges the advanced high vacuum fluidics of the AMO Prestige unit (Allergan, Irvine, California, USA) with the burst and occlusion mode programmability of the AMO Diplomax (Allergan, Irvine, California, USA). The Sovereign has an on-board fluidic computer that allows the pump to rotate forward and backward, which helps surgeons to control the release of vacuum. Microprocessors sample vacuum and flow parameters 50 times a second, create a "virtual" anterior chamber model. At the moment of surge, the machine's computer senses the increase in flow and instantaneously slows or reverses the pump to stop surge production.

Series 20000 Legacy (Alcon, Fort Worth, USA) has a pump system called TurboStalticTM pump that is a very smooth system, having a floating head so there are no pulsations as the pump speed and vacuum build-up takes place. It has non-compliant fluidic channels to allow for higher vacuum with fewer pulsations. The tubing in the cassette (MaxVacTM) has been replaced with rigid plastic fluidic channels that are totally non-compliant. It has the option of smaller aspiration tubing lumen, which providing increased fluidic resistance reduces total flow from the eye; that tubing has a thicker wall to reduce the compliance, and these features help to obtund surge, even using high vacuum. Author has found that this machine has a very good control of the surge phenomenon, but the Infiniti System (Alcon, Forth Worth, USA) possesses even superior fluidic capabilities: all fluid pathways in the instrument are composed of a rigid elastomeric membrane that improves fluid compliance. It features a noninvasive pressure sensor that provides real-time vacuum information to the computer, making it possible to use higher vacuums. The Infiniti's Fluid Management System (FMS) samples the vacuum precisely and responds to both directional and quantitative changes in pressure by altering the flow rate. The system can drop the flow rate from 100 cc/min to zero in several milliseconds. When no nuclear material is on the phaco tip, having a great deal of flow and vacuum is counterproductive and excessive turbulence is created for no purpose. This unique feature of the Infiniti increases the safety of the phacoemulsification procedure and also dramatically improves surgical efficiency.[26] The irrigation/ infusion sensor automatically compensates for the slight compliance that remains in the system. Infiniti also has a very useful capability, which lets surgeons know when the irrigation bottle is running dry.

The Storz Millenium® and Premiere® (Bausch & Lomb, Claremont, California, USA) also achieve low system compliance via the use of lower compliance tubing.[24] Moreover using the Millennium®, the dual linear foot pedal can be programed to separate both the flow and vacuum from power similar to Premiere on its posterior settings. In this way, flow or vacuum can be lowered before beginning the emulsification of an occluding fragment. The emulsification therefore occurs in the presence of a lower vacuum or flow so that surge is minimized. Separating simultaneous linear control of vacuum and ultrasound into two planes of pedal movement, with linear control of vacuum in phaco mode, the surgeon can approach material with safer lower vacuum levels and increase it only after desired material is positively engaged. Storz Millennium and Premiere machines pumps′ allow the surgeon to set a time delay for full commanded vacuum buildup which starts when the surgeon enters foot pedal position 2. However, once this delay has elapsed, any subsequent engagement of material will be exposed to a typically rapid vacuum pump rise time.[24]

Changes in phaco needle designs, to make them safer and more effective, have been developed as other alternatives to avoid or minimize surge. The standard 19 gauge phaco needle has an outer diameter of 1.12 mm and an inner diameter of 0.91 mm. It has a good holding power due to its large surface area, especially if beveled. However when the occlusion is broken, there is possibility of surge. To diminish this problem the Standard Microtip 20 gauge was designed, with 0.9 mm of outer diameter and 0.66 mm of inner diameter. The MicroFlow® tip (Bausch & Lomb, Claremont, California, USA) designed by Barrett[7] has an outer diameter of 1.07 mm (similar to a standard phaco needle), and although it has also an inner diameter of 0.9 mm at the end of the tip (again, similar to a standard phaco needle), it has a smaller shaft inner diameter (0.5 mm). This tip has a good holding force, but unlike a standard 1.12 phaco needle, it provides a fluidic resistance due to its smaller shaft inner diameter, avoiding sudden increment in flow levels, after breaking the occlusion, when emulsifying fragments.[24] It reduces this flow by about 40%. Moreover since the Microflow® design has an internal ring surface within the tip, perpendicular to the long axis of the needle and therefore to the direction of the movement of the tip while applying ultrasonic energy, produces additional cavitation.[24] It is possible, however, that after emulsifying some lens material, and when returning to position 2 in the foot pedal, the emulsified material plugs the shaft, which is only 0.5 mm in diameter, and aspiration may become compromised. When the surgeon notes that situation, it is necessary to apply a small amount of ultrasound energy (even if there is not lens material visible at the tip), just to make the tip vibrate, and solve the obstruction. Author's experience using the Microflow® has been very good in regard to surge control.

Other tip designs using a similar principle are the flared tips, like the MicroSeal®. There are two kinds of those, the Standard tip and Microtip, the outer diameter at the tip are 1.32 mm and 1.02 mm, and inner diameter are 1.07 mm and 0.82 mm respectively; the difference is that this needle has a smaller outer shaft diameter (0.76 mm) and a larger inner shaft diameter (0.57 mm) than the MicroFlow®.

Other approaches to the issue of surge have been to design a bypass port on the side of the phaco tip [Aspiration Bypass System—(ABS®)].The ABS® tips have 0.175–0.230 mm (depending if it is the microtip or standard tip) holes drilled in the shaft of the needle. During occlusion, the hole provides for a continuous alternate fluid flow, yielding a 4–11 cc/min, depending in the tip diameter and vacuum level. This will cause dampening of the surge on occlusion break. The ABS® port remains inactive as long as the main port is not occluded.

Currently surgeons also have options such as a high infusion sleeve (Alcon) to increase the inflow.

In order to avoid surge, manufacturers have resort to other approaches related with tubing. Since the amount of fluid that surges into the aspiration port is a function of the device's compliance, any fluid circuit component which was changed in volume by the high vacuum needs equilibration, for instance decreased tubing volume.[24]

If the tubing becomes constricted during the occlusion, it then expands on occlusion break, and this expansion is an additional source of vacuum production. This fluid may not be replaced rapidly enough by infusion to prevent shallowing of the anterior chamber. Thus having tubes reinforced to prevent collapse, with minimal compliance, will help to avert surge.

Of course they should still allow an ergonomic manipulation of the tubing/handpiece, as well as (in peristaltic pumps) allow the adequate functioning of the pump mechanism.[24] Some manufacturers have designed other especial tubing system to diminish the flow, coiled tubing that can help to slow the flow in the aspiration line, thus keeping the anterior chamber deep and stable. The outflow exiting from the eye is slowed by the resistance of the curvature of each concentric spiral in the tubing. Staar (Monrovia, California, USA) uses this system (UltraVac V1®).

Other options to obtund surge include devices designed to be placed in the way of the aspiration line. One of these is the Vacuum Surge Suppressor (VSS) (Surgin Inc., Tustin, California, USA). It is incorporated in the aspiration line and adjacent to the phaco handpiece, and regulates fluid flow out of the eye. As vacuum increases, VSS constricts, thereby limiting fluid outflow and maintaining a deep and stable anterior chamber.

The other device is the Cruise Control®, which has a very clever design developed by Staar (Monrovia, California, USA) featuring a flow restricting segment, 2 cm long with a 0.3 mm internal lumen, which reduces the vacuum surges generated during phaco. A micropore cylindrical filter captures nuclear material and removes all debris from the aspirated fluid before they can enter and clog the flow restricting segment. It increases the safety in standard phaco cases, making the procedure more forgiving for inflow/outflow imbalances, and so it is a very nice tool for the beginning surgeon, especially when entering in the field of chopping techniques, which present a higher risk of surge. It has also demonstrated to be very useful to perform the transition to microincisional bimanual phacoemulsification, where the surge issue is more critical.[27-30] It easily attaches to aspiration port on the phaco handpiece, and is compatible with peristaltic or venturi phaco machines. Cruise Control limits the flow in a non-linear manner such that only excessive flows are limited. Regular flow rates, below 50 cc/min, are not affected. Cruise Control works regardless of the size and configuration of phaco tips or tubing.

Of course it is possible to combine any anti-surge system with any tip, thus adding capabilities.

One important concept is that the surgeon should be changing settings throughout the course of the case.

As more of the nuclear material is removed and the posterior capsule is exposed, surge becomes a greater concern. The vacuum should be lowered for this phase. Beware of weak zonules, however, even the lower epinuclear vacuum setting may be too high if the zonules are lax. This is because the posterior capsule is able to "trampoline" toward the phaco tip if the weakened zonules do not keep it taut, and vacuum must be lowered even further in this event.[30, 31]

Zonular Problems

Weakened zonules will dehisce more easily. Forceful maneuvers of the nucleus may shear zonules. Aspirating the anterior capsule or adherent lens material may break the zonules in that location. Stripping the cortex tangentially rather than radially helps to distribute this force upon as large an area of zonules as possible. Moreover inadequate zonular tension allows trampolining of the flaccid posterior capsule during epinuclear and cortical cleanup.

Hydrodissection is a crucial step in avoiding stress applied to zonules, and cortical cleaving as described by Fine,[32] loosens the adhesion of the cortex to the capsule. The more easily the cortex separates from the capsule, the less likely a floppy capsule will be pulled toward the aspirating instrument tip.

Insertion of a capsular tension ring (CTR) is of tremendous help in the presence of zonular laxity. The CTR is available from two different sources (Morcher Capsular Tension Ring, FCI Ophthalmics; StabilEyes, Advanced Medical Optics Inc.). A simple ring of PMMA with an eyelet at either end, the ring may be inserted into the capsular bag to enhance stability and centration. This can be done at any point in the procedure following completion of the requisite capsulorhexis. Ring insertion can be accomplished using either forceps or a specially designed injector (Geuder).[33] In the presence of a focal zonular dehiscence or weakness, the ring redistributes capsular forces to areas of stronger zonular support. Another benefit is that the centrifugal pressure it applies makes the flaccid capsular bag tauter. To enjoy the intraoperative benefits of having the ring it should be inserted early following the rhexis, especially if the zonule is compromised.[34] However inserting it at the end will still bring benefits in the long term because it limits the postoperative capsule retraction and phimosis, which eyes with weak zonules are predisposed. There is also some evidence that CTRs may also retard posterior capsule opacification by mechanically blocking lens epithelial cell migration.[35] One drawback is that the presence of the CTR during phacoemulsification increases difficulty of cortical clean-up since the ring holds the cortex against the equatorial capsule and creates a counterforce to aspiration. In most cases this situation can be solved by stripping cortex tangentially rather than radially and using a 0.2 mm aspiration port to facilitate and maintain occlusion. The increased stability of the bag with the ring in place permits the use of fairly aggressive I/A without compromise to the capsule. Bimanual I/A works particularly well in this situation because it eliminates the uniquely challenging subincisional cortex removal process.

The CTR is helpful in any situation in the integrity of the zonular apparatus is in doubt. Pseudoexfoliation syndrome represents a primary indication, as do traumatic zonular dialysis and developmental subluxation of the lens (e.g. Marfan Syndrome). Axial length greater than 26 mm also is a relative indication due to potential instability of the posterior capsule and lower scleral rigidity; vitrectomized eyes may also benefit from placement of a CTR during cataract surgery.

CTRs should never be inserted if the capsulorhexis or posterior capsule is torn, since it can be directed out of the bag.

In the presence of zonular dialysis or extremely loose zonules, flexible microhook iris retractors can also be used to stabilize the capsular bag. Retractors are inserted through paracentesis openings in each of four quadrants to hook and fixate the capsulorhexis.[36,37]

Mackool, has designed titanium capsule retractors with hooked ends, which are elongated enough to support the peripheral capsular fornix as well as the capsulorhexis. Unlike CTRs, the capsule retractors provide excellent support in the anterior-posterior direction and do not trap the cortex (each retractor applies only point pressure to the capsular fornix without ensnaring the cortex). Called the capsule support system, these hooks are available in a reusable (Duckworth and Kent Ltd., Hertfordshire, England) or a single-use design (Impex, Staten Island, NY).[38] The usage of retractors may permit to delay the ring insertion until after the cortex has been removed, facilitating this step.[39]

In complex cases with very large zonular defects, a CTR that may be sutured to sclera has been designed.[40,41]

It is important to employ a technique that minimizes zonular and capsular stress. The firmer and larger the nucleus, the greater the degree to which sculpting forces are transmitted to the capsular bag. To reduce movement if the surgeon chooses cracking techniques, during sculpting, he should sculpt at a slower rate, to emulsify lesser amounts of nucleus with each pass, and use enough phaco power for the tip to cut, rather than push the nucleus.

Several techniques exist that avoid intracapsular sculpting altogether and may be preferable for higher risk cases. The supracapsular flip technique, as popularized by Maloney,[42] displaces and flips the endonucleus out of the capsular bag prior to emulsification. If accomplished, this prevents the phaco instrumentation forces from being borne by the capsular bag. The ease with which this flipping maneuver can be achieved varies depending upon the size of the endonucleus relative to the capsulorhexis diameter. A nucleus that is too large or a capsulorhexis that is too small would limit the suitability of this technique. One of the best techniques for complicated cases is phaco chop. "Stop and chop"[43] and phaco chop techniques are good options, but latter are preferable because eliminate sculpting. Options in "non stop"-phaco includes horizontal Nagahara-style chop, vertical "quick-chop"[44] and Vejarano´s Safe chop. Phaco chop reduces stress on the zonules and capsule. In sculpting, the nucleus is fixated by the capsular bag. In chopping, it is immobilized instead by the phaco tip.

Pseudoexfoliation syndrome, especially when significant zonular instability is present, poses a challenge in regard with long term stability. Several reports of significant capsule phimosis despite ring placement in pseudoexfoliation cases reveal that the ring may not protect from this complication and underscore the need for a large capsulorhexis in these patients.[45]_Furthermore, reports of late IOL/capsule subluxation in patients with severe Pseudoexfoliation suggest a need for re-evaluating IOL fixation techniques.[46-47] Whether ring placement will lower the incidence of this serious late complication remains to be demonstrated.

In regard with the IOL insertion if the capsular bag is intact despite a focal zonular dialysis, the bag-fixated IOL should be positioned so that the haptic axis points toward the area of zonular dehiscence, since the haptics serve as a partial capsular tension ring to outwardly expand the quadrant of the bag that is lacking centrifugal zonular tension. In the presence of a CTR it is not indispensable.

Posterior Capsule Rents

Maintaining the integrity of the posterior capsule is important not only to support the IOL but to diminish the incidence of retinal complications like cystoid macular edema and retinal detachment. Even in the best hands, rupture of the posterior capsule and vitreous prolapse occur in 0.5–1% of cataract operations.[15] Conditions that increase the risk of posterior capsule rupture during phacoemulsification include ergonomic problems, which make it difficult for the phaco tip to safely access the nucleus. They may be related to extraocular conditions such as severe esotropia, a deep-set eye, a Bell's phenomenon, patient eye movement, and an inability to position the head properly because of respiratory or musculoskeletal problems. Intraocular conditions that decrease the surgical working space include a small pupil, a small capsulorhexis, and a shallow anterior chamber. On the other hand, too deep anterior chamber that may be present in high axial myopia or in cases with history of posterior vitrectomy, forces the phaco needle to approach the lens from a very steep vertical angle, which compromises both visualization and access.

Fluctuation in IOP may result from insufficient inflow (inadequate bottle height, or when the bottle becomes empty without noticing; too tight incisions compressing the irrigation sleeve); from excessive outflow (too high vacuum/flow parameters, too large incisions with leakage); from post-occlusion surge or from a combination of these factors. It will reflect in chamber depth and may cause trampolining of the posterior capsule. The amplitude of this movement is increased in young patients and in myopes with thin sclera because of decreased scleral rigidity, and in older patients or cases with weak zonules because the zonular apparatus is not stretching firmly the capsule. To avoid damaging the posterior capsule either with the phaco needle or with the chopper, it is important to avoid these sudden changes.

Increased nuclear size and density elevates the risk of posterior capsule rupture. Maneuvers such as sculpting, rotation, and cracking all generate some lateral displacement of the nucleus, which applies stress to the capsule and the zonules. The epinucleus helps to cushion the posterior capsule against these forces. However, as the endonucleus becomes larger, the epinucleus becomes proportionately thinner and may even be absent. The larger nucleus of a mature cataract is more difficult to bisect, and frequently has a leathery posterior plate, which requires to perform maneuvers much closer to the posterior capsule.

Posterior polar cataracts (especially if calcified) are among high risk cases, due to an increased incidence of posterior capsular holes attributable to adherence of the cataract to the posterior capsule.[48] In these cases it is preferable to perform a very good hydrodelineation instead of performing hydrodissection. Following the emulsification of the nucleus, the epinucleus will be easier to separate from the posterior plaque using viscodissection. If when removing the plaque surgeons find a big hole in the posterior capsule, never react removing the handpiece, fill the anterior chamber with viscoelastic and aspirate the cortex in a dry manner to avoid the vitreous prolapse.

A small capsulorhexis poses a higher risk of aspirating the capsule edge with the phaco tip, and moreover during hydrodissection, resistance to flow created by the small rhexis may lead to fluid accumulation deep in the nucleus and precipitate a posterior capsular tear.

Early diagnosis and management of posterior capsule rupture is particularly critical while there is still nucleus present within the eye because of the risk of a dropped nucleus.

Once a posterior capsular tear occurs, subsequent surgical maneuvers and forces tend to expand its size, sometimes very quickly.

Chang outlined six signs of early posterior capsule rupture or zonular dehiscence[49]:

1. Sudden deepening of the chamber, with momentary expansion of the pupil
2. Sudden, transitory appearance of a clear red reflex peripherally
3. Newly apparent inability to rotate a previously mobile nucleus
4. Excessive lateral mobility or displacement of the nucleus
5. Excessive tipping of one pole of the nucleus
6. Partial descent of the nucleus into the anterior vitreous space

Author would add that the nucleus falls away from and does not move toward the phaco tip, and sometimes a more subtle sign is present: deepening of the posterior chamber.

Management of a torn posterior capsule depends on when the tear occurs; the amount and density of the remaining nucleus; the presence of other accompanying risk factors (e.g. small pupil, loose zonules, etc.), and the individual surgeon's level of confidence and experience.

When suspecting or discovering a posterior capsule tear, what the surgeon should do first is to inject viscoelastic (or air) through the side port, avoiding with this maneuver an abruptly withdraw the phaco or I/A tip, and so a sudden collapse of the anterior chamber will cause the posterior capsule bulges forward and the anterior hyaloid face ruptures, which will allow vitreous to prolapse through the defect toward the wound.

If vitreous is present immediately after the capsular tear, it should not be removed until after the nucleus or nuclear fragments are emulsified, because it may provide support to keep the nucleus from falling posteriorly.

If the nucleus is soft, and only a small residual amount remains, the procedure may be continued preventing additional vitreous prolapse into the anterior chamber or to the wound. Reduce the parameters: lowering aspiration flow rate and decreasing the vacuum will eliminate surge and allow the bottle to be lowered. A slow motion phaco must be done (e.g. bottle height 55 mm, flow 18 cc/min and vacuum 100 mm Hg). Use dispersive viscoelastics to tamponade the defect, and to move fragments away from it. Place cohesive viscoelastics below the lens nucleus to elevate it into the anterior chamber. It may be necessary to create a paracentesis opposite the incision, through which a hook can loosen and manipulate nuclear fragments into the proper position. A Sheet's Glide can be placed beneath the phaco tip (sometimes surgeons have to enlarge slightly the main incision to avoid excessive movement of the glide when moving the phaco tip) and, if possible, into the opposite residual capsular bag equator or ciliary sulcus, to prevent small nuclear fragments from descending through the capsular defect (narrow glides are available from Visitec or can be manually fashioned to the appropriate width for a small incision).[50] The nucleus should then be emulsified in the anterior chamber using two instruments, if possible in one piece. The second instrument is used to feed the edge of the nuclear fragment into the phaco tip. It is best to avoid creating multiple nuclear fragments that might fall through the posterior capsule rent into the posterior segment. Foot pedal positions 2 and 3 should be used only when the nucleus is adjacent to the phaco tip to avoid aspirating vitreous. It is preferable to use separate, bimanual I/A hand pieces through 1 mm clear corneal incisions to remove the epinucleus and cortex. The lack of incisional fluid leak will reduce fluctuations in chamber depth. The surgeon should avoid working directly above the capsular tear. Cortex should never be stripped directly away from the capsular tear, as this will enlarge the tear. A unimanual, nonautomated technique may offer the most control for cortical aspiration using a 23 gauge cannula or a Simcoe cannula. First, viscodissection is performed between residual cortex and the posterior capsule. Cannula placed on a syringe filled with balanced salt solution is then inserted through various paracentesis incisions to gain 360° access to lens material. Gentle infusion first loosens cortex; then, with the sensitivity afforded by this manual technique, cortical strands may be stripped from the capsular fornix and brought up into the anterior chamber. Complete removal may be deferred until after the IOL is positioned and the pupil is miotic.[51]

Viscoexpression of the remaining fragments, enlarging the incision to 4.0–6.0 mm, and performing manual small incision extracapsular cataract extraction and the claw vectis technique using the dry technique, also have been advocated and may be an option to removal residual lens material, if surgeons have the instruments and the experience.[52]If there is a sizeable amount of residual nucleus, and particularly if it is brunescent, or other surgical risk factors are present, it is advisable to convert to a large incision extracapsular cataract extraction (ECCE). Viscoelastic should be injected underneath the nucleus to support it. Suture the temporal corneal or scleral incision and perform a scleral wide superior incision, err on the side of an overly generous incision size with respect to the nuclear material remaining. Avoid bimanual expression, use an irrigating vectis serrated or a serrated lens loop to extract the nucleus with the help of a generous amount of viscoelastic.

Once nuclear emulsification or extraction is completed, a bimanual vitrectomy should be performed. This is accomplished by establishing irrigation through a separate 23 gauge cannula through the paracentesis. The irrigation bottle is positioned at the appropriate height to maintain the anterior chamber during vitrectomy. A vitrectomy cutter is then placed through a newly created paracentesis and through the rent in the posterior capsule to draw vitreous back through the rent toward the posterior segment. It is better if the vitrectomy is not performed through the main incision. Because this incision is much larger than the vitrectomy instrument, the fluid outflow may cause vitreous to wash out of the wound and vitreous prolapses alongside the instrument shaft through the wound. As more and more vitreous is drawn forward by both the vitrector and this prolapse, mobile residual lens material will tend to fall posteriorly due to loss of support. If the phaco incision is not self-sealing, it should be hydrated or sutured. Vitrectomy should be performed with a high cutting rate (400–750 cuts per minute), an aspiration flow rate of 20 cc/min, and a vacuum of 100–200 mm Hg. The vitrectomy is continued until no vitreous remains anterior to the plane of the posterior capsule. If lens material must be removed, the cutting rate should be reduced and the vacuum power gradually increased, or surgeons can use the dry cortical

17. Jeng BH, Hoyt CS, McLeod SD. Completion rate of continuous curvilinear capsulorhexis in pediatric cataract surgery using different viscoelastic materials. J Cataract Refract Surg. 2004;30(1):85-8.
18. Arshinoff SA. Dispersive-cohesive viscoelastic soft shell technique. J Cataract Refract Surg. 1999;25:167-73.
19. Horiguchi M, Miyake K, Ohta I, et al. Staining of the lens capsule for circular continuous capsulorrhexis in eyes with white cataract. Arch Ophthalmol. 1998;116:535-7.
20. Melles G, de Waard P, Pameyer J, Beekhuis W. Trypan blue capsule staining to visualize the capsulorhexis in cataract surgery. J Cataract Refract Surg. 1999;25:7-9.
21. Dada V, Sharma N, Sudan R, et al. Anterior capsule staining for capsulorhexis in cases of white cataract Comparative clinical study. J Cataract Refract Surg. 2004;30:326-33.
22. Arshinoff SA. Using BSS with viscoadaptatives in the ultimate soft-shell technique. J Cataract Refract Surg. 2002;28:1509-14.
23. Conner C. Rescuing an errant capsulorrhexis. [online] Available from www.ophthalmic.hyperguides.com [Access on January 2012].
24. Seibel BS. Phacodynamics: Mastering the tools and techniques of Phacoemulsification Surgery, 3rd edition. Thorofare: Slack Inc.; 1999.
25. Wilbrandt H. Comparative analyses of the fluidics of the AMO Prestige, Alcon, Fort Worth.USA, Fort Worth.USA Legacy, and Storz Premiere phacoemulsification system. J Cataract Refract Surg. 1997;23:766-80.
26. Mackool R. Advancing phaco technology:an overview of the new infiniti lens removal system. Cataract and Refractive Surgery Today. 2003.
27. Chang DF. Transition to bimanual microincisional phaco. Highlights of Ophthalmology. 2005.
28. Vejarano LF, Tello A, Vejarano A. The safest and most effective technique for cataract surgery. Highlights of Ophthalmology. 2004;32(2):13-9.
29. Vejarano LF, Tello A. Fluidics in phakonit. In: Agarwal A (Ed). Bimanual Phaco: Mastering the Phakonit /MICS Technique. Thorofare: Slack Inc.; 2004.
30. Chang DF. 400 mm Hg High Vacuum Bimanual Phaco Attainable with the Staar Cruise Control Device. J Cataract Refract Surg. 2004;30:932-3.
31. Chang DF. Phaco chop: mastering techniques, optimizing technology, and avoiding complications. Thorofare: Slack Inc.; 2004.
32. Fine IH. Cortical cleaving hydrodissection. J Cataract Refract Surg. 1992;18:508-12.
33. Witschel BM, Legler U. New approaches to zonular cases; the capsular ring. Audiovisual. J Cataract Implant Surg. 1993;9(4).
34. Bayraktar S, Altan T, Kucuksumer Y, et al. Capsular tension ring implantation after capsulorhexis in phacoemulsification of cataracts associated with pseudoexfoliation syndrome. Intraoperative complications and early postoperative finding. J Cataract Refract Surg. 2001;27:1620-8.
35. D'Eliseo D, Pastena B, Longanesi L, et al. Prevention of posterior capsule opacification using capsular tension ring for zonular defects in cataract surgery. Eur J Ophthalmol. 2003;13:151-4.
36. Merriam JC, Zheng L. Iris hooks for phacoemulsification of the subluxated lens. J Cataract Refract Surg. 1997;23:1295-7.
37. Lee V, Bloom P. Microhook capsule stabilization for phacoemulsification in eyes with pseudoexfoliation-syndrome-induced lens instability. J Cataract Refract Surg. 1999;25:1567-70.
38. Mackool RJ. Capsule stabilization for phacoemulsification. J Cataract Refract Surg. 2000;26:629.
39. Chang DF. Capsular tension rings versus capsule retractors. stabilizing the weakened capsular bag during phacoemulsification. Cataract and Refractive Surgery Today. 2004.
40. Cionni RJ, Osher RH. Management of profound zonular dialysis for weakness with a new endocapsular ring designed for scleral fixation. J Cataract Refract Surg. 1998;24:1299-306.
41. Cionni RJ. Suture fixation of the capsular bag. Cataract and Refractive Surgery Today. 2004.
42. Maloney WF, Dillman DM, Nichamin LD. Supracapsular phacoemulsification: a capsule-free posterior chamber approach. J Cataract Refract Surg. 1997;23(3):323-8.
43. Koch PS, Katzen LE. Stop and chop phacoemulsification. J Cataract Refract Surg. 1994;20:566-70.
44. Chang DF. Phaco chop techniques: comparing horizontal vs vertical chop. Highlights of Ophthalmology. 2004.
45. Faschinger CW, Eckhardt M. Complete capsulorhexis opening occlusion despite capsular tension ring implantation. J Cataract Refract Surg. 1999;25:1013-5.
46. Masket S, Osher RH. Late complications with intraocular lens dislocation after capsulorhexis in pseudoexfoliation syndrome. J Cataract Refract Surg. 2002;28:1481-4.
47. Jehan FS, Mamalis N, Crandall AS. Spontaneous late dislocation of intraocular lens within the capsular bag in pseudoexfoliation patients. Ophthalmology. 2001;108:1727-31.
48. Masket S. Posterior polar cataract: an "invitation" to posterior capsular rupture. Supplement to Cataract & Refractive Surgery Today. 2003.
49. Chang DF, Conquering capsule complications: a video primer, American Academy of Ophthalmology/PAAO Join Meeting, Orlando 2002.
50. Michelson MA. Use of a Sheets' glide as a pseudo-posterior capsule in phacoemulsification complicated by posterior capsule rupture. Eur J Implant Refract Surg. 1993;5:70-2.
51. Louis D. "Skip" Nichamin. Management of a broken posterior capsule and advanced vitrectomy technique. [online]. Available from www.ophthalmic.hyperguides.com [Accessed on January 2012].
52. Akura J, Hatta S, Kaneda S, et al. Management of posterior capsule rupture during phacoemulsification using the dry technique. J Cataract Refract Surg. 2001;27:982-9.
53. Lu H, Jiang YR, Grabow HB. Managing a dropped nucleus during the phacoemulsification learning curve. J Cataract Refract Surg. 1999;25:447-50.
54. Kelman C. New PAL method may save difficult cataract cases. Ophthalmology Times. 1994;19:51.
55. Packard R. Technique prevents nucleus drop through capsular tear. Ocular Surgery News 19:14, 2001.
56. Chang DF, Packard R. Posterior assisted levitation for

nucleus retrieval using Viscoat after posterior capsule rupture. J Cataract Refract Surg. 2003;29:1860-5.
57. Lal H, Sethi A, Bageja S, et al. Chopstik technique for nucleus removal in an impending dropped nucleus. J Cataract Refract Surg. 2004;30:1835-9.
58. Neuhann TT, Neuhann T. "The Rhexis-Fixated Lens," film methods of IOL optic capture through a capsulorhexis presented at the ASCRS Symposium on Cataract, IOL and Refractive Surgery, Boston, Massachusetts, USA, April 1991.
59. Worst JGF. L'implantation d'un cristallin artificiel (Iris Clip Lens de Binkhorst), Bull. et Mém. Soc. Française d'Ophtalm. 1971;84:547-62.
60. Menezo JL, Martinez MC, Cisneros AL. Iris-fixated Worst claw versus sulcus-fixated posterior chamber lenses in the absence of capsular support. J Cataract Refract Surg. 1996;22(10):1476-84.
61. Hara T, Hara T. Ten-year results of anterior chamber fixation of the posterior chamber intraocular lens. Arch Ophthalmol. 2004;122(8):1112-6.
62. Oshima Y, Oida H, Emi K. Transscleral fixation of acrylic intraocular lenses in the absence of capsular support through 3.5 mm self-sealing incisions. J Cataract Refract Surg. 1998;24(9):1223-9.
63. Zetterstrom C, Laurell CG. Comparison of endothelial cell loss and phacoemulsification energy during endocapsular phacoemulsification surgery.J Cataract Refract Surg. 1995;21(1):55-8.
64. Kreisler KR, Mortenson SW, Mamalis N. Endothelial cell loss following "modern" phacoemulsification by a senior resident. Ophthalmic Surg. 1992;23:158-60.
65. O'Brien PD, Fitzpatrick P, Kilmartin DJ, et al. Risk factors for endothelial cell loss after phacoemulsification surgery by a junior resident. J Cataract Refract Surg. 2004;30:839-43.
66. Sugar J, Mitchelson J, Kraff M. Endothelial cells trauma and intraocular lens insertion. Arch Ophthalmol. 1978;96:449-50.
67. Balyeat HD, Nordquist RE, Lerner MP, et al. Comparison of endothelial damage produced by control and surface modified poly(methyl methacrylate) intraocular lenses. J Cataract Refract Surg. 1989;15(5):491-4.
68. Werner LP, Legeais JM, Durand J, et al. Endothelial damage caused by uncoated and fluorocarbon-coated poly(methyl methacrylate) intraocular lenses. J Cataract Refract Surg. 1997;23(7):1013-9.
69. Kraff MC, Sanders DR, Lieberman HL. Endothelial cell loss and trauma during intraocular lens implantation: a specular microscopic study. Am Intraocular Implant Soc J. 1978;4(3):107-9.
70. Balazs EA, Freeman MI, Kloti R, et al. Hyaluronic acid and replacement of vitreous and aqueous humor. Mod Prob Ophthalmol. 1972;10:3-21.
71. Miller D, Stegmann R. Use of sodium hyaluronate in human IOL. Implantation. Ann Ophthalmol. 1981;13:7:811-5.
72. Stegmann R, Miller D. Extracapsular cataract extraction with hyaluronate sodium. An Ophthalmology. 1982;14(9):813-5.
73. Soll DB, Harrison SE. The use of chondroitin sulfate in protection of the corneal endothelium. Ophthalmology. 1981;88(suppl):51.
74. Aron-Rosa D, Cohn HC, Aron JJ, et al. Methylcellulose instead of Healon in extracapsular surgery with intraocular lens implantation. Am Acad Ophthalmol. 1983;90:1235-8.
75. Miller D, Stegmann R. Use of Na-hyaluronate in anterior segment eye surgery. Am Intra-Ocular Implant J. 1980;6:13-5.
76. Kerr Muir MG, Sherrard ES, Andrews V, et al. Air, methylcellulose, sodium hyaluronate and the corneal endothelium. Endothelial protective agents. Eye. 1987;1 (Pt 4):480-6.
77. Harfstrand A, Stenevi U, Schenholm M, et al. Sodium hyaluronate on the corneal endothelium. Implant Ophthalmol. 1990; 4:83-7.
78. Rafuse PE, Nichols BD. Effects of Healon vs. Viscoat on endothelial cell count and morphology after phacoemulsification and posterior chamber lens implantation. Can J Ophthalmol. 1992;27(3):125-9.
79. Holzer MP, Tetz MR, Auffarth GU, et al. Effect of Healon 5 and 4 other viscoelastic substances on intraocular pressure and endothelium after cataract surgery. J Cataract Refract Surg. 2001;27:213-8.
80. Holmen JJB, Lundgren B. Scheimpflug photography study of ophthalmic viscosurgical devices during simulated cataract surgery. J Cataract Refract Surg. 2003;29(3): 568-74.
81. Kiss B, Findl O, Menapace R, et al. Corneal endothelial cell protection with a dispersive viscoelastic material and an irrigating solution during phacoemulsification: low-cost versus expensive combination. J Cataract Refract Surg. 2003;29(4):733-40.
82. Miyata K, Namamoto T, Maruoka S, et al. Efficacy and safety of the soft-shell technique in cases with a hard lens nucleus. J Cataract Refract Surg. 2002;28:1546-50.
83. Behndig A, Lundberg B. Transient corneal edema after phacoemulsification: comparison of 3 viscoelastic regimens. J Cataract Refract Surg. 2002;28:1551-6.
84. Kim H, Joo CK. Efficacy of the soft-shell technique using Viscoat and Hyal-2000. J Cataract Refract Surg. 2004;30:2366-70.
85. Kim EK, Cristol SM, Geroski DH, et al. Corneal endothelial damage by air bubbles during phacoemulsification. Arch Ophthalmol. 1997;115:81-8.
86. Kim EK, Cristol S, Kang SJ, et al. Viscoelastic protection from endothelial damage by air bubbles. J Cataract Refract Surg, 2002;28:1047-53.
87. Kraff MC, Sanders DR, Lieberman HL. Specular microscopy in cataract and intraocular lens patients: A report of 564 cases. Arch Ophthalmol. 1980;98:1782-4.
88. Alió JL, Mulet ME, Shalaby AMM, et al. Phacoemulsification in the anterior chamber. J Cataract Refract Surg. 2002;28:67-75.
89. Pirazzoli G, D'Eliseo D, Ziosi M, et al. Effects of phacoemulsification time on the corneal endothelium

using phacofracture and phaco chop techniques. J Cataract Refract Surg. 1996;22(7):967-9.
90. Bourne RR, Minassian DC, Dart JK, et al. Effect of cataract surgery on the corneal endothelium: modern phacoemulsification compared with extracapsular cataract surgery. Ophthalmology. 2004;111(4):679-85.
91. Mannis MJ, Miller RB, Carlson EC, et al. Effect of hypothermic perfusion on corneal endothelial morphology. Br J Ophthalmol. 1983;67:804-7.
92. McCarey BE, Edelhauser HF, Van Horn DL. Functional and structural changes in the corneal endothelium during in vitro perfusion. Invest Ophthalmol. 1973;6:410-7.
93. Edelhauser HF, Van Horn DL, Hydiuk RA, et al. Intraocular irrigating solutions: Their effect on the corneal endothelium. Arch Ophthalmol. 1975;93:648-57.
94. Araie M. Barrier function of corneal endothelium and the intraocular irrigating solutions. Arch Ophthalmol. 1986;104(3):435-8.
95. Samuel MA, Desai UR, Strassman I, et al. Intraocular irrigating solutions. A clinical study of BSS Plus and dextrose bicarbonate fortified BSS as an infusate during pars plana vitrectomy. Indian J Ophthalmol. 2003;51(3):237-42.

21 Management of Incomplete Capsulorhexis Cases with Biaxial Approach

Arturo Pérez-Arteaga (Mexico)

Introduction

To deal with an incomplete capsulorhexis is a situation affecting directly toward the knowledge, skills and health of the operative doctor; every surgeon that has faced this situation, knows about the terrible complications that can occur if an appropriate management is not achieved.[1-4] It is a singular situation, maybe a particular intraoperative feature occurring frequently during a lens extraction but that can overcome to potential nightmare complications like vitreous loss, nuclear and epinuclear fragments dislocated to the vitreous, a complete luxation of the nucleus to the vitreous cavity and problems in intraocular lens (IOL) placement that can go from descentration until a complete dislocation.[5-7] This is the interesting feature of this state; it is almost a complication, but it is not a complete one, and the good management of it will avoid the surgeon to deal with truly nightmare complications.[8-11]

It is also a situation that cannot be involved in a single term, because to describe "Incomplete Capsulorhexis" can include a wide variety of situations going from a single inappropriate tear occurred in the anterior capsule that can be corrected in a very simple fashion like performing a wider capsulorhexis, until a bigger tear involving even the posterior capsule that will change the entire phacoemulsification management; the versatility in the wide range of clinical presentations is the interesting feature of this situation.[12-20]

The biaxial approach has showed to us during many years of work on it, that this surgical management of the anterior capsule has many advantages in comparison with the coaxial approach, not only during the routine performance of the microcapsulorhexis, but evermore, during the management of the surgical complications that can occur during its performance.[21-28] The objective of this chapter is to describe some particular variations to the biaxial phacoemulsification approach that must be put in practice in these particular cases, pointing the advantages of biaxial phaco over the coaxial style, encouraging so to more surgeons worldwide to adopt these techniques in benefit of their patients.

Avoiding Complications During Biaxial Phaco with an Incomplete Capsulorhexis

Once surgeons are sure that they have an incomplete capsulorhexis and don´t know exactly if it has run to the posterior capsule, the golden rule is to avoid transmission of forces to the capsular bag. It must be an "in the air surgery" or maybe called a "floating surgery"; it means a complete procedure at the iris plane.[17-20]

Some years ago, Prof Keiki Mehta from Mumbai, India, described what he called, "The Lens Salute Technique" (please see the Biaxial Prechop Chapter in this Textbook), that consists in a hemi-luxation of the nucleus to the iris plane, during the hydrodissection and hydrodelineation. Author agrees, that this maneuver helps to decrease the transmission of forces to the capsular bag and to the zonule; even in non-complicated cases (it means complete and nice capsulorhexis). In cases of incomplete capsulorhexis, this maneuver can be the safer way to perform a non-complicated phacoemulsification; it is the key to work at the iris plane.

Surgical Technique

Once surgeons are sure that their capsulorhexis is incomplete, surgeons have to change their mind to a "floating surgery". In this chapter the pictures presented show a case where an intentional "can opener" was performed to the anterior capsule of the lens, instead of a

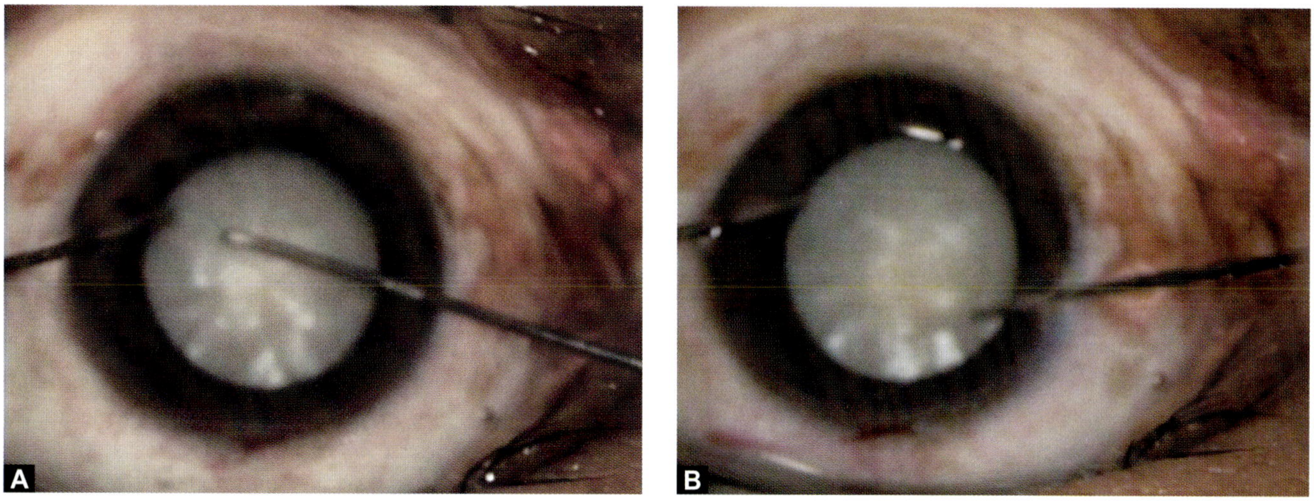

Figs 1A and B: Can opener to the anterior capsule

capsulorhexis; this was decided for demonstrative reasons. With this kind of anterior capsule opening, surgeons are completely sure that their capsulorhexis is incomplete (Figs 1A and B).

Now author will describe the surgical technique to solve this situation:

1. **Perform Gentle Hydrodissection (**Figs 2A and B): Because in many cases surgeons can`t know exactly the state of the capsular bag when a capsulorhexis is not complete, surgeons must be very careful when performing hydrodissection and hydrodelamination; surgeons have to perform soft maneuvers in an incomplete mode separating only the layers adjacent to the anterior capsule in the meridians where surgeons are able to see it very well; this maneuvers of hydrodissection and hydrodelamination should be very similar to those cases of Posterior Polar Cataracts. "To be gentle" is the key factor for this surgical step; avoid maneuvers like vigorous injection and rotation of the nucleus. Even so, the goal will be to take the nucleus outside from the capsular bag, so a small amount of rotation just to be sure that the nucleus is free, can be performed.
2. **Searching for an Easy "Lens Salute Position"** (Fig. 3): Because surgeons don`t know about the integrity of the posterior capsule, it will be a tremendous mistake to perform the phacoemulsification procedure inside the capsular bag. Maneuvers like prechop, vigorous chopping and stop and chop in the bag must be avoided. The key factor to control their phacoemulsification procedure is to work outside the capsular bag, it means "a floating surgery"; it is in these

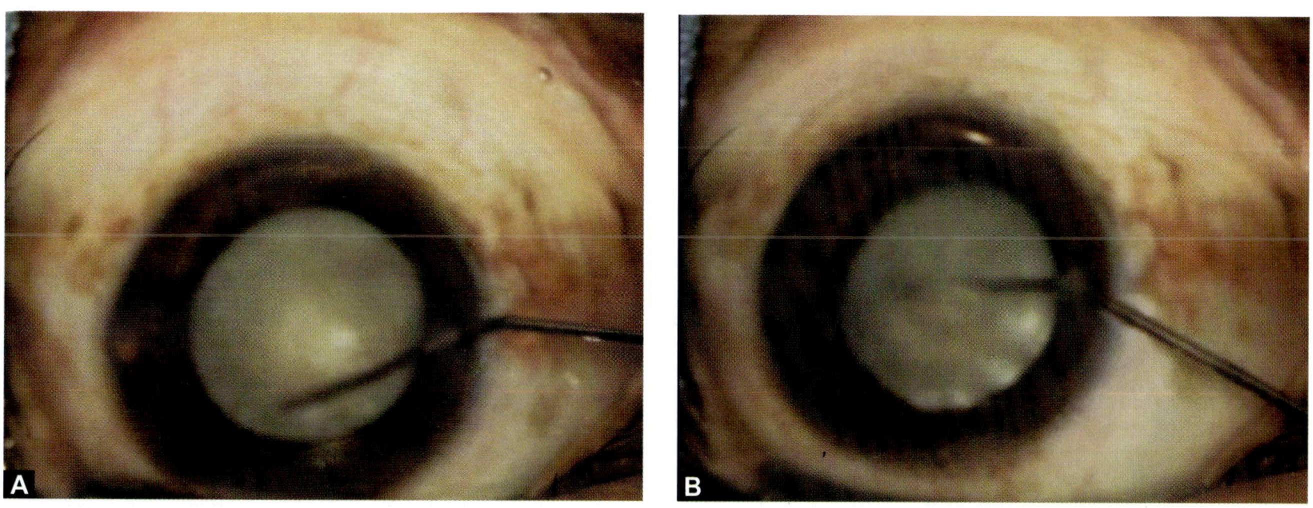

Figs 2 A and B: (A) Gentle hydrosurgery, (B) Gentle nuclear rotation

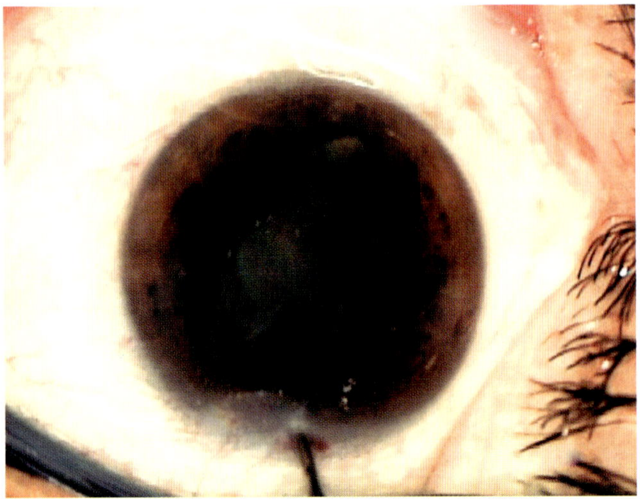

Fig. 3: Nucleus being placed in lens salute position

kind of cases where surgeons can apply the concept that the safest place to work for a cataract surgeon is the iris plane. Once the nucleus has reached the iris plane, surgeons are able to avoid the transmission of forces to the "incomplete" capsular bag, posterior capsule and the ciliary zonule; but furthermore, because surgeons are working in a biaxial approach, they can place their irrigating cannula (or irrigating chopper) behind the nucleus, helping with this maneuver to separate with the irrigation, the nucleus from the posterior capsule or in definitively complicated cases, with the hyaloid face. This situation is impossible if surgeons are working in a coaxial approach, because they do not have irrigation available at their non-dominating hand and even worst, their coaxial irrigation pushes the nucleus back to the possible incomplete capsular bag. The main concept that surgeons must learn to work with in these particular cases, is that surgeons have to believe that the posterior capsule is broken, even if they have some particular signs that it is not, with the objective to avoid initial or subsequent damage. There are two ways to take the nucleus outside the capsular bag:

(a) **Perform the "Lens Salute Technique"** during the Hydroprocedures (please see the chapter of Biaxial Prechop in this Textbook): If well surgeons are not quite sure about the integrity of the posterior capsule and they have to be gentle during the hydrosurgery, without rotation of the nucleus inject a small amount of solution behind the anterior capsule in the best place where surgeons can see it; while injecting, gentle press down the equator of the nucleus in this same position; do not press the nucleus in the center or in the mild periphery, it has to be at the extreme periphery, otherwise surgeons can push it into the vitreous cavity; while injecting at the same time then pressing, the saline solution will run behind the nucleus to the opposite side, creating a posterior wave that pushes the nucleus forward, because the wave moves between the nucleus and the posterior capsule; even if there is absence of a posterior capsule, the wave will move between the nucleus and the hyaloid face, pushing anyway the nucleus forward; this is why this maneuver will not work if surgeons push the nucleus in another location different from the extreme periphery; disaster consequences can be obtained in this maneuver if not performed properly. Remember that the final position that the nucleus reaches with this maneuver is a "tilt" position, a plane of inclination (Fig. 3), that will allow surgeons to collocate their irrigating chopper or cannula behind the nucleus, at the site where it reaches the iris plane (Fig. 4). Remember, the key factor is to take it out from the capsular bag, the nucleus will withdraw in an easy way because surgeons do not have a small continuous curvilinear capsulorhexis that can retain it in the capsular bag; maybe author can call it an advantage of an incomplete capsulorhexis. Once the nucleus has reached the "Lens Salute" position surgeons can maintain the irrigating cannula behind the nucleus while placing the phaco needle with the dominant hand; once surgeons have these two instruments holding the nucleus (Fig. 4), they can perform a bi-axial prechop technique, by pressing the nucleus with both instruments (Figs 5A and B). Notice that

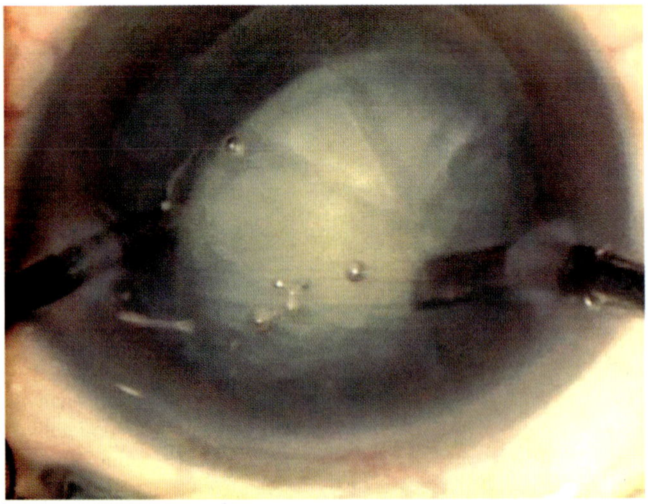

Fig. 4: Irrigating cannula behind the nucleus and phaco needle at the front

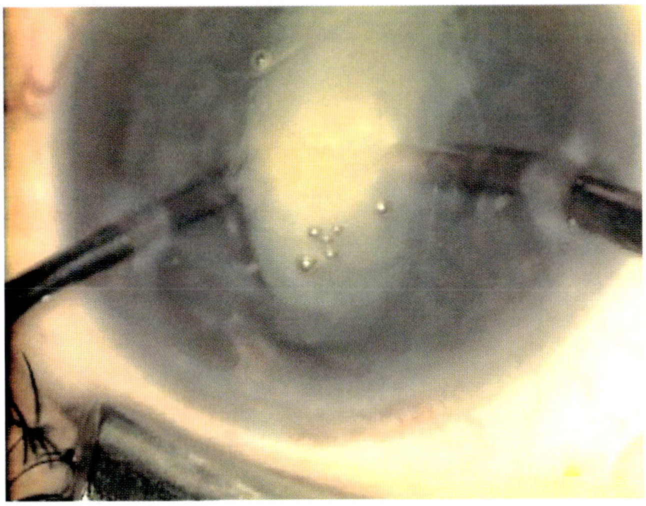

Fig. 5A: Biaxial prechop performed with irrigating cannula and phaco needle

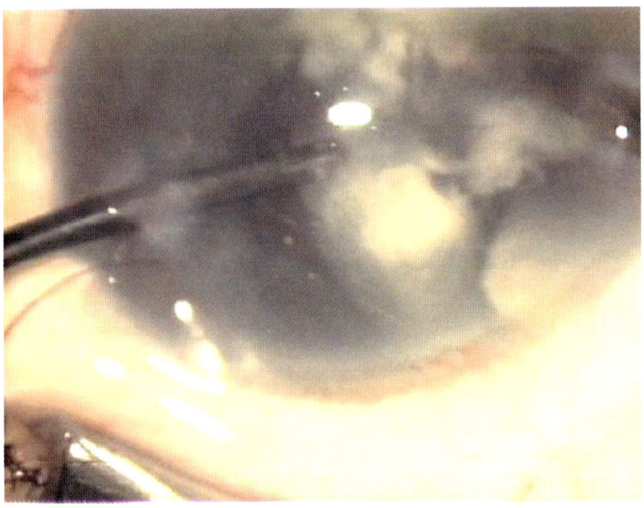

Fig. 5B: Nuclear fragmentation with both instruments

author is describing a technique of biaxial prechop at the iris plane, as was described in the chapter of Biaxial Prechop in this Textbook; nevertheless the Biaxial Prechop technique can be performed with the irrigating cannula and the phaco needle, as well as with two cannulas, as was described in the respective chapter.

(b) ***Another Possible Technique*** to avoid the performance of the "Lens Salute technique", avoiding the pressure over a weak capsular bag is described as follows. Perform gentle and soft hydrodissection, without or with very gentle nuclear rotation (Figs 2A and B), followed by the insertion of the irrigating chopper (or cannula) and the phaco needle to the anterior chamber (Fig. 6); be sure to have enough amount

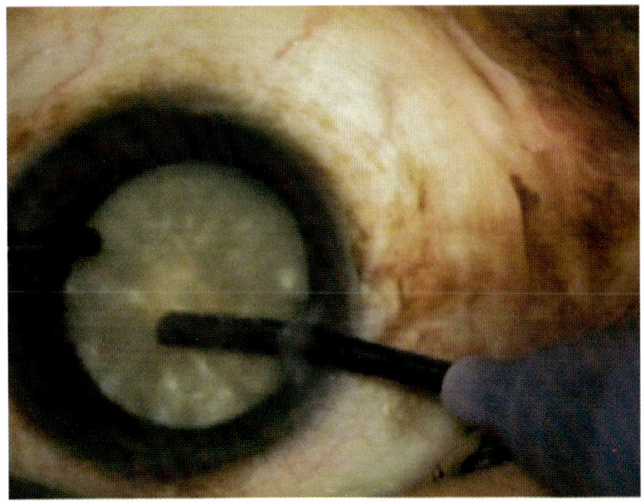

Fig. 6: 700 double ended irrigating cannula and 0.9 Kelman Phaco tip, inserted in the eye

of fluid (active or passive infusion according to the gauge of preference) to avoid surge and high vacuum (according to surgeons' phaco needle and their phaco-machine parameters); start the irrigation and embed the phaco needle with a small amount of ultrasonic power inside the center of the nucleus (Fig. 7); beware not to push the nucleus during this maneuver, surgeons are not sure about the integrity of the posterior capsule; do not create a groove! Once their phaco needle is deep enough in the nucleus, stop ultrasonic force but do not stop the vacuum—do not perform a groove, remember that surgeons need to work outside the capsular bag—keep the vacuum

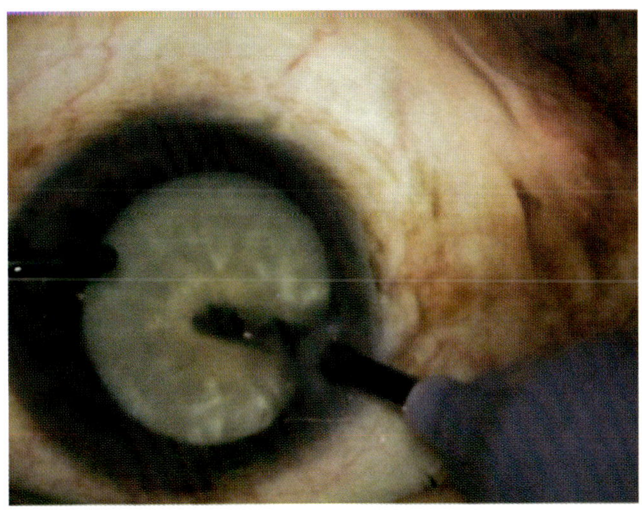

Fig. 7: Nucleus embed with the phaco needle. Do not create a groove!

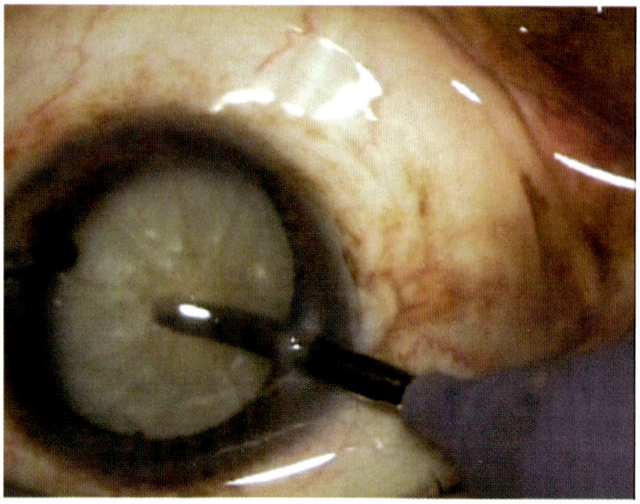

Fig. 8: Nucleus held firmly with vacuum

active, do not loose the nucleus (Fig. 8), keep it holding firmly with only the vacuum force and in a single but gentle movement, pull the unit phaco needle-nucleus outside the capsular bag, in a maneuver just like in the old times of the intracapsular surgery, when the unit cryo probe-cataract were moved in a single but gentle movement to withdraw the cataract from the eye (Fig. 9). In this case, the movement is just to put the nucleus at the iris plane. Once surgeons are at the iris plane they are not still done; do not miss the vacuum, keep holding the nucleus firmly (surgeons are not sure if behind the nucleus they have a posterior capsule or the hyaloid anterior face; keep holding it with their vacuum and gently move their irrigating chopper (or cannula) behind the nucleus with nondominant hand (Fig. 10); this instrument has irrigation, so it is easy

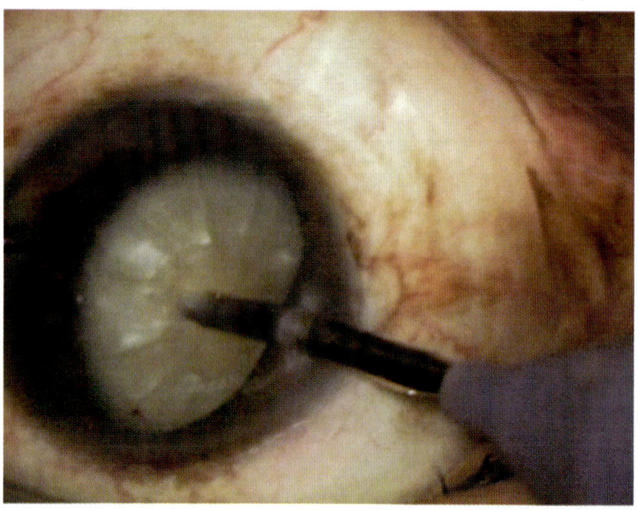

Fig. 9: Nucleus pulled with vacuum

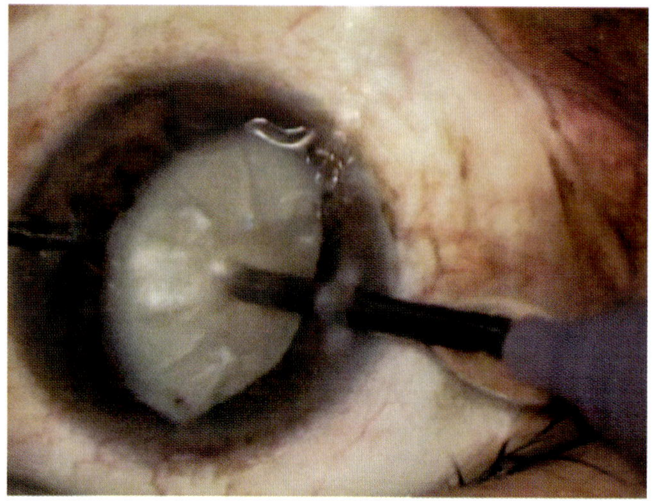

Fig. 10: Irrigating cannula placed behind the nucleus

to know that it is surgeons who place it properly just behind the nucleus, this irrigation, acting as a third hand—situation impossible to obtain in a coaxial approach—will separate the nucleus from the capsular bag, possible broken posterior capsule or possible hyaloid face. Once surgeons' irrigating device is behind the nucleus, keep holding it with vacuum, do not miss it, and simply move their irrigating device to cut the nucleus—sustained with vacuum at the iris plane—from the rear to the front (Figs 11A and B). Surgeons will obtain a nice division in two halves at the iris plane, far away from the corneal endothelium and from the possible damaged capsular bag (Fig. 12). Keep fragmenting the two halves of nucleus into quadrants at the same iris plane (Figs 13A to D). Then when surgeons have enough divided the nucleus they can start to phaco at the iris plane (Figs 14A and B).

3. **Maintaining a Positive Intraocular Pressure with Irrigation:** Because to work at the iris plane is the objective, the maintenance of wide spaces in the anterior and posterior chambers plays a particular important role; if somehow surge is present, the possible damage to the intraocular structures is feasible; if well surge can convert in reality a virtual damage to the posterior capsule, with the nightmare consequences of nuclear material in the vitreous cavity, surgeons should think that it can also decrease in an important manner the speed of recovery of a patient suffering of corneal edema because of endothelial touch. Be sure that surgeons have enough fluid to work that will help them to create space of maneuver, avoid touch of intraocular structures and support high vacuum

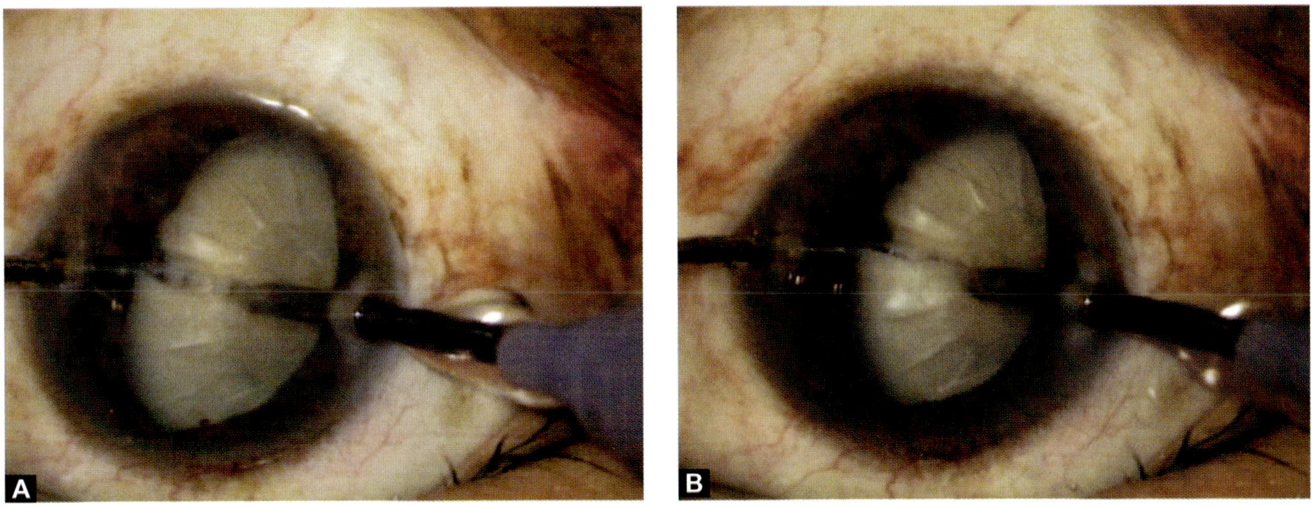

Figs 11A and B: Prechop with irrigating cannula and phaco tip

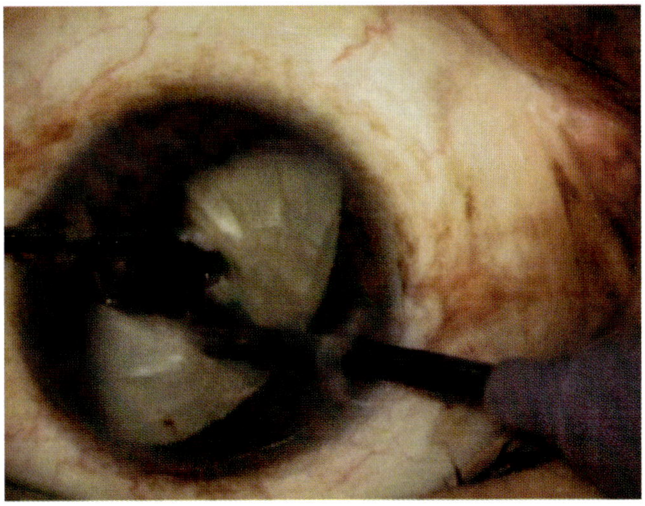

Fig. 12: Nucleus divided

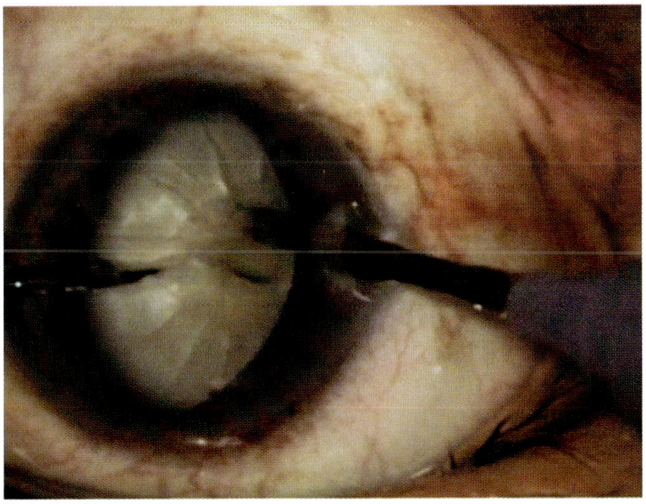

Fig. 13A: Nucleus starting fragmentation with vacuum and irrigating cannula

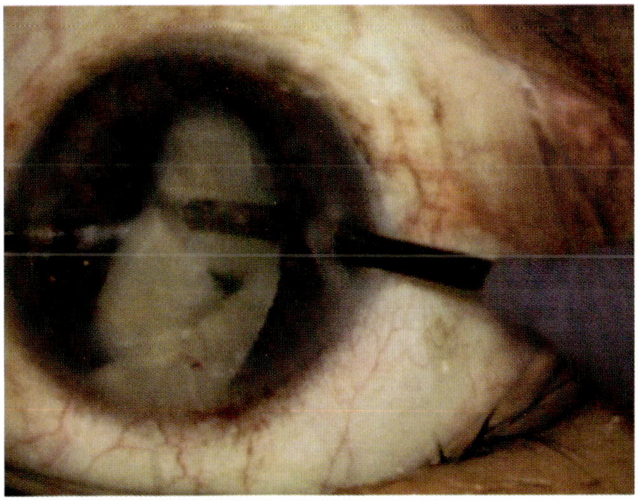

Fig. 13B: Notice the pressure between both intruments to cause nuclear fragmentation

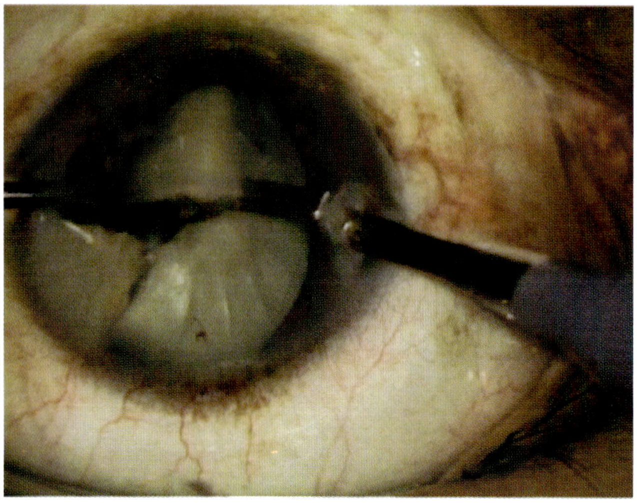

Fig. 13C: Three pieces nuclear fragmentation

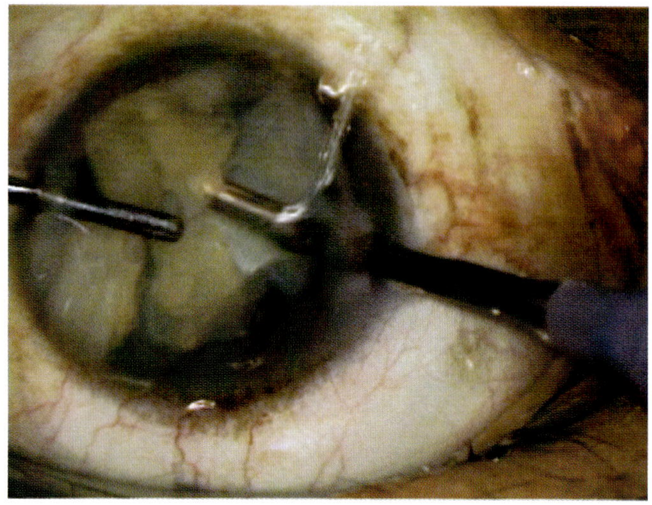

Fig. 13D: Starting phaco in some intermittent mode for multiple nuclear pieces

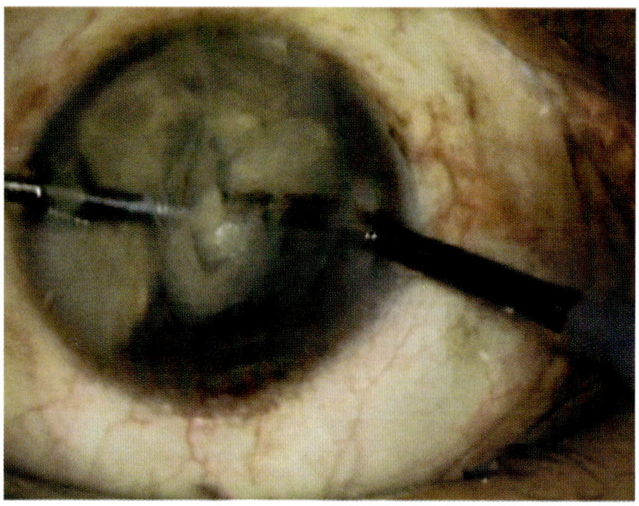

Fig. 14A: Phacoemulsification of nuclear pieces

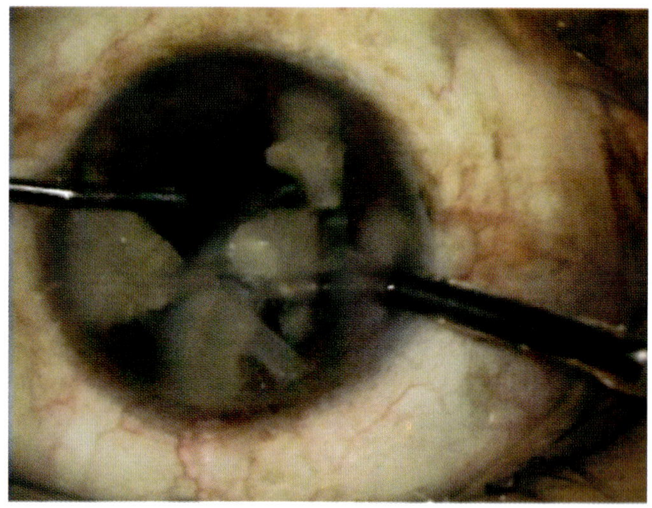

Fig. 14B: Notice that the phaco tip is not moving during phaco

levels during their phaco maneuvers. As a general rule, if surgeons are using an irrigating device of 19 gauge or wider, surgeons can trust in passive infusion (gravity force); but if surgeons are using diameters of 20 gauge or smaller, do not let the possibility or not of surge to "Lady Luck", use forced infusion—internal or external—it is their assurance to success in these complicated cases.

4. **Biaxial Prechop Technique at the Iris Plane (with "Lens Salute" or with "Pull the Nucleus Technique"):** Anyhow surgeons have placed the nucleus at the iris plane, a mechanical fracture of the nucleus performed between the phaco needle (placed in the front part of the nucleus) and some irrigating device either chopper or cannula (placed in the rear part of the nucleus) is the key to success; surgeons have the following advantages:
   - They are working outside the capsular bag.
   - They have the irrigating force separating the nucleus from the posterior chambers structures, and remember that surgeons are not quite sure about their anatomical integrity of them.
   - They are cutting all the nuclear strands from the back to the rear, so an incomplete chop is difficult to obtain, unless surgeons lose their vacuum force.

- They are holding the nucleus with vacuum, so it functions as a unit, as a single piece that can be managed in single movements.
- They have the irrigation posterior to the nucleus, so the pieces are pushed forward, never to the posterior chamber

Avoid the use of prechopper forceps, prechopper maneuver inside the capsular bag, coaxial irrigation, stop and chop techniques, and all the techniques that take surgeons' surgery again to the posterior chamber; also beware for the corneal endothelium, work at the iris plane, not at the anterior chamber. Fragment as much as possible their pieces at the iris plane; divide many times the nucleus with the same technique, vacuum force applied to the nucleus and vertical chop applied at the same time from the rear to the front.

5. **Avoiding Work at the Capsular Bag. Pulling the Fragments to the Iris Plane:** Because surgeons are not sure about the anatomical integrity of the posterior capsule to work at the iris plane, placing their irrigation behind the nucleus is the key factor; surgeons have a third hand helping to keep their nuclear fragments at the iris plane, but also helping to maintain the possible broken posterior capsule or the vitreous body far away from their working area. Nevertheless some surgeons recently have pointed the benefits of a mechanical device that should be placed behind the nucleus to have a safe phacoemulsification when there is a possibility of damaged posterior capsule (artificial posterior capsule); the future will tell us about their real benefits and possible complications. Nevertheless, they share with us the same way of thinking, that in cases of phacoemulsification performed with an incomplete capsulorhexis, the working place must be the iris plane, and some physical force (either mechanic or fluidic) must be collocated behind the nucleus, to avoid the loose of nuclear fragments to the vitreous cavity, but also to avoid more damage to the structures located in the posterior chamber.
6. **Maintaining a Positive Intraocular Pressure while Switching to Irrigation/Aspiration Mode:** Because surgeons are working in a biaxial approach, they have the tremendous advantage that can switch from phaco mode to irrigation/aspiration mode, without the need to stop irrigation (Fig. 15). In a coaxial approach, once surgeons have finished the phacoemulsification of the nucleus they have to switch from one handpiece to another, so surgeons have to stop the irrigation between both steps, unless they inject viscoelastic material through a second incision to maintain wide open the anterior and posterior chambers; but if this is the case, surgeons are very near to convert from coaxial to a biaxial surgeon. With the biaxial approach surgeons only need to switch from their phaco probe to aspirating cannula with the dominating hand (and with the help of their assistant) keeping the irrigating device active inside the eye, holding it with their nondominant hand, maintaining this way the anterior and posterior chambers wide open, and the possible damaged capsule, hyaloids face or vitreous body far away from their incisions; it is a tremendous advantage of a microincision surgery in a biaxial approach.

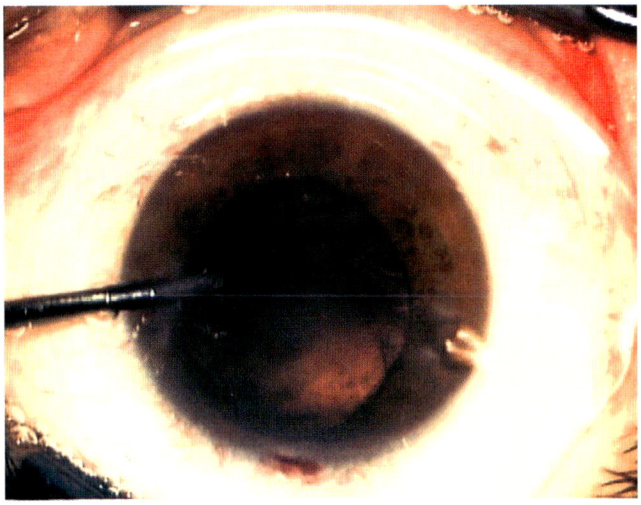

Fig. 15: Irrigating cannula maintained inside the eye to avoid negative intraocular pressure

Conclusion

Many advantages have been observed when performing biaxial lens surgery in cases of complicated capsular management. These advantages can be noticed since the first maneuvers when surgeons start to feel the capsular tissue and the maneuvers that can be performed in order to avoid entering to a more complicated case. But furthermore, these advantages go along the case during the management of the chop maneuvers, phacoemulsification, irrigation/aspiration and biaxial anterior vitrectomy when needed. It is completely true that MICS is not a matter of incision size, is a matter of management of new tools, new maneuvers, new forces, new fluidics inside the eye that helps the surgeon to decrease the possible complications of cataract surgery, but furthermore, of great value in solving complex and challenging cases like the presented in this chapter.

References

1. Stefan Sacu, Rupert Menapace, Oliver Findl. Effect of optic material and haptic design on anterior capsule opacification and capsulorrhexis contraction. Am J Ophthalmol. 2006;141(3):488-93.
2. Deborah S Jacobs, Terry A Cox, Michael D Wagoner, et al. Capsule staining as an adjunct to cataract surgery: a report from the American Academy of Ophthalmology. Ophthalmology. 2006;113(4):707-13.
3. Jorge Alió, José Luis Rodríguez-Prats, Ahmed Galal, et al. Outcomes of microincision cataract surgery versus coaxial phacoemulsification. Ophthalmology. 2005;112(11):1997-2003.
4. Roberto Pinelli, Fazio P. Dynamics of capsulorrhexis. In: Ashok Garg (Ed). Mastering the Phacodynamics (Tools, Technology and Innovations). New Delhi: Jaypee Brothers Medical Publishers.
5. Sabine Kurz, Frank Krummenauer, et al. Biaxial micro-incision versus coaxial small-incision clear cornea cataract surgery. Ophthalmology. 2006;113(10):1818-26.
6. Navneet Brar, Sandra Lora Cremers. Assesing surgery skills. Ophthalmology. 2007;114(8):1587.
7. Mahiul MK Muquit, Milch J Menage. Intraoperative floppy iris syndrome. Ophthalmology. 2006;113(10):1885-6.
8. Suzuki T, Hayakawa K, Kawai K. The 23 gauge capsulorrhexis forceps having a cystotome function. J Exp Clin Med. 2005;30(1):11-3.
9. Kawai K. Comparison of 23 gauge and 25 gauge anterior capsulotomy forceps. Tokai J Exp Clin Med. 2004;29 (3): 105-10.
10. Packer M, Hoffmann R, Fine H. Refractive lens surgery. Ophthalmology Clinics N Am. 2006;19(1):77-88.
11. Wasserman D, Apple DJ, Castaneda VE, et al. Anterior capsular tears and loop fixation of posterior chamber intraocular lenses. Asia. Ophthalmology. 1991;98(4):425-31.
12. Castaneda VE, Legler UF, Tsai JC, et al. Posterior continuos curvilinear capsulorrhexis. An experimental study with clinical applications. Ophthalmology. 1992;99(1):45-50.
13. Ahmed Sallam, Hooman Sherafat. Intraocular lens implantation in cases with anterior capsule tears extending to the posterior capsule. J Cataract Refract Surg. 2007;33(6):938-9.
14. Marques FF, Marques DM, Osher RH, et al. Fate of anterior capsular tears during cataract surgery. J Cataract Refract Surg. 2006;32(10):1638-42.
15. Fishkind WJ, Gimbel HV, Sun R. Ferensowics M. Intraoperative management of capsular tears in phacoemulsification and intraocular lens implantation. Ophthalmology. 2001;108;2190-2.
16. Gimbel HV, Teuhann T. Development, advantages and methods of continuos curvilinear capsulorhexis technique. J Cataract Refract Surg. 1990;16:31-7.
17. Assia EI, Apple DJ, Tsai JC, et al. Mechanism of radial tear formation after anterior capsulectomy. Ophthalmology. 1991;98:432-7.
18. Vajpayee RB, Sharma N, Dada T, et al. Management of posterior capsule tears. Surv Ophthalmol. 2001;45(6):473-88.
19. Gimbel HV, Sun R, Ferensowicz M, et al. Intraoperative management of posterior capsule tears in phacoemulsification and intraocular lens implantation. Ophthalmology. 2001;108(12):2186-9.
20. Assia EI, Apple DJ, Barden A, et al. An experimental study comparing various anterior capsulectomy techniques. Arch Ophthalmol. 1991;109(5):642-7.
21. Hettlich HJ, El-Hifnawi ES. Scanning electron microssopy studies of the human lens after capsulorhexis. Ophthalmologe. 1997;94(4):300-2.
22. Hamada S, Low S, Walters BC, et al. Five-year experience of the 2.incision push-pull technique for anterior and posterior capsulorhexis in pediatric cataract surgery. Ophthalmology. 2006;113(8):1309-14.
23. Oner FH, Durak I, Soylev M, Ergin M. Long term results of various anterior capsulotomies and radial tears on intraocular lens centration. Ophthalmic Surg Lasers. 2001;32(2):118-23.
24. Sallam A, Sherafat H. Intraocular lens implantation in cases with anterior capsule tears extending to the posterior capsule. J Cataract Refract Surg. 2007;33(6):938-9.
25. Osher RH. Inraocular lens implantation in cases with anterior capsule tears extending to the posterior capsule. J Cataract Refract Surg. 2007;33(6):939-40.
26. Wilson ME. Anterior lens capsule management in pediatric cataract surgery. Trans Am Ophthalmol Soc. 2004;102:391-422.
27. Kwartz J. Implantation of foldable intraocular lenses in the presence of anterior capsular tears. Eye. 1996;10 (Pt 4):529-30.
28. Arturo Perez-Arteaga. Step by Step to Biaxial Lens Surgery. New Delhi: Jaypee Brothers Publishers; 2008.

22

Micro-Biaxial Cataract Surgery Combined with 25 Gauge Transconjunctival Sutureless Vitrectomy

Arturo Pérez-Arteaga (Mexico)

Introduction

It is well known by retinal surgeons that pars plana vitrectomy (PPV) generates cataract. This induction of the lens opacity can be produced with or without direct lens touch during the PPV procedure. If there is lens touch during the vitrectomy, there is damage to the lens capsule and this is the direct mechanism of cataract induction; if this the case the capsule rupture creates a challenge for the anterior segment surgeon, who in a second procedure, must beware the fact of a lens extraction with a previous damage posterior capsule and the lack of a vitreous cushion during the surgery. If there is no damage to the posterior capsule, the mechanism of cataract formation corresponds to the break up of the intraocular physiological barriers, and the change in the intraocular physiology and metabolism. Maybe in this second case (the rupture of the intraocular barriers) the opacity of the lens may occur in low speed rather than in the case of the capsule damage, and may also the challenge for the cataract surgeon be minor, in comparison of cases of capsular rupture.[1-5]

For these reasons, during the last years, there is a growing tendency to perform lens extraction during the PPV, in particular in patients who are in the presbyopic age.[6-10] Authors believe that in young patients, who still have accommodation, may be they can better perform only the PPV with extreme care to keep the integrity of the posterior capsule, and indicate a further lens extraction when the cataract formation produces an impaired visual function. But in the presbyopic patient, in whom there is not accommodation, the combined procedure of anterior and posterior segments can be the correct criteria to follow.

When authors are talking about microincisions, JW Hwang was the first to report in an excellent article, the technique to perform combined phacoemulsification and 25 gauge transconjunctival sutureless vitrectomy (TSV25); this article shows by the first time the performance of no-stitches phaco combined with no-stitches posterior vitrectomy.[2] The method to perform phacoemulsification was a standard technique, so authors can be agree that only the posterior segment surgery was truly a microincisional procedure.[11-16] Prof. Amar Agarwal is the first surgeon in the world to describe micro-biaxial technique for lens extraction (700 micron biaxial phaco) combined with the TSV25 system, in the same surgical time in one eye. This was reported in the Journal of Cataract and Refractive Surgery, in November, 2007.[17] This is a truly amazing technique and the one that authors describe in this chapter, because it really uses incisions of less than 1 mm and completely sutureless; this combination of microphakonit with TSV25 makes the combined procedure more rapid and minimally invasive and may be a very useful procedure in vitreoretinal pathologies without dense fibrous proliferation.[18]

Physical Basis

The objective for the anterior segment surgeon must not only to perform the lens extraction but also to facilitate the vitreoretinal surgeon his subsequent work, leading only smooth conditions and avoiding obstacles. To perform this objective the cataract surgeon must keep in mind that four important conditions must exist at the end of the phacoemulsification.

1. Clear view of the posterior segment: It means to achieve the transparency of the structures in the anterior segment.
2. Stability of the anterior chamber: Sometimes the posterior segment surgeon can work with noncontact lenses; even so the stability of the anterior chamber

is quite important. But many times the only available tool for a clear view of the posterior segment is the contact lenses (pre-corneal lens). In these cases, the stability of the anterior chamber and the absence of leakage are of particular importance. Only a chamber with complete stability will be able to support the pressure of a contact lens over the cornea, in order to visualize the posterior segment (Fig. 10).

3. Nice dilated pupil: As wider the pupil diameter after the phacoemulsification procedure, much more visualization of the vitreoretinal structures during the posterior segment surgery. Taking care of the uveal tissue during phacoemulsification is a considerable detail (Fig. 10).
4. Integrity of posterior capsule: The posterior segment surgical procedure will become easier if there is integrity of the posterior capsule. During the PPV there will be a closed environment in the vitreous cavity; this helps to exclude the structures of the anterior segment in the mechanical surgical maneuvers, the fluidics management and the intra and postoperative issues regarding the vitrectomy procedure.
5. If there is a rupture in the posterior capsule, there will not only be an increase in the difficulty of performing PPV but also in the possible damage to anterior segment structures like corneal endothelial cells; this possibility can take place sometimes during the surgery and some other time in the postoperative period; in those conditions, silicone oil or recurrent hemorrhage can directly touch to the cornea.
   Anyway, silicone oil is able to migrate to the anterior segment even without a rupture in the posterior capsule, but the risk increases when there is lack of integrity of this intraocular structure.

The single formula with the objective to facilitate the posterior segment surgeon to perform his/her work after he/she finished the phacoemulsification procedure is to obtain a stable anterior chamber with transparent structures (Fig. 13).

Coaxial Versus Biaxial

Maybe many surgeons worldwide are agree that intraocular lens (IOL) implantation must be performed after the PPV has been done, because the anterior surgeon is able to know about the intraoperative conditions of the posterior segment procedure, like use or not to use of silicone oil, and so the compensation in the power of the IOL can be assumed in the same surgical act. For this reason, maybe the ideal state to perform the PPV in a combined procedure should be aphakia. Another reason supporting the aphakia, as an intermediate state in these cases, is to avoid the enlargement of the incision that must be done in most of the cases for the IOL implantation, and so the minimal leakage that can be obtained with smaller incisions. Nevertheless the discussion still exists.

In coaxial and microcoaxial surgery the incisions are longer than in biaxial surgery and much more in comparison to micro-biaxial techniques (microphakonit). Smaller incision means less leakage, and so, more stability of the anterior chamber with the only objective to help the posterior segment surgeon during the intraoperative maneuvers.

Because, “less invasive means more stability”, maybe 700 micron techniques (micro-biaxial cataract surgery) can be a good option to achieve aphakia just before a PPV procedure. Sutureless is feasible, and chamber stability will work really fine this way even with the use of a pre-corneal contact lens while performing PPV.[17]

Amar Agarwal described first time in the world, the combined technique of microphakonit (micro-biaxial) followed by minimally invasive PPV (25 G) with very good results. All the variations, like suture or sutureless PPV, contact or noncontact pre-corneal lens can be used; but in all these variations the constant must be to keep the stability of the anterior chamber. The variation, authors like to introduce in this chapter regarding the Agarwal`s technique, is the performance of the scleral incisions and the stoppers placement for 25 G instrumentation before starting micro-biaxial phacoemulsification.[17]

Step by Step

Authors suggest the surgical steps in this order:

1. Perform the 25 G sclerotomies and place the 25 G stoppers in each incision.
2. Perform biaxial cataract (or clear lens) extraction with 700 micron technique.
3. Perform 25 G transconjunctival sutureless PPV.
4. IOL implantation with model and power calculation according to the required conditions of previous PPV.

The biaxial phaco and the IOL placement are performed first then the scleral incisions and the 25 G sutureless transconjunctival vitrectomy are performed. So the steps can be different, nevertheless the micro-phaco incisions allow the surgeon to maintain a good intraocular pressure (IOP) for the complete performance of the 25 G vitrectomy.

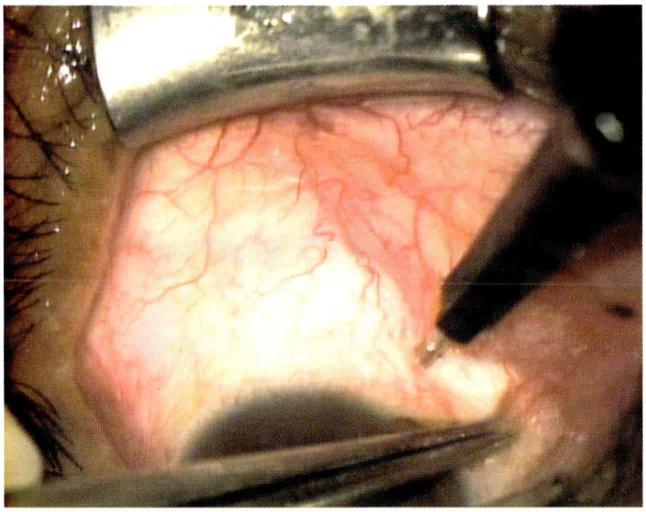

Fig. 1: Performance of scleral tunnel incisions prior to clear corneal incisions

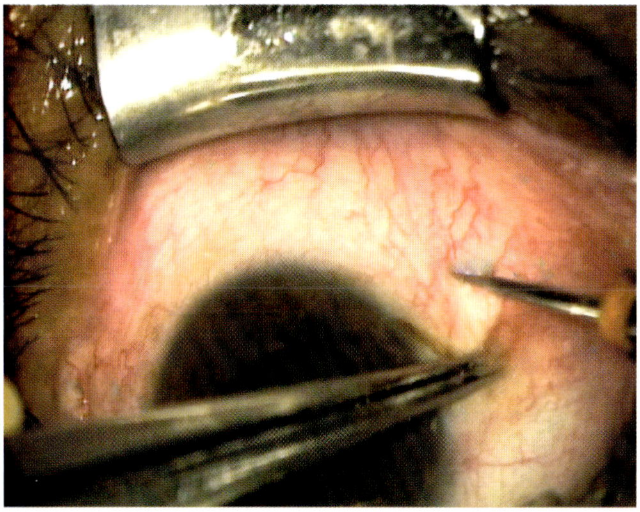

Fig. 2: First step in collocation of scleral stoppers

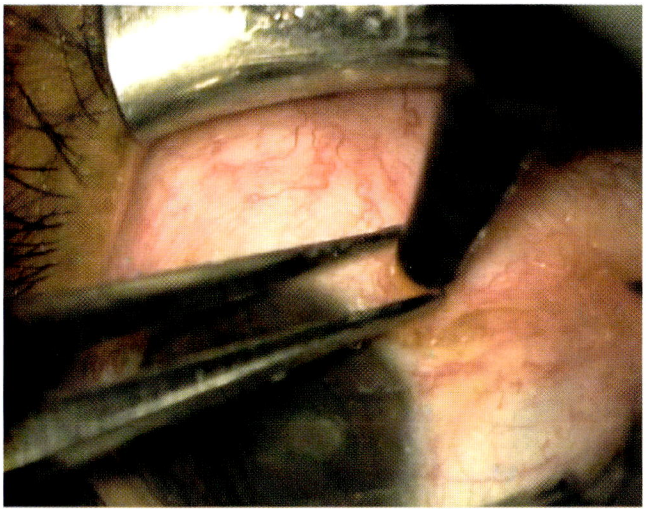

Fig. 3: Second step in collocation of scleral stoppers

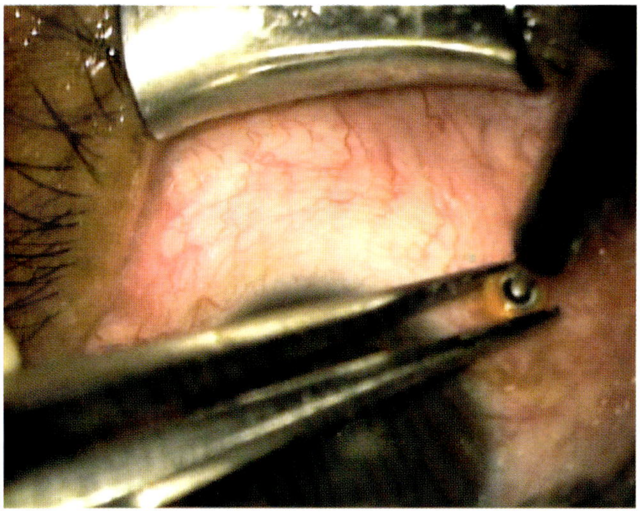

Fig. 4: Third step in collocation of scleral stoppers

Incisions

1. Perform the scleral tunnel incisions (Fig. 1).
2. Place the 25 G scleral stoppers in the three incisions in order to avoid leakage (Figs 2 to 7).
3. Perform the 700 micron clear corneal incisions (Fig. 8).
4. Perform first the nondominant hand incision. Fill the anterior chamber with viscoelastic and perform the incision with the dominant hand.
5. Do not perform any other incision. Less the invasive, best is the behavior of the anterior chamber; maybe the best time to perform the incision for the IOL placement is after both procedures have been finished.

Capsulorhexis

1. Perform all the maneuvers with both hands. Because these kinds of eyes sometimes have absence of red reflex, the surgeon must search the point of reflection of the capsule with the microscope light, and place the eye in this axis to obtain a better view. While performing the capsular surgery with bimanuality, surgeon's nondominant hand is directing the eye to the best light angle and the dominant hand is performing the capsular movements.
2. Hold the eye with the visco-cannula by the nondominant hand incision (surgeon can inject visco any time

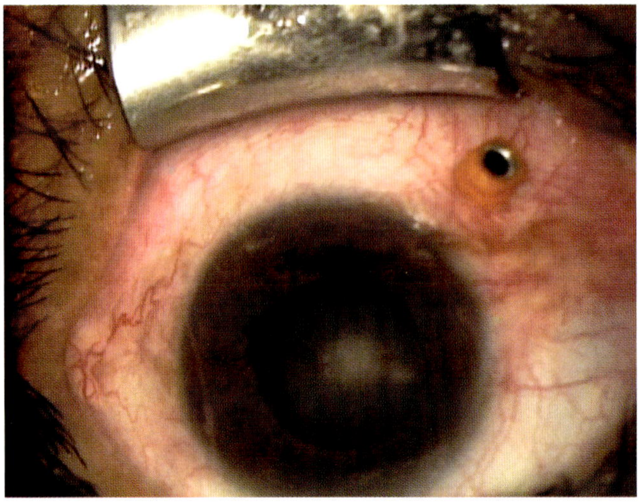

Fig. 5: First scleral stopper in place

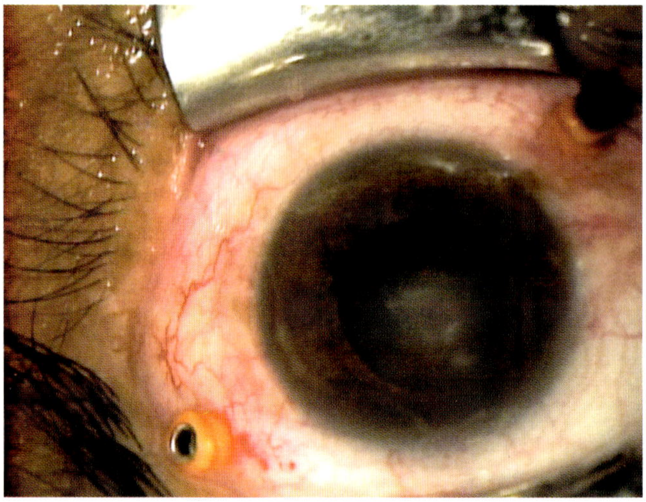

Fig. 6: Two pockets in place. Notice that one has stopper and another has not

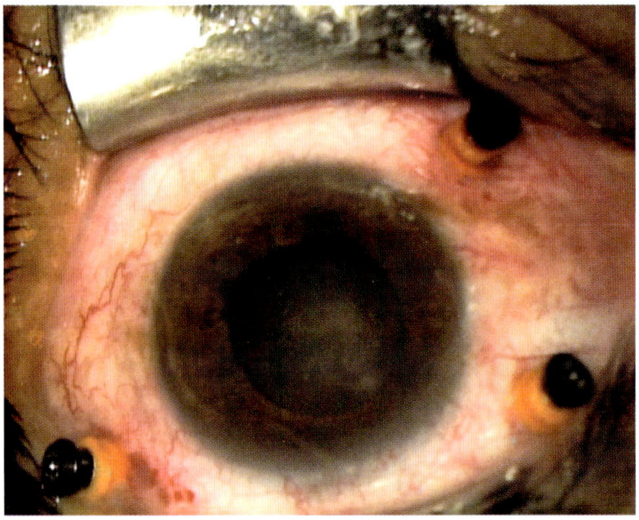

Fig. 7: Three scleral stoppers in site

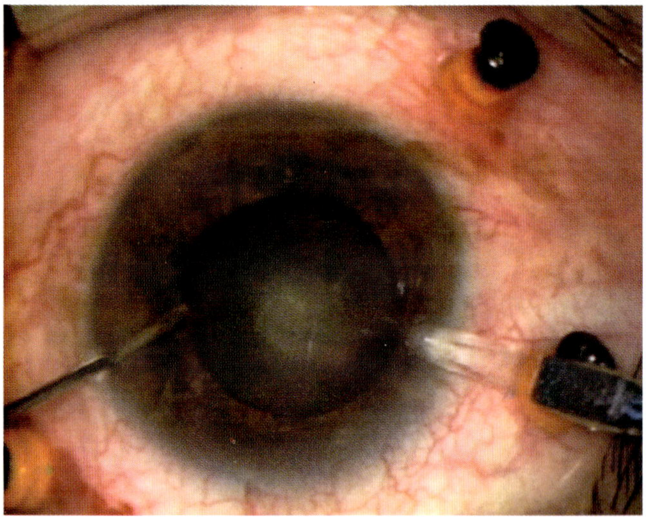

Fig. 8: Clear corneal incisions are being performed with scleral tampons

she needs) and insert cystitome with your dominant hand. Be sure to look always the light reflex over the anterior capsule.

3. Perform microcapsulorhexis using both hands. Learn to use the light reflex to see the capsule. Use nondominant hand to hold the eye, orient it to the best angles of light source and to inject visco. Try to forget about the need of red reflex.

Hydrodissection

1. Use both incisions in order to have two different angles of attack.
2. Move the eye to see with light reflex of capsulorhexis margin.
3. Be careful; avoid too much pressure. surgeons are not able to see the posterior wave because there is no red reflex. Surgeons can feel comfortable when they are able to rotate the nucleus.

Phacoemulsification

1. Try to perform all the maneuvers outside the capsular bag at the iris plane. There is no red reflex to be used as reference (Fig. 9).

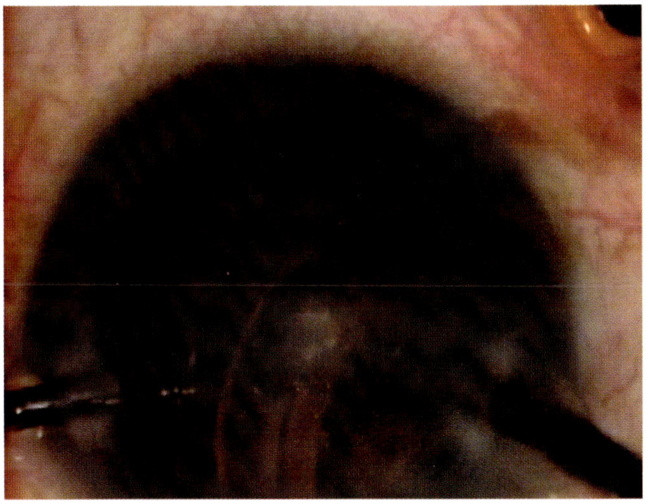

Fig. 9: Micro-Biaxial phaco is performed as usual

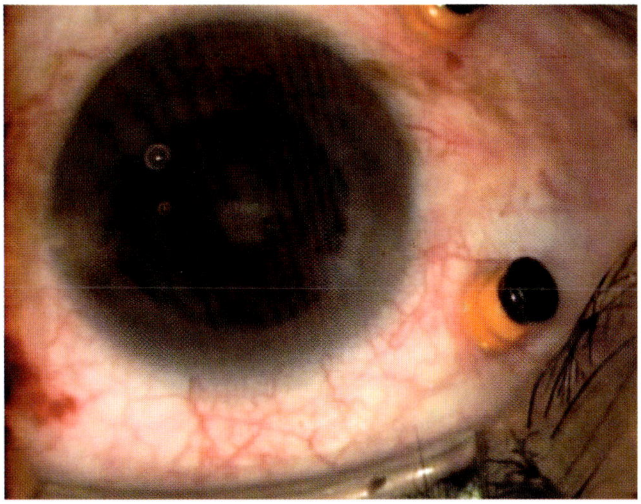

Fig. 10: Eye in aphakia ready to start pars plana vitrectomy. Notice the vitreous hemorrhage

2. If surgeon finds difficulties to perform phaco outside the capsular bag, beware of the depth or his/her movements and instruments because the posterior capsule is difficult to see.
3. Move the eye with bimanuality searching the light reflex.

Irrigation/Aspiration

1. When finish phacoemulsification change to irrigation/ aspiration (I/A) instruments avoiding a collapse of the anterior chamber. A lack of stability in the anterior segment can lead to some posterior segment complications undesirable for the posterior segment surgeon.
2. I/A maneuvers are difficult because of absence of red reflex. Again move the eye with both hands to the best place to visualize the cortical material and the posterior capsule. Take advantage of bimanuality and of the anterior chamber stability.
3. Close the incisions with stromal edema and place visco in the anterior chamber. High-density visco can be a good option if the surgeon notices some leakage. Be aware to cause any chamber collapse.
4. Be sure about the chamber stability before starting PPV (Fig. 10).

Pars Plana Vitrectomy

1. The posterior segment surgeon will find very easy to start to work if the eye has a good IOP. With low IOP there are many difficulties, meanwhile the good IOP is the key to success. (Fig. 10). The 25 G sclerotomies with stoppers placed during phaco, and the 700 micron clear corneal incisions are basic for achieving this goal.
2. Retire the stoppers from scleral incisions and allow the entry of instrumentation for vitrectomy through it (Fig. 11).
3. Be sure that the anterior chamber remains wide open without any leakage while starting PPV; be aware of this before the collocation of pre-corneal lens, in cases when needed (Fig. 12).
4. Be sure about the eye stability while performing complete PPV (Fig. 14).
5. Take care about the integrity of the posterior capsule in particular if silicone oil is implanted in the vitreous cavity.

Intraocular Lens Implantation

1. Choose the IOL power and model according the events during PPV.
2. Fill again the anterior chamber with visco until surgeon feels comfortable with the amplitude of the anterior segment and the IOP.
3. Try to use the smallest incision size.
4. Be gentle with the eye. Keep in control the IOP. The eye has not now the “cushion” of the vitreous body.
5. It may be better to implant with forceps, in order to avoid increase the IOP with injector.

Final Steps

1. It is surgeon`s choice to place stitches at the IOL implantation incision.

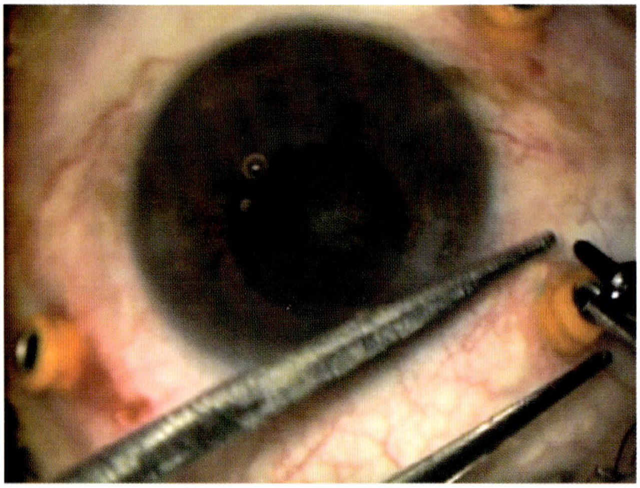

Fig. 11: Stoppers are retired to start pars plana vitrectomy

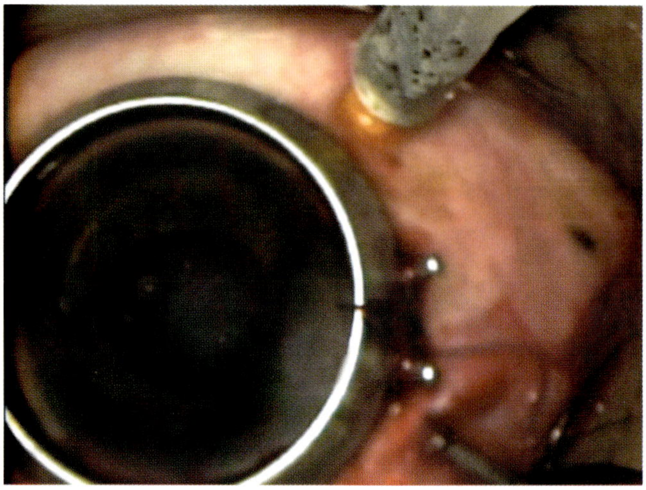

Fig. 12: Precorneal lens and irrigation cannula in place. Notice the stability of the anterior chamber

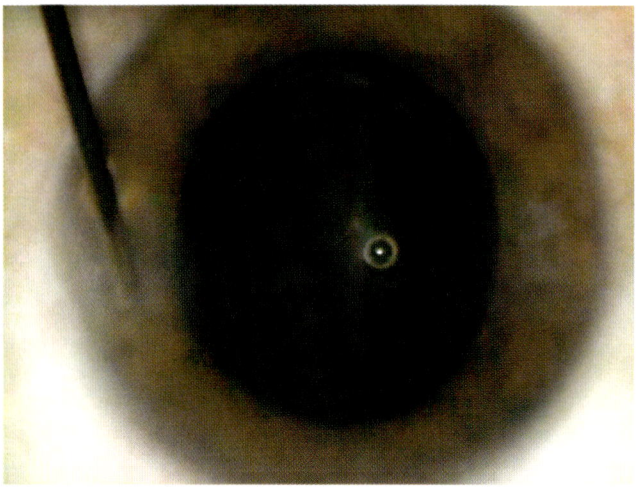

Fig. 13: Eye in aphakia after 700 micron lens extraction, ready to start the posterior vitrectomy

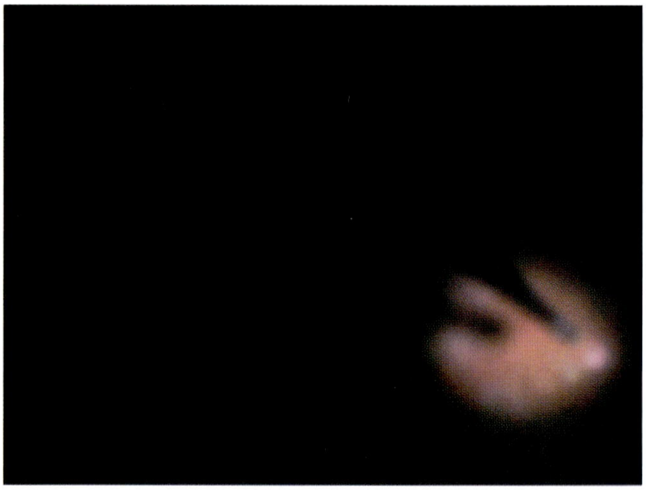

Fig. 14: Endolaser application through contact lens and 700 micron phaco

2. Create again stromal edema in all incisions (Fig. 13).
3. Check the IOP before finish (Fig. 13). Check it frequently in the postoperative period.

Conclusions

The microincisions made in the proper way are self-sealing; therefore, they provide ideal anterior chamber resistance without sudden changes in pressure or leakage for the manipulation of the globe during the vitrectomy stage. This anterior chamber stability allows greater precision during the most risky surgical maneuvers, such as creating the anterior capsulorhexis, cleaning the capsule and implanting the IOL, helping to prevent impairment of the ensuing stages of vitrectomy. The collocation of 25 G stoppers before starting phaco, avoid the manipulation of scleral incisions in an eye with aphakia.

As the vitrectomy may induce a change in intraocular fluid circulation and thus strengthen oxidative damage to the proteins of the crystalline lens, the combined operation should be considered preferable when complete vitrectomy is planned in eyes with initial lens opacity or even in the presbyopic patient, according to some surgeons. As part of the combined procedure, bimanual microphacoemulsification to extract the cataract offers potential advantages in terms of the procedure's safety and effectiveness regarding anatomical and functional outcomes, adding support for the concept of combining lens removal and vitrectomy. 25 G sutureless vitrectomy is another advantage for this technique. The combination of microphakonit with TSV25 makes the combined procedure more rapid and minimally invasive and may be a very useful procedure in vitreoretinal pathologies without dense fibrous proliferation.

The author likes to give his acknowledgments to the Retinal Surgeons that work at his Ambulatory Surgery Center, Yuri Axayacatl Flores Fuentes M.D. & Juan Jose Luis Parra Limón MD for their formidable work with the patients and their particular contributions that made this chapter possible.

References

1. Gian Maria Cavallini, Alessandro Pupino, Cristina Masini, et al. Bimanual microphacoemulsification and Acri.Smart intraocular lens implantation combined with vitreoretinal surgery. J Cataract Refract Surg. 2007;33(7):1253-8.
2. Jong-uk Hwang, Young Hee Yoon, Deok-Soo Kim, et al. Combined phacoemulsification, foldable intraocular lens implantation, and 25-gauge transconjuntival sutureless vitrectomy. J Cataract Refract Surg. 2006;32(5):727-31.
3. Cheng-Jong Chang, Yun-Hsiang Chang, Shang-Yi Chiang, et al. Comparison of clear corneal phacoemulsification combined with 25-gauge transconjuntival sutureless vitrectomy and standard 20-gauge vitrectomy for patients with cataract and vitreoretinal disease. J Cataract Refract Surg. 2005;31(6):1198-1207.
4. Demetriades AM, Gottsch JD, Thomsen R, et al. Combined phacoemulsification, intraocular lens implantation, and vitrectomy for eyes with coexisting cataract & vitreoretinal pathology. Am J Ophthalmol. 2003;135:291-6.
5. Lam DCS, Young AL, Rao SK, et al. Combined phacoemulsification, parsplana vitrectomy, and foldable intraocular lens implantation. J cataract Refract Surg. 2003;29:1064-9.
6. Sofia Androudi, Muna Ahmed, Tito Fiore, et al. Combined pars plana vitrectomy and phacoemulsification to restore acuity in patients with chronic uveitis. J Cataract Refract Surg. 2005;31(3):472-8.
7. David HW Steel. Phacovitrectomy:Expanding indication. J Cataract Refract Surg. 2007;33(6):933-6.
8. Ling R, Simcock P, McCoombes J, et al. Presbyopic phacovitrectomy. Br J Ophthalmol. 2003;87:1333-5.
9. Chaughry NA, Cohen KA, Flynn HW, et al. Combined pars plana vitrectomy and lens management in complex vitreoretinal disease. Semin Ophthalmol. 2003;18:132-41.
10. Heiligenhaus A, Holtkamm A, Koch J, et al. Combined phacoemulsification and pars plana vitrectomy: clear corneal versus scleral incisions: prospective randomized multicenter study. J Cataract Refract Surg. 2003;29:1106-12.
11. Nawrocki J, Michalewska Z, Cisiecki S. Cool phaco in combined phacoemulsification and vitrectomy surgery. Klin Oczna. 2006;108:16-9.
12. Giacomo Panozzo, Barbara Parolini. Cataracts associated with posterior segment surgery. Ophthalmol Clin North Am. 2004;17(4):557-68.
13. Aravind Haripriya, Srinivasan Aravind, Kavitha Vadi, et al. Bimanual microphaco for posterior polar cataracts. J Cataract Refractive Surg. 2006:32(6):914-7.
14. Patrick Watts, James Hunter, Catey Bunce. Vitrectomy and lensectomy in the management of posterior dislocation of the lens fragments.. J Cataract & Refract Surg. 2000; 26(6):832-7.
15. Tanuj Dada, Sanjeev Kumar, Ritu Gadia, et al. Sutureless single-port transconjunctival pars plana limited vitrectomy combined with phacoemulsification for management of phacomorphic glaucoma. J Cataract Refract Surg. 2007;33(6):951-4.
16. Agarwal A, Agarwal S, Agarwal A, et al. Antichamber collapser. J Cataract Refract Surg. 2002;28:1085-6.
17. Agarwal A, Jacob S, Agarwal S. Combined microphakonit and 25-gauge transconjunctival sutureless vitrectomy. J Cataract Refract Surg. 2007:33:1839-40.
18. Step by Step for Bi-Axial Lens Surgery. Pérez-Arteaga A. Jaypee Brothers Publishers, India. 2008.

23 Biaxial: The Best Choice in Pediatric Cataracts

Luis Felipe Vejarano-Restrepo (Colombia)

Introduction

Cataract surgery has been evolving at a very rapid way during the last decades, passing from extracapsular extraction to ultrasonic phacoemulsification, which has become progressively the standard method for cataract surgery around the world, because it affords less-astigmatism induction, rapid-astigmatism stabilization, less-postoperative inflammation and less possibility of postoperative complications than extracapsular cataract extraction.[1-6] One of the latest crucial breakthroughs in phacoemulsification has been to perform the phacoemulsification surgery through a microincision with a bimanual approach, using a sleeveless phaco tip. The idea of removing the crystalline lens through two microincisions has been proposed since the 1970s,[7-8] however it was not until that independently Agarwal in India and Tsuneoka in Japan began that technique in 1998 and 1999 respectively;[9,10] it gained popularity, although it is still practiced by a small percentage of the world's surgeons. Agarwal coined the term "Phakonit", which initially stood for phacoemulsification (phaco) performed with a needle opening (N) via an ultra-small incision (I) with the sleeveless ultrasound tip (T).[11] Originally Agarwal described an incision as small as 0.9 mm,[9] using a standard sleeveless microtip. Although initially the theoretical possibility of a possible thermal burn was a concern, this fear was dispelled by several studies; Tsuneoka showed experimentally in a porcine eye that using a sleeveless ultrasound tip, the temperature of the cornea at the incision elevated only 8.4°C without developing thermal burns.[10] In other experiments, Olson et al. demonstrated that clinically unusual parameters were necessary to produce a wound burn in bimanual phaco and moreover, when using "cold phaco" with a bare 19 gauge aspiration needle in human cadaver eyes, a wound burn could not be produced at the highest energy settings unless all flow into the eye and all aspiration were occluded. These settings are well beyond clinically applicable conditions. The author's explanation is that it is difficult to completely occlude a linear stab incision with a metal circular instrument, unlike the situation in standard coaxial phaco, where a flexible irrigation sleeve fills the wound and reduces the flow around the sleeve, particularly in a tight wound. The combinations of a tight wound, filled by a flexible irrigation sleeve, and complete occlusion of aspiration, and therefore complete blockage of irrigation, results in a wound burn. So in fact, the risk of thermal burn may be less in phakonit than in coaxial phaco.[12,13]

Agarwal initially reported 305 eyes that underwent the technique successfully. He had the assistant continuously pouring cooled balanced salt solution (BSS®) over the phaco needle. The original incision had to be enlarged in order to implant the intraocular lens (IOL). Not a case of thermal wound occurred.[14] Tsuneoka and coauthors[15] also initially reported 637 cases that underwent cataract surgery through a 1.4 mm incision without a case of thermal burn. Likewise author and colleague have not found any case of corneal wound burn in their cases.[16]Around the world several other surgeons, including the author and colleague, have reported their results using bimanual microincisional surgery with different phaco machines.[16-27] Alió, coined the term Microincision Cataract Surgery (MICS)[23] and has reported good visual performance of two availables IOLs, which may be implanted through microincisions.[24,25] In a prospective randomized consecutive case series, he reported that MICS significantly lowered mean phacoemulsification time, mean total phacoemulsification percent, mean effective phaco time and surgically induced astigmatism when compared with coaxial phacoemulsification.[26] Fine has highlighted the advantages of maintaining a more stable intraocular environment during lens removal.[27] This advantage may be especially important in high myopes who are at a greater risk for retinal detachment following lens extraction[27] or high hyperopes decreasing the possibility of an expulsive hemorrhage.

In 2002, Olson, was the first to use a 0.8 mm phaco needle and a 21 gauge irrigating chopper in bimanual cataract surgery and called this technique microphaco.[13,14,28]These techniques of performing phacoemulsification through incisions around 1.0–1.5 mm have been spreading around the world. Other names given to these techniques are bimanual phacoemulsification and sleeveless phaco. Recently, Agarwal reported the microphakonit, a similar technique, but using a 0.7 mm needle and a 0.7 mm irrigating chopper through a sub 1 mm incision [28-30]For match all the names that this technique has, author and colleague prefer to use MICS when they use only aspiration through microincision with no phaco needle, like in pediatric cataracts, where with only aspiration surgeons can remove it; but if surgeons going to use ultrasound power then called phakonit, microphakonit if the incision is smaller, microphaco or bimanual phaco so indicates that the removal of the cataract is going to be by ultrasound (phaco power).

Going from a 0.9 mm phaco needle to a 0.7 mm needle diminished the aspiration flow rate, the holding power and in general the efficiency of the tip, so in order to have a feasible procedure, a modified 30 degree tip was developed by Microsurgical Technology (MST), Redmond, USA, with thinner walls, allowing for an increased inner diameter thereby increasing efficiency close to that of a 0.9 mm tip. Agarwal uses his end-opening sharp irrigating chopper and gas forced infusion, initially he employed an external air pump and then the Anterior Vented Gas Forced Infusion (AVGFI) system of the Alcon's Accurus equipment, with the infusion pump preset to 100 mm Hg.[28,31] Author has been using the phakonit technique for more than 4 years (since September 2002), with a personal chopping technique, the "Vejarano's safe chop"[16,32-34] and the Vejarano's irrigating chopper.[33,34] Author and colleague have already published results with a phakonit technique through 1.2–1.5 mm, using the 20 gauge Microtip, or 19 gauge Standard or MicroFlow® tips.[16] Now author and colleague have available the special designed 0.7 mm Nanotip (MST) that allows them to perform the surgery through 0.8 mm incision. Because of the good results of these techniques author and colleague are using it in all their adult and pediatric cataract patients and they show their technique on these cases.

Surgical Technique

Biaxial

Before surgery, the pupil is dilated with tropicamide 1% and phenylephrine 10%. Povidone-iodine 10% is applied on the lashes and eyelids margins and povidone-iodine 5% is applied in the conjunctiva and washed out 3–5 minutes later, if the pupil doesn't dilate good enough, then use Epinephrine 1/10000 U in the anterior chamber.

In regard with the side port incision, it must be as watertight as possible when the instrument (irrigating chopper or irrigating device) is in position, but without compromising its maneuverability, and this is a very important issue, since in phakonit this is the instrument that makes most of the movement necessary to emulsify the nucleus and in pediatric cataract to mobilize the opacified crystalline. For this reason, author and colleague use a trapezoidal shape side port incision, which internally maintains very good water tightness, and externally has more room for a wider arch of movement of the instrument; if you feel the instrument gets stuck at the incision is a good idea to apply a small amount of viscoelastic on the chopper to make its movement easier.

Author and colleague have found that performing a trapezoidal 0.8/1.2 mm (inner/outer size) incision let them to use the Vejarano's Irrigating Chopper® (AC7340, Accutome, Malvern, USA) (Fig. 1), which for phakonit has 20 gauge (approximately 0.9 mm diameter), with almost no leakage and very good maneuverability. To achieve a good architecture, author and colleague use a 0.8/1.2 mm diamond knife (Accutome, Malvern, USA) (Fig. 2) to perform this incision, but an alternative is to use 20 gauge vitreoretinal blades or 1.2/1.4 mm steel blades (MicroSurgical Technology, Redmond, USA).

When performing the main incision, author and colleague use 1.2 mm diamond lancet or the same 0.8/1.2 mm diamond knife to avoid additional expenses (both Accutome, Malvern, USA) if they are going to use a 20 gauge microtip, and a 1.5 mm diamond blade (Natural Clear Cornea Vejarano's Microincision Knife, AK6018;

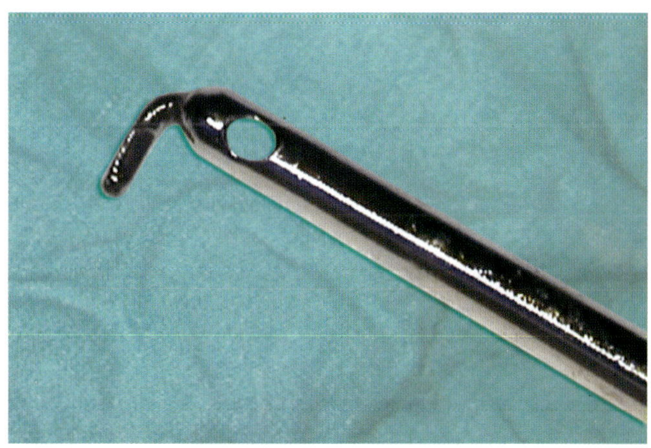

Fig. 1: Vejarano's irrigation chopper for phakonit. It has 0.9 mm diameter, and two irrigation holes close to the tip

Accutome, Malvern, USA) when using a 19 gauge Standard or MicroFlow® tip. Author and colleague think that it is not indispensable that the main incision has a trapezoidal shape because, in phakonit, the phaco needle does not move considerably, just back and forth. Moreover, in the wider (1.5 mm) incision a trapezoidal shape could lead to excessive leakage.

The incision width is not determined arbitrarily but is contingent upon the needle diameter. A common misconception is that a 0.9 mm diameter instrument will fit in a 0.9 mm incision. This will cause excessive stretching of the incision and may tear it, compromising its water-tightness and due to the too tight contact between the tissue and the phaco tip, will increase the risk of thermal damage because the fluid going out helps to cool the needle's shaft. On the other hand a too big incision will increase the leakage and will compromise the anterior chamber stability. According to the gauges of the irrigating instrument and the phaco needle that surgeons normally use, they can determine the proper size of incisions. Surgeons can calculate the circumference length of the instrument, using the formula $[2(\pi \times r)]$; where, **r** means radius of the instrument in mm. Then, since each lip of the incision covers a half, not the whole length of the instrument's circumference is needed (and the incision length corresponds to one incision's lip length), surgeons have to divide the result by two (in order to find out how long is half of the circumference of the instrument and therefore the incision length). Moreover, the cornea has elastic properties and so surgeons have to take in account the tissue compliance that empirically, according with the true incision length measured in our procedures, author and colleague have calculated in 20%. Thus the final formula to decide upon the right length of the incision is:

$[2(\pi r)/2] - 20\%$. This may be simplified as: $\pi \times r \times 0.8$.

For instance for a 0.9 mm tip (approximately 20 gauge), the incision length should be:

$\pi \times r \times 0.8 = \pi \times 0.45 \text{ mm} \times 0.8 \approx 1.1 \text{ mm}$.

For a 1.1 mm tip (approximately 19 gauge), the incision length should be:

$\pi \times r \times 0.8 = \pi \times 0.55 \text{ mm} \times 0.8 \approx 1.4 \text{ mm}$.

Generally, author and colleague use DuoVisc® (Alcon, Fort Worth, Texas, USA) with the Arshinoff's Soft Shell technique;[35] in all the pediatric cases, author and colleague stain the anterior capsule with trypan blue before viscoelastic in regular cataracts with zonular integrity and after viscoelastic in those cases with anomalies in the shape of the crystalline as Marfan syndrome, agenesia and others in order to avoid the stain of the vitreous with the dye; this stain makes the capsulorhexis easier and gives a better sensation of control, also this dye gives to the capsule more rigidity and less elasticity.

A 5.0 mm or less continuous curvilinear capsulorhexis (CCC) is created because of the features of the capsule it increases its diameter, using the Micro Incision Capsulorhexis Forceps, 23 gauge (Accutome, Malvern, USA) or DUET Capsulorhexis Forceps with Fine grasping tip, 23 gauge (MicroSurgical Technology, Redmond, USA), through microincisión the stability of the anterior chamber is amazing avoiding the draining of the viscoelastic material through the incisions and of course controlling the positive pressure of the vitreous in these infants cases preventing capsulorhexis lost, also surgeons can use the vitrector to try to get a similar shape of CCC but with its edges won't be really continuous.

In cases where there is not good red reflex (white pediatric cataracts) author and colleague always use trypan blue as described by Melles,[36] but diluting the commercially available 0.1% solution to a 0.05% solution, with very good results in contrast and visualization.

Hydrodissection is performed using the Gimbel or Chang cannulae, previously depressing lightly the posterior lip of the incision, to allow that a small amount of viscoelastic goes out from the anterior chamber, thus avoiding a sudden arise of intraocular pressure during hydrodissection; hydrodelineation, may be performed rarely, according with surgeon's personal preferences but with only hydrodissection surgeon obtains the luxation of the nucleus, so go underneath anterior capsule and direct toward the periphery of the crystalline; inject the BSS there and in other different places and immediately the nucleus goes to the anterior chamber where surgeon can aspirate or emulsify it avoiding any contact with the posterior capsule.

The Vejarano's Irrigating Chopper® 20 gauge (Accutome, Malvern, USA), or 22 gauge (MicroSurgical Technology, Redmond, USA) is entered through the side port, in order to maintain adequate space in the anterior chamber. The features of the 20 gauge chopper are shown in Figure 1. It has an outer diameter of 0.9 mm (approximately 20 gauge) that fits rather tightly in the 0.9/1.2 mm side port incision. Author and colleague have found it to be very useful, and with a high safety profile in cases performed using the Infiniti Vision System (Alcon, Fort Worth, Texas, USA).

A partially sleeveless phaco tip is entered to the anterior chamber through the main incision (in those cases that surgeons believe will need phaco power). A cut sleeve is used in the phaco needle, according to the description by Prakash,[37] and author and colleague found that it is useful to diminish the amount of fluid splashed from the phaco needle during the application of ultrasound energy (like rain). Author and colleague do not use any additional external fluid to cool the wound.

The parameters used in the phaco machines are related with the hardness of the nuclei, which in these cases is very low just to try to unclog the tip. Author and colleague use gas forced infusion with the systems that have it incorporated, but they have found that with the Vejarano´s irrigating chopper they can perform the surgery with a stable anterior chamber, using the bottle with passive (gravitatory) infusion at an enough height, even in these cases where the vitreous push anteriorly in the whole procedure.

The parameters can be summarized as follows:

Infiniti® Vision System

Fixed flow rate : 25–30 cc/min

Lineal vacuum : 250–300 mm Hg

Dynamic rise : 3–4 Lineal power: 10%

Mode : Pulsed, 20–50 pps

Modulation power : 20% ON

Mode : Burst, 50 msec

Bottle high : 180 cm above the patient's head

Bimanual irrigation/aspiration (I/A) of cortical remnants using bimanual handpieces and, if necessary, posterior capsule polishing are done also the aspiration and cleaning of the anterior capsule epithelial cells to try to avoid its fibrosis, in cases with soft nuclei (as the majority of them); since the beginning author and colleague use this bimanual I/A to remove the whole crystalline avoiding any use of ultrasound.

Previously to the IOL insertion in every case, author and colleague implant a capsular tension ring (CTR) to gives scleral support in these cases with not enough rigidity and try to stop the growth of the lens cells from the equator and the capsule contraction too; author and colleague had been doing this since two-and-a-half years with excellent results avoiding that.

Author and colleague prefer to make a new tunnel incision through the sclera superiorly to implant the IOL to prevent any leakage, anterior chamber collapse postoperatively and infection because the lack of rigidity in this young eyes, and author and colleague always use 10-0 nylon suture to close the wound.

The decision of the IOL is still a point of discussion. Usually author and colleague implant acrylic hydrophobic IOLs [Acrysof SA60A, Acrysof Natural single-piece or Acrysof IQ IOLs (Alcon, Fort Worth, Texas, USA)] using a Titanium Single Hand Injector EL-30 (Epsilon, Montclair, California, USA), which makes possible the implantation through an 1.8–2.2 mm incision. It is important that the injector is a single hand instrument (with a plunger), since the second hand is use to exert contra-pressure with a second instrument through the side port incision, fixating the eye and the injection through the incision must be fast and always in the bag.

At the end of the case, author and colleague always leave a 0.3 cc of Kenalog (4.5 mg) which can help to see any leakage through the incisions, and they notice a big advantage in decreasing the postoperative inflammation, non any pupillary membrane and always a reactive pupil at next day, with this concentration author and colleague didn't have had any elevation of the intraocular pressure.

Micro-Biaxial

The microphakonit technique is very similar, but obviously the incisions' length is smaller. Author and colleague use instruments 22 gauge, even irrigating choppers [Agarwal or Vejarano or Verges (Microsurgical Technology, Redmond, USA] or I/A tips.

According with the formula explained above, for a 0.7 mm instrument (approximately 22 gauge), the incision length should be:

$$\pi \times r \times 0.8 = \pi \times 0.35 \text{ mm} \times 0.8 \approx 0.9 \text{ mm}.$$

Author and colleague construct a 0.9 mm side port incision with the 0.9–15 degree side port Diamod Knife (Accutome, Malvern, USA) (Fig. 2) to introduce the microphakonit 22 gauge Vejarano's irrigating chopper (Microsurgical Technology, Redmond, USA) (Fig. 3) which is approximately 0.7 mm in external diameter and 0.65 mm in internal diameter. Like Dr Agarwal's microphakonit

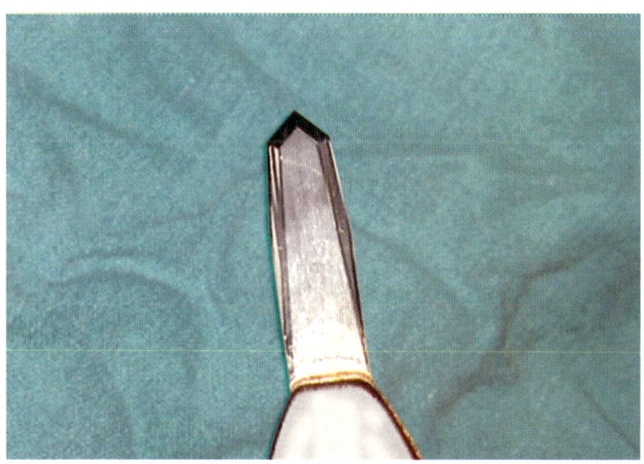

Fig. 2: A 0.9/1.2 mm diamond knife (Accutome)

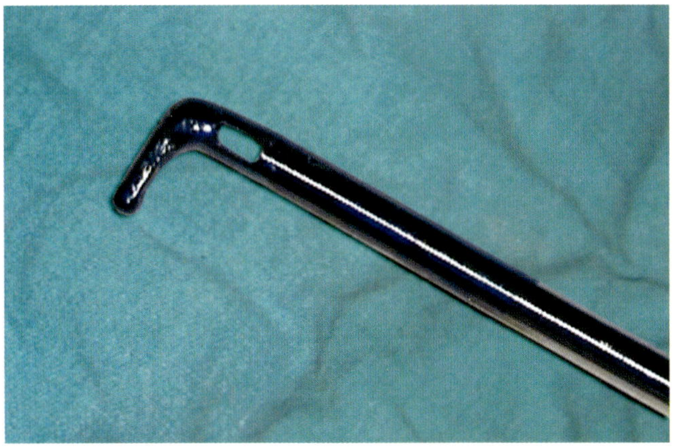

Fig. 3: Microphakonit 22 gauge Vejarano's irrigating chopper, (Microsurgical Technology)

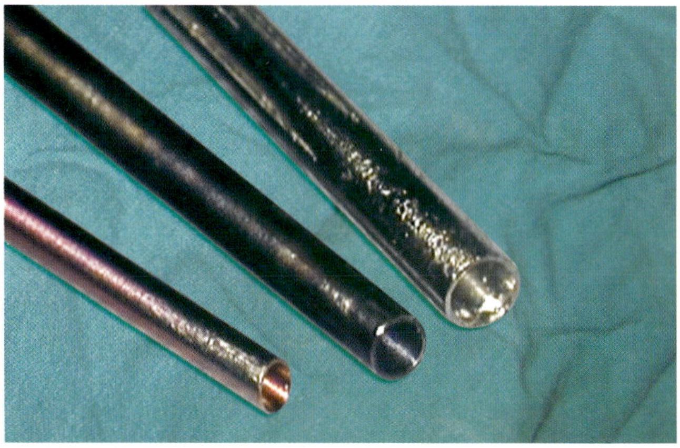

Fig. 4: Comparison of phaco needles from MicroFlow (standard tip) (Bausch & Lomb), MicroTip (Alcon) and NanoTip (Microsurgical Technology)

chopper, this instrument has thinner walls, allowing for an increased inner diameter, and moreover it features two lateral very elongated irrigation holes, thereby increasing inflow.

Main incision of 0.9 mm is performed using the same diamond blade or using the new MST 0.8 mm disposable lancets but with these the 23 gauge. Microutrata forceps fits very tightly which its mobility difficult. Author and colleague use the MST nano tip, 0.7 mm diameter (Fig. 4), and the Infiniti® system (Alcon, Fort Worth, Texas, USA). Author and colleague have found that this tip has a very good performance and efficiency in emulsifying and aspirating the nuclear material, despite its very small outer diameter, because of its design of a very thin wall.

The parameters used on the Infiniti® system are the same ones as for Phakonit.

When finishing the pediatric cases author and colleague prefer to put a suture in both, the main incision (always) and paracentesis if leakage is noted. Moreover, in order to diminish the possibility of capsular opacification, and hence the necessity of a posterior YAG-laser capsulotomy, and also to minimize the anterior capsule retraction as in phakonit, author and colleague always use a CTR in these pediatric cases. Their experience after two-and-a-half years of follow-up is that 94% of the capsules are transparent, and they have not had any case of capsular phimosis.

Also as in phakonit, author and colleague always use the Kenalog at the end of the case.

Conclusion

There is an evident trend between leading ophthalmologists all around the world to perform microincision techniques, because of its advantages more in these pediatric cataracts where the inflammation is an issue to think. Author and colleague think that smaller incisions are in fact safer, since they are working in an almost closed system. Using the right parameters the anterior chamber is much more stable than in coaxial phaco with much less turbulence, endothelial cells trauma and less BSS. Moreover during the phaco it is evident of an improved followability, since currents rejecting fragments far from the phaco tip, such as in coaxial phacoemulsification, are avoided. In addition, the incoming irrigation flow can be used as a third intraocular instrument, which helps in directing fragments to the phaco tip and pulling structures away from it like posterior capsule or iris.

The availability of better instruments, including the MST nanotip designed with the cooperation of Dr Agarwal and MST, along with the Vejarano's irrigating choppers (20 gauge and 22 gauge) and bimanual I/A tips (20 gauge and 22 gauge) (Fig. 5), let the surgeons to safely perform microincision cataract surgery, and even break the 1 mm

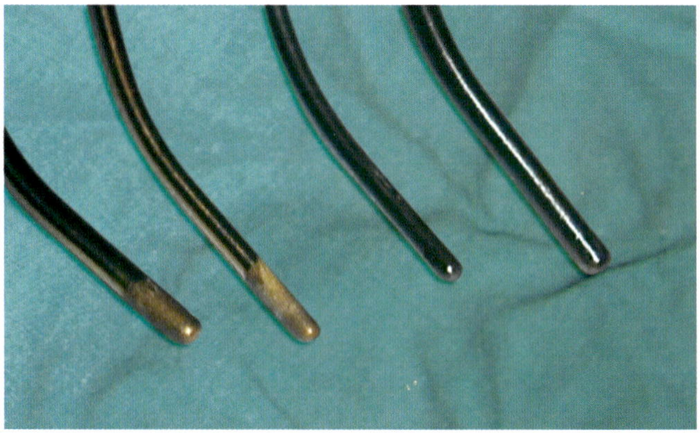

Fig. 5: Bimanual irrigation/aspiration tips (20 gauge and 22 gauge) (Microsurgical Technology)

frontier with the microphakonit, a really nano-surgery technique. Author and colleague think that these several advantages make microincisional phacoemulsification techniques ideal also for pediatric cases.

The use of a CTR has improved their results in the sense that the posterior capsule is kept transparent and the anterior capsule retraction is avoided and the use of Kenalog has reduced the inflammation postoperatively and improves the velocity of visual recovery.

References

1. Minassian DC, Rosen P, Dart JK, et al. Extracapsular cataract extraction compared with small incision surgery by phacoemulsification: a randomized trial. Br J Ophthalmol. 2001;85:822-9.
2. Cavallini GM, Lugli N, Campi L, et al. Surgically induced astigmatism after manual extracapsular cataract extraction or after phacoemulsification procedure. Eur J Ophthalmol. 1996;6:257-63.
3. Watson A, Sunderraj P. Comparison of small-incision phacoemulsification with standard extracapsular cataract surgery: post-operative astigmatism and visual recovery. Eye. 1992;6(Pt 6):626-9.
4. Chee SP, Ti SE, Sivakumar M, et al. Postoperative inflammation: extracapsular cataract extraction versus phacoemulsification. J Cataract Refract Surg. 1999;25:1280-5.
5. Francis PJ, Morris RJ. Post-operative iris prolapse following phacoemulsification and extracapsular cataract surgery. Eye. 1997;11(Pt 1):87-90.
6. Linebarger EJ, Hardten DR, Shah GK, et al. Phacoemulsification and modern cataract surgery. Surv Ophthalmol. 1999;44:123-47.
7. Girard LJ. Ultrasonic fragmentation for cataract extr-action and cataract complications. Adv Ophthalmol. 1978;37:127-35.
8. Shearing SP, Relyea RL, Loaiza A, et al. Routine phacoemulsification through a one-millimeter non-sutured incision. Cataract. 1985;2(2):6–11.
9. Agarwal A, Agarwal S, Agarwal A. Phakonit: lens removal through a 0.9 mm incision. J Cataract Refract Surg. 2001;27:1531-2.
10. Tsuneoka H, Takuya S, Takahashi Y. Feasibility of ultrasound cataract surgery with a 1.4 mm incision. J Cataract Refract Surg. 2001;27:934-40.
11. Agarwal A, Agarwal S, Agarwal A. Phakonit and laser phakonit: lens removal through a 0.9 mm incision. In: Agarwal S, Agarwal A, Sachdev MS, et al. (Eds). Phacoemulsification, Laser Cataract Surgery and Foldable IOLs, 2nd edition. New Delhi: Jaypee Brothers Medical Publishers; 2000. pp. 204-16.
12. Soscia W, Howard JG, Olson RJ. Bimanual phacoe-mulsification through 2 stab incisions. A wound-temperature study. J Cataract Refract Surg. 2002;28(6): 1039-43.
13. Soscia W, Howard JG, Olson RJ. Microphacoemulsification with WhiteStar A wound-temperature study. J Cataract Refrac Surg. 2002;28,(6):1044-6.
14. Agarwal A, Agarwal S, Agarwal A. Phakonit: Phacoemulsification through a 0.9 mm corneal incision.J Cataract Refract Surg. 2001;27:1548-52.
15. Tsuneoka H, Shiba T, Takahashi Y. Ultrasonic phacoemulsification using a 1.4 mm incision: clinical results. J Cataract Refract Surg. 2002;28:81-6.
16. Vejarano L Felipe, Tello A. Outcomes with the ThinOptx IOL. Using the lens as part of Microincisional Cataract Surgery. Cataract Refract Surg Today. 2004;84.
17. Centurion V, Caballero JC, Lacava AC. The time is now for MICS Technique and technology align to permit ultrasmall cataract incisions. Ocular Surgery News. 2003.
18. Carreño E. Cirugía por microincisión realizada con faco estándar. Ocular Surgery News Latin America Edition. 2003;5:2.
19. Chang DF. 400 mm Hg high-vacuum bimanual phaco attainable with the Staar Cruise Control device. J Cataract Refract Surg. 2004;30(4):932-3.
20. Pandey SK, Werner L, Agarwal A, et al. Phakonit: cataract removal through a sub-1.0 mm incision and implantation of the ThinOptX rollable intraocular lens. J Cataract Refract Surg. 2002;28(9):1710-3.
21. Braga-Mele R, Liu E. Feasibility of sleeveless bimanual phacoemulsification with the Millennium microsurgical system. J Cataract Refract Surg. 2003, 29(11): 2199-203.
22. Pérez-Arteaga A. Anterior vented gas forced infusion system of the Accurus Surgical System in Phakonit. J Cataract Refract Surg. 2004;30(4):933-5.
23. Alió JL. Microincision Cataract Surgery [MICS] Improves Safety, Surgeon Says. Ocular Surgery News. 2001.
24. Alió JL, Schimchak P, Montés-Micó R, et al. Retinal image quality after microincision intraocular lens implantation. J Cataract Refract Surg. 2005;31(8):1557-60.
25. Alió JL, Rodriguez-Prats JL, Vianello A, et al. Visual outcome of microincision cataract surgery with implantation of an Acri.Smart lens. J Cataract Refract Surg. 2005;31(8):1549-56.
26. Alio L, Rodriguez-Prats JL, Galal A, et al. Outcomes of microincision cataract surgery versus coaxial phacoemulsification. Ophthalmology. 2005;112(11):1997-2003.
27. Fine IH, Hoffman RS, Packer M. Optimizing refractive lens exchange with bimanual microincision phacoemulsification. J Cataract Refract Surg. 2004;30:550-4.
28. Agarwal A. How small can you go? Ophthalmology Times Europe. 2006.
29. Agarwal A, Agarwal A, Agarwal S. A look at Microphakonit Phaco. Eyeworld Magazine. 2005.
30. Agarwal A, Agarwal A, Agarwal S. Microphakonit surgery performed with 0.7-mm tip. Ocular Surgery News Europe/ Asia-Pacific Edition; 2005.
31. Agarwal A, Agarwal S, Agarwal A, et al. Antichamber collapser. J Cataract Refract Surg. 28;7:1085-6.
32. Vejarano LF, Tello A. Safe chop: a safer technique. In: (Ed). New Outcomes in Cataract Surgery. Panamá: Highlights of Ophthalmology; 2005.

33. Vejarano LF, Tello Alejandro. Vejarano's safe chop technique: a safer chopping. Tech Ophthalmol. 2005;3(3):109-15.
34. Vejarano L Felipe, Tello A. Vejarano safe chop makes transition to chopping easier. Ocular Sugery News. 2005;23(5):10-1.
35. Arshinoff SA. Dispersive-cohesive viscoelastic soft shell technique. J Cataract Refract Surg 1999;25:167-73.
36. Melles G, de Waard P, Pameyer J, et al. Trypan blue capsule staining to visualize the capsulorhexis in cataract surgery. J Cataract Refract Surg. 1999;25:7-9.
37. Prakash DP. Cutting phaco sleeve permits ultrasmall-incision surgery: Using a cut sleeve without irrigation eliminates water splashing and improves visibility during surgery. Ocular Surgery News Europe/Asia-Pacific Edition; 2003.

24 Micro-Biaxial Posterior Capsule Cleaning

Arturo Pérez-Arteaga (Mexico)

Introduction

This is a very small chapter because of its content, but not because of its importance. It describes a powerful utility that the micro-biaxial irrigation/aspiration technique has in cases of posterior capsule opacity (PCO), in particular those cases where there is not a fibrotic process; instead of fibrosis what happens is cell proliferation, it means that the opacity is formed by Elschnig's pearls (clear, pearl-like clusters formed by proliferation of epithelial cells that grow on the lens capsule in secondary cataract formation)[1] (Fig. 1). For many surgeons worldwide, the formation of Elschnig's pearls the indication is the neodymium YAG laser posterior capsulotomy; nevertheless surgeons have to remember that the posterior capsulotomy, performed by any method, increases the rate of retinal detachment, in different percentage according to many published series, in particular in the myopic eye. To keep the integrity of the posterior capsule, avoiding the communication between the aqueous and the vitreous cavity; it can be a key point to decrease the incidence of posterior segment troubles in some groups of patients.

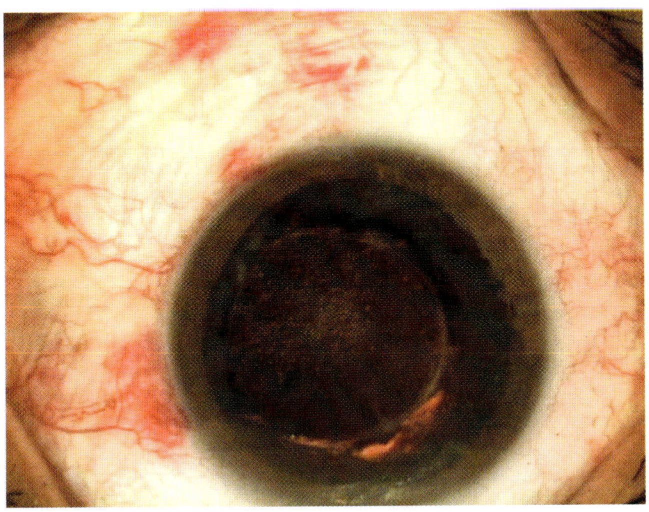

Fig. 1: Elschnig pearls

The cleaning of the Elschnig´s pearls can be a very important procedure in cases where the surgeon wants to keep the integrity of the posterior capsule. For these particular cases, the micro-biaxial irrigation/aspiration technique can give a safe and fast visual recovery, in particular because it can be performed under topical anesthesia, allowing the patient immediate visual improvement, as in cases of neodymium YAG laser posterior capsulotomy, but with the advantages of the integrity of the posterior capsule.

Advantages of Bimanuality

In this same textbook, Prof. Mark Packer, has pointed the advantages of bimanuality as follows:[2-6]

1. Enhanced chamber stability thanks to a more nearly perfectly closed system.
2. Better followability due to separation of infusion and aspiration.
3. Access to 360 degrees of the anterior segment with either infusion or aspiration by switching instruments from one hand to the other.
4. It permits using the flow of irrigation fluid as a tool to move material within the capsular bag or anterior chamber.
5. Prevention of iris billowing and prolapse in cases of intraoperative floppy iris syndrome.
6. Significantly decreased chance of vitreous prolapse in the case of a posterior capsular tear, zonular dialysis or subluxed cataracts, thanks to maintenance of a pressurized stream of irrigation from above.[8]

These same advantages describe for bimanuality can be found in this technique of pearls aspiration. The surgeon has a complete control of what is happening at the anterior chamber and has complete access to all the sectors and meridians of the posterior capsule for the complete aspiration of the pearls; it means a complete cleaning. In cases of an eventual rupture of the posterior capsule during the aspirating procedure, the surgeon knows that it has a complete closed environment, and the hyaloid face (or the vitreous body) will be pushed back into the vitreous cavity because of the maintenance of the pressurized system in a closed environment given by the irrigation. So, a severe complication can be reduced in consequences.[7-12]

Maybe the most important disadvantage of the procedure of pearls aspiration, is the fact itself of the conservation of the integrity of the posterior capsule in comparison with capsulotomy procedure. If well, the vitreoretinal complications are reduced in incidence; the possibility of new formation of pearls and the consequent new opacity of the posterior capsule is not reduced by this procedure. Nevertheless a well informed patient (in particular the one with increased potential of vitreoretinal disease) can understand that a new clean up process in a future is possible, but with the procedure there is not an increase in the possibility of developing vitreoretinal complications.

Surgical Technique

1. Preparation and drape anterior segment surgery under topical anesthesia.
2. Perform two 700 micron incisions with the appropriate instrumentation. Authors have found much better to separate both incisions something between 120 degrees and 180 degrees; this increases the range of maneuver and the access to all meridians of the chamber (Figs 2A and B). The good performance and the good size of the incisions are mandatory to allow an easy entrance of the instrumentation and avoid leakage.
3. Utilize intra-cameral anesthetic if surgeon feels comfortable according their patient.
4. Check your parameters of irrigation and aspiration in phaco machine. Test the functioning of the system outside the eye. Good parameters for 700 micron system are 110 cm H_2O of forced infusion and 300–400 mm Hg of vacuum; these parameters allow the surgeon to keep a formed anterior chamber, avoiding the surge, because irrigation is more than aspiration. Introduce both cannulas, irrigation and aspiration, to the anterior chamber (Fig. 3).
5. Perform bimanual (biaxial) irrigation/aspiration, searching for all the pearls at the posterior capsule (Figs 4A to C). Remember that surgeon has a closed environment and has access to all the meridians. In case of the presence of an intraocular lens (IOL), maintain the irrigating cannula at the anterior chamber and the aspirating cannula between the IOL and the posterior capsule. If the IOL is trapped at the capsular bag, sometimes is necessary to perform some anterior capsulectomy with the objective to make room enough to introduce the cannula behind the IOL.
6. Once surgeons are sure that the posterior capsule is clean, make a final review searching for a place for nice red reflex to observe the structures of the anterior chamber (Fig. 5).
7. Surgeons can maintain the irrigating cannula inside the eye, withdraw the aspirating cannula and introduce viscoelastic material through the dominant incision, with the objective of keeping a positive intraocular pressure; avoiding this way the collapse and so negative pressure transmitted to the vitreous body. This maneuver has been discussed in some other chapters.

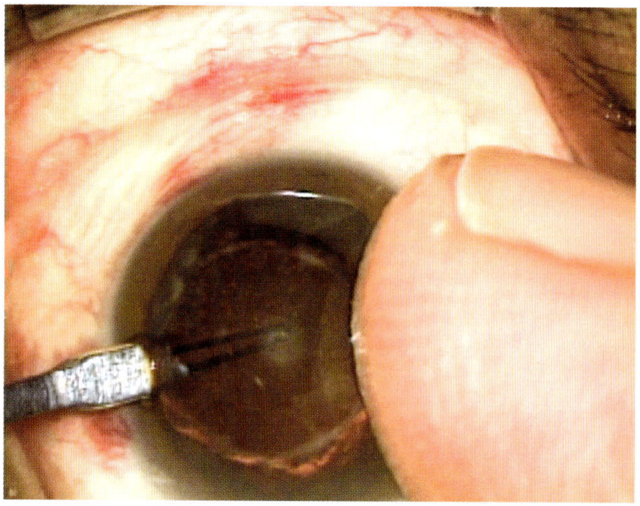

Fig. 2A: Nondominant hand 700 micron incision

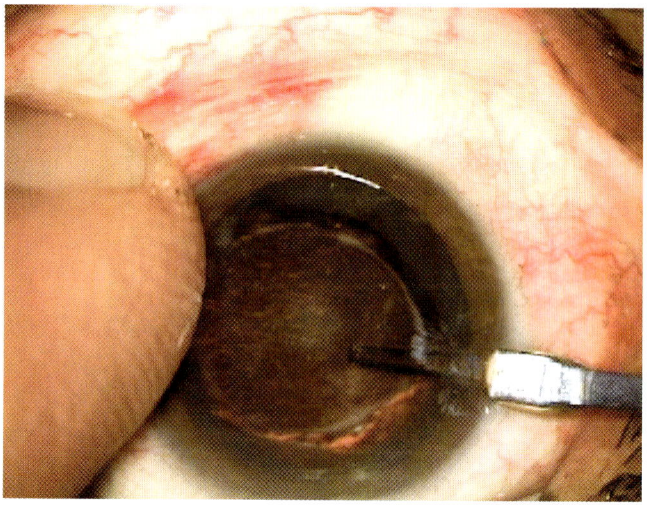

Fig. 2B: Dominant hand 700 micron incision

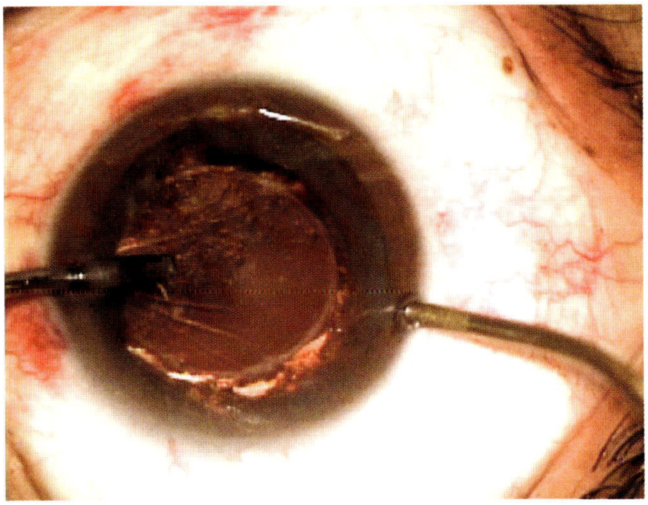

Fig. 3: Introduction of 700 micron irrigation/aspiration cannulas

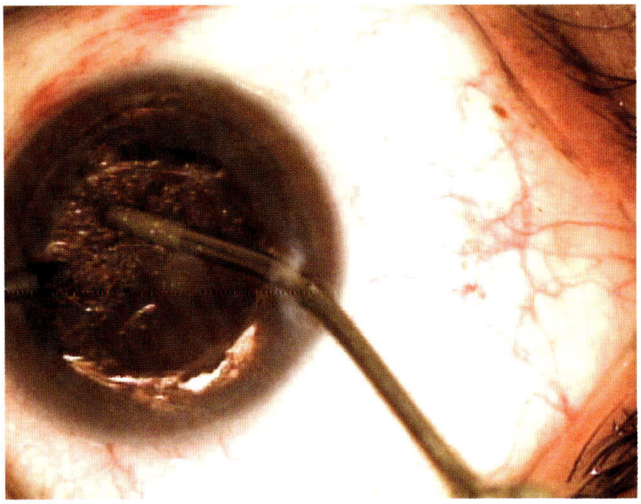

Fig. 4A: Aspiration process starting

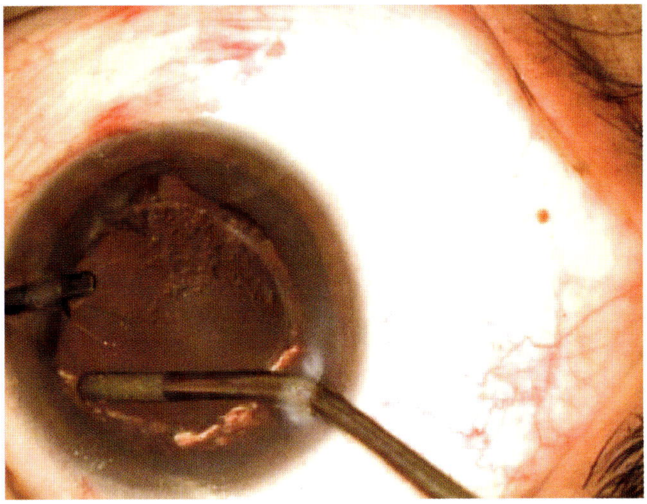

Fig. 4B: Aspiration process in progress

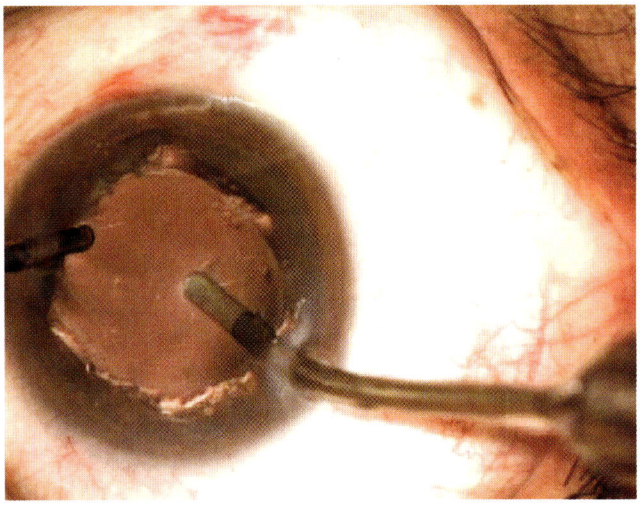

Fig. 4C: Finishing the aspirating process

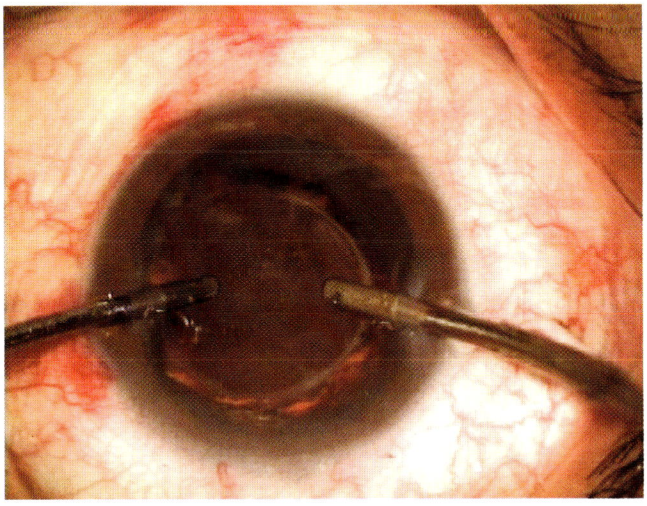

Fig. 5: Ready to withdraw instruments from the eye

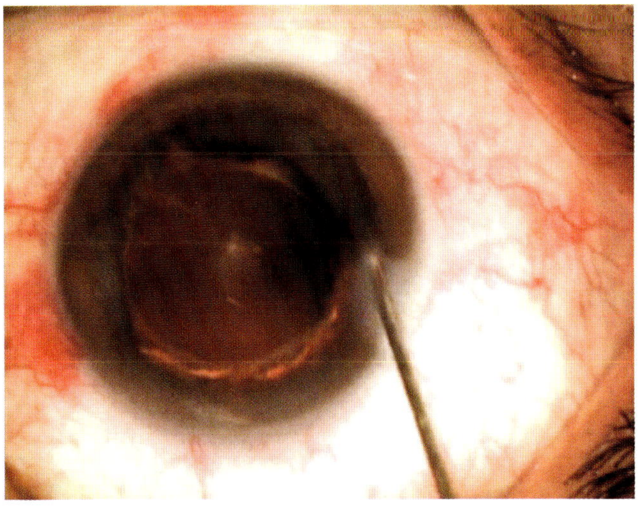

Fig. 6: Incisional edema

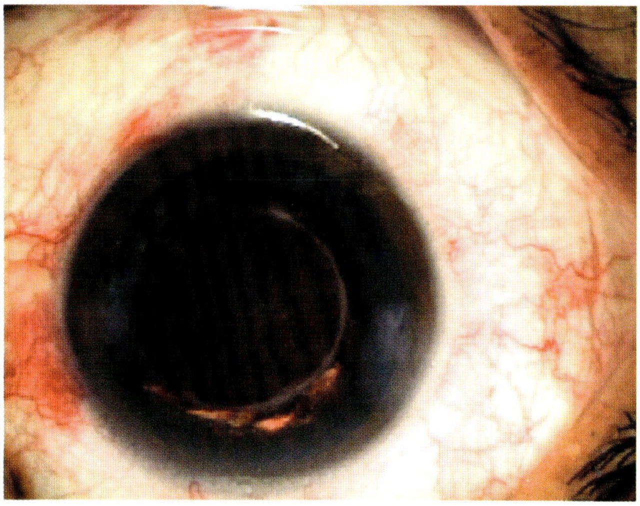

Fig. 7: Procedure finished

8. Finally the surgeon is able to produce some transitorily edema at both incisions sites to close by complete the anterior chamber (Fig. 6).
9. Once surgeons are sure about the intraocular pressure, the procedure is finished. Surgeons can inject prophylactic antibiotic solution if they want (Fig. 7).

References

1. Shearing S, Relyea R, Loaiza A. Routine phacoemulsification through a one-millimeter non-sutured incision. Cataract. 1985;2(2):6-10.
2. Jeng BH, Huang D. Anterior chamber stability during bimanual irrigation and aspiration: Theoretical and experimental analysis. J Cataract Refract Surg. 2001;27:1670-8.
3. Mehta C, Mehta K. Irrigation/aspiration techniques in phaco. In: Garg A. Mastering the Phacodynamics (Tools, Technology and Innovations). New Delhi: Jaypee Brothers Medical Publishers (P) Ltd.; 2007;24:199-205.
4. Alió J, Rodríguez-Prats JL, Galal A, et al. Outcomes of microincision cataract surgery versus coaxial phacoemulsification. Ophthalmology. 2005;112(11):1997-2003.
5. Tognetto D, Sanguinetti G, Sirotti P, et al. Visualization of fluid turbulence and acoustic cavitation during phacoemulsification. J Cataract Refract Surg. 2005;31(2):406-11.
6. Sinha R, Sharma N, Vajpayee RB. Intralenticular bimanual irrigation: aspiration for subluxated lens in Marfan´s syndrome. J Cataract Refract Surg. 2005;31(7):1283-6.
7. Haripriya A, Aravind S, Vadi K, et al. Bimanual microphaco for posterior polar cataracts. J Cataract Refract Surg. 2006;32(6):914-7.
8. Packer M, Fine IH, Hoffman RS. Refractive Lens Surgery. Ophthalmol Clin North Am. 2006;19(1):77-88.
9. Kanellopoulos AJ, Photolysis Investigative Group. Laser cataract surgery: A prospective clinical evaluation of 1000 consecutive laser cataract procedures using the Dodick photolysis Nd:YAG system. Ophthalmology. 2001;108(4):649-54.
10. Khng C, Osher RH. Surgical options in the face of positive pressure. J Cataract Refractive Surg. 2006;32(9):1423-5.
11. Cernák A, Cuvala J, Trnavec B, et al. Bimanual irrigation/aspiration. Cesk Slov Oftalmol. 1999;55(1):21-3.
12. Brauweiler P. Bimanual irrigation/aspiration. J Cataract Refract Surg. 1996;22(8):1013-6.

25

Refractive Lensectomy with 700 Micron System

Arturo Pérez-Arteaga (Mexico)

Introduction

In this chapter author has described how to perform a complete lens extraction avoiding by complete use of ultrasonic energy and using only vacuum and infusion as the forces to apply inside the eye to complete the entire surgery.

This technique is useful for many kinds of lens surgeries, not only for refractive lensectomy. The condition is the feature that the nucleus can be soft enough in order to avoid any kind of ultrasonic power (linear, torsional or other) and some other technologies for lens fragmentation (e.g. Aqualase, Photolysis), performing so the entire lens extraction using only aspiration of the lens material; irrigating force and vacuum force.[1]

Lens Features

The main feature in order to perform this technique is the lens softness. For hard nucleus, aspiration won´t be enough to produce a complete lens fragmentation and so a successful extraction; in these cases ultrasonic energy will be mandatory. The concept of lens softness can have variations according to the surgeon and some established criteria, maybe all the nucleus that are able to be emulsified through technologies, like Aqualase and Photolysis, are capable to be operated with biaxial phacoaspiration, avoiding so by complete any other physical force inside the eye.

Some examples of crystalline lens that can reach the softness needed to perform this technique are:[2-5,11]

- Congenital cataracts
- Traumatic cataracts
- Posterior polar cataracts
- Intumescent cataracts
- Milky cataracts
- Cataracts in young patients (developmental cataracts)

Advantages

The main advantages of this technique, in comparison to any other phaco technique that author can mention in this chapter, regarding the use of biaxial phacoaspiration for soft nucleus are:[6-10]

1. Less physical forces applied inside the eye. Because no ultrasonic energy is applied, no laser forces, no changes in the tissues temperature, the surgeon utilizes only the irrigating force and the vacuum. This means less trauma to the intraocular structures, in particular for the corneal endothelial cells.
2. Less instrumentation utilized. The surgeon only needs knife, viscoelastic material, micro-capsulorhexis forceps, irrigation/aspiration cannulas and the instrumentation needed to the IOL implantation. No phaco handpieces are in use. As much as a technique is simple, more reliable it becomes.
3. No need to switch between instrumentation during lens extraction, so less trauma to the tissues. There is no need to switch from one handpiece to another; with only the biaxial irrigation/aspiration handpieces, the complete surgery can be performed; this gives the opportunity to surgeon to decrease the number of intraoperative maneuvers.
4. The advantage of the "invisible surgical tools" is the irrigating force by one side and the vacuum by the other in a closed environment. This allows the surgeon to perform the phacoaspiration technique with minor movements; the instrumentation inside the eye barely moves; the "invisible forces" do almost all the work. This is the followability.
5. The advantages in fluidics of biaxial surgery including the low amount of irrigation (even with the use of forced infusion) through a 700 micron irrigating cannula.

Why in Biaxial and not in Coaxial

There are important differences of biaxial phacoaspiration versus coaxial or micro-coaxial phacoaspiration:[9-11]

1. Surgeons are working in a complete closed environment. No surge at all is occurring.
2. As the irrigation force goes inside, there is only one way to go outside is the aspirating cannula; there is no leakage, it means the followability.
3. The use of forced infusion and vacuum as operating tools decreases the amount of movements performed by the surgeon inside the eye.
4. Less amount of irrigation is in use in comparison with coaxial and micro-coaxial. Even less with 700 micron instrumentation; a complete biaxial phacoaspiration procedure can be performed with this technology utilizing no more than 40–50 cc of balanced salt solution.
5. Access to all meridians. No problem with subincisional epinucleus or cortical material, as in coaxial technology.
6. No need to switch instruments during the entire procedure of aspirating nucleus, epinuclear material and cortical material.

Surgical Technique

1. Be aware of your instrumentation, in particular regarding the diameter of your cannulas. Remember that wider diameters do not need forced infusion, but when using smaller diameters (like the 700 micron technology) forced infusion is recommended, this way avoiding surge.

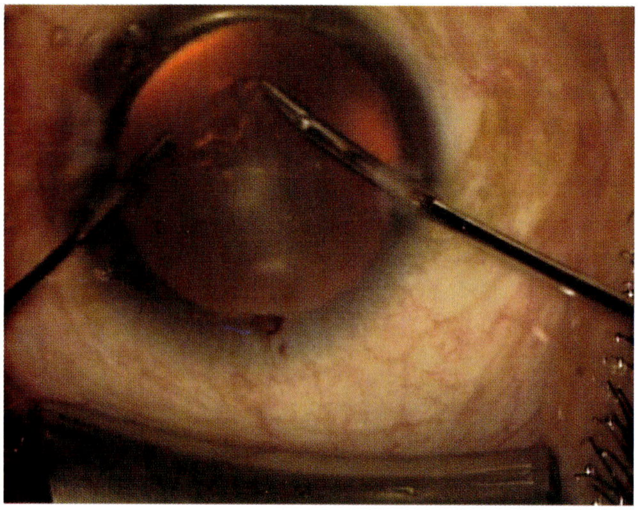

Fig. 1: Starting micro-biaxial capsulorhexis

2. Be aware of parameters; if using 700 micron cannulas apply between 90 cm H_2O and 120 cm H_2O of infusion and something between 300 mm Hg and 400 mm Hg of vacuum. Change parameters according to skills of surgeon, instrumentation and learning curve. Try to move to small diameter instrumentation as part of surgeons' learning curve, it increases the advantages in fluidics that the biaxial techniques give to them.
3. Perform two incisions with the proper knife taking care of the wound architecture. A closer environment is mandatory for the correct work of the "invisible forces".
4. Perform bimanual micro-capsulorhexis as surgeons have learned in the previous chapters. The size is surgeon`s choice (Figs 1 to 3).
5. Perform hydrodissection and hydrodelineation in a bimanual mode; then surgeons are able to feel the real softness of the nucleus and can help themselves to decide if it is a good case for biaxial phacoaspiration (Figs 4 and 5).
6. If the nucleus is too soft it withdraws outside the capsular bag in an easy way and then surgeons are ready to prechop before start to aspirate (Fig. 6). Try to perform mechanical fragmentation in all cases; they are soft nucleus very easy to prechop.
7. If the nucleus is a little harder, it will remain inside the capsular bag. Nevertheless a soft nucleus is easy to aspirate without the use of prechopping maneuvers.
8. If surgeon likes to prechop, place the nucleus in a "lens salute mode" with the hydrodissection cannula (Fig. 6).
9. If the nucleus is in "lens salute" position, the prechop maneuvers will not be able to transmit the force to the capsular bag or zonula. There is no case to perform the prechop maneuvers inside the capsular bag if surgeons can avoid risks with this maneuver, in particular in soft nucleus.
10. Perform prechop maneuvers with two viscoelastic cannulas (25 gauge); one entering the eye through each incision (Figs 7 to 10). It is very easy to perform if surgeon places one cannula behind the nucleus and another in the front then just press the nucleus to switch between them, it means, take the cannula that is at the front to the rear and the cannula that is behind the nucleus to the front. Then surgeons are sure that they are fragmenting the nucleus in a safe way.
11. Once the nucleus has been divided in multiple pieces surgeons are ready to start phacoaspiration (Fig. 10).
12. Enter first the irrigating cannula and then press the foot pedal to start irrigation. If the incisions were

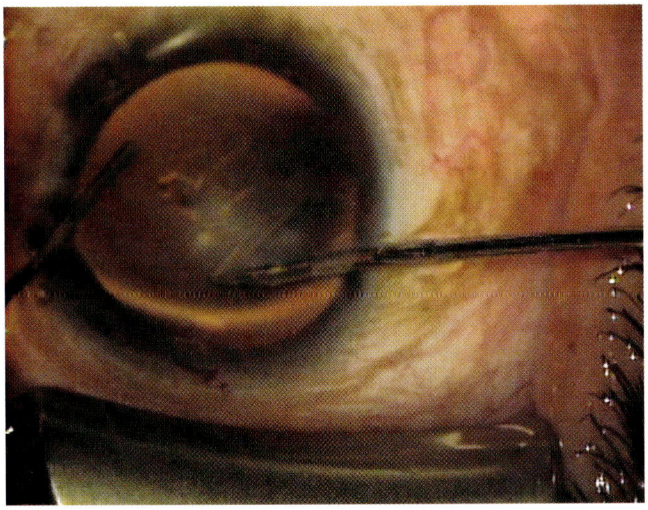

Fig. 2: Middle micro-capsulorhexis

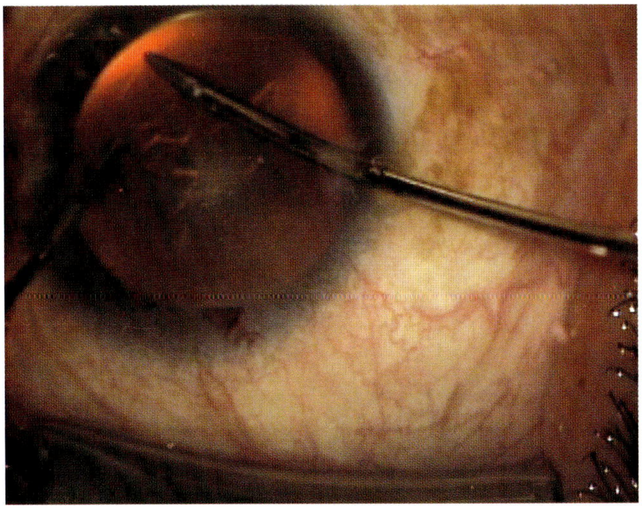

Fig. 3: Finishing microcapsulorhexis

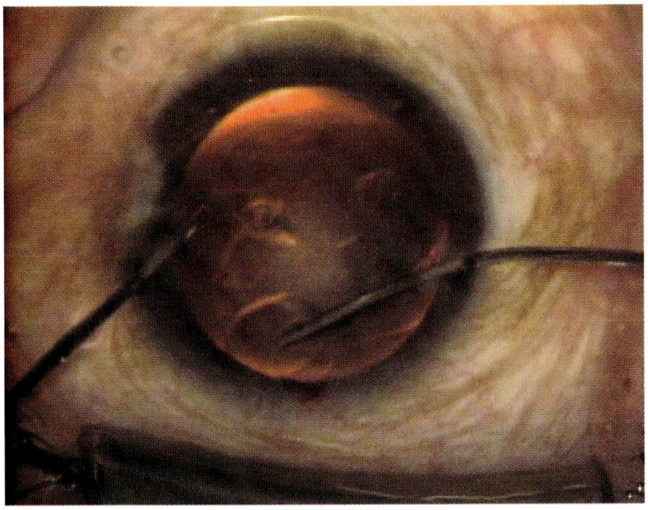

Fig. 4: Initial hydrodissection wave

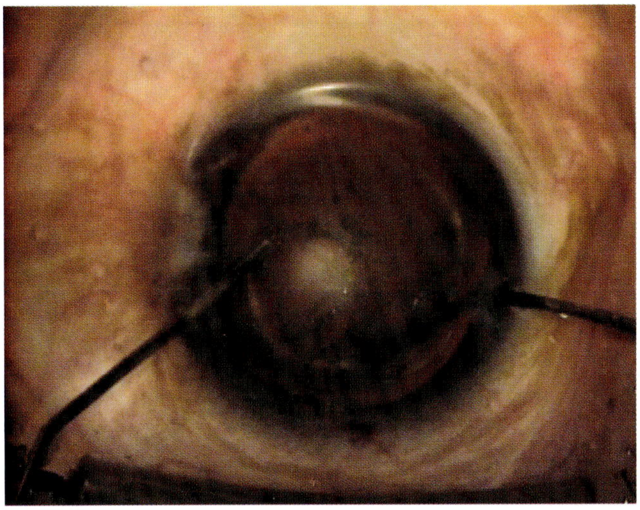

Fig. 5: Hydrodelamination. Notice the golden ring

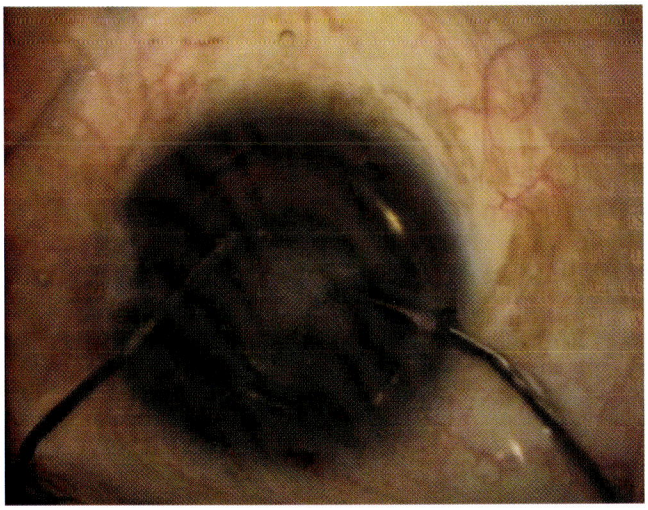

Fig. 6: Soft nucleus outside the capsular bag

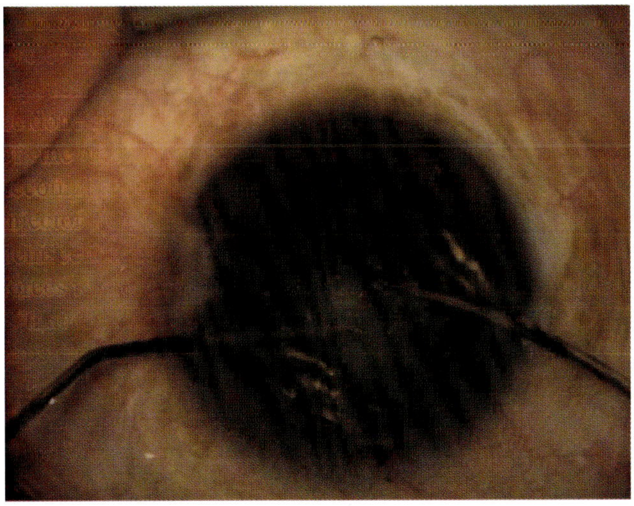

Fig. 7: Cannulas in position ready for prechop at the iris plane

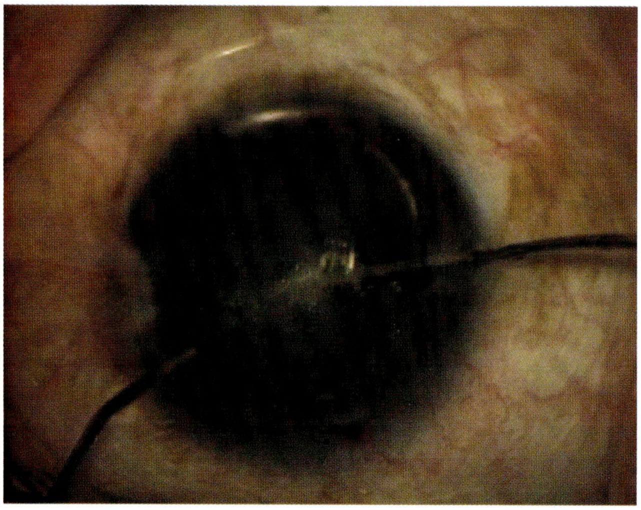

Fig. 8: Cannulas performing nucleus fragmentation

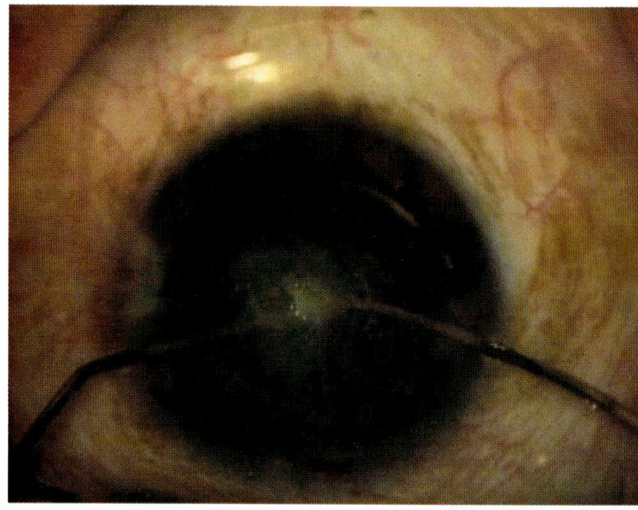

Fig. 9: Nuclear fragmentation

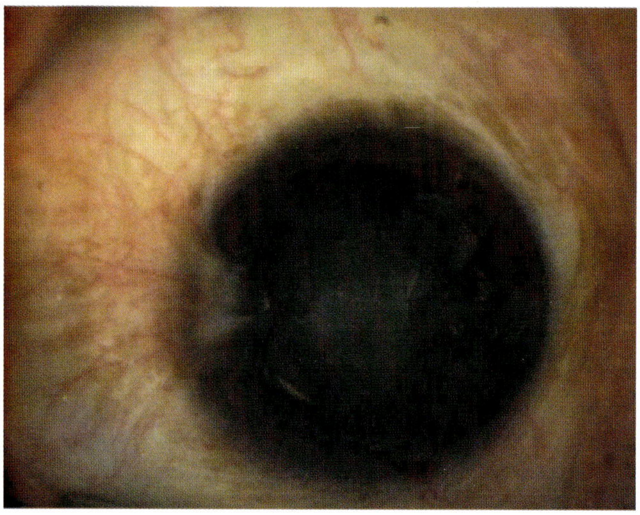

Fig. 10: Nucleus fragmented

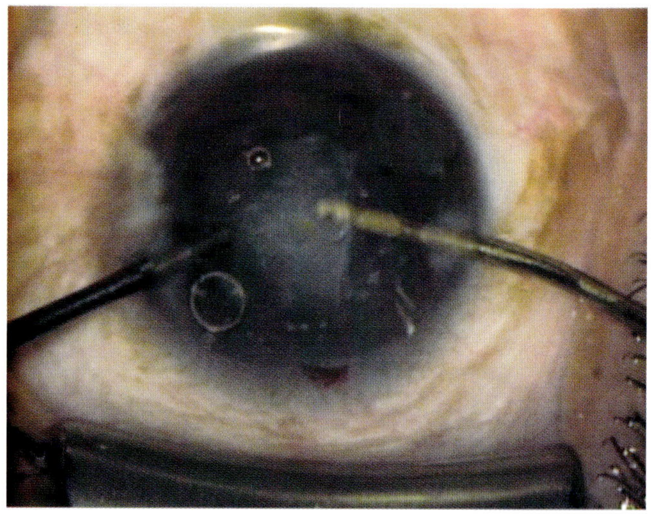

Fig. 11: 700 micron irrigating and aspirating cannulas inside the eye

made in the correct mode, even your cannula is inside the eye with the irrigation on, a balance of pressures will occur and no leakage at all will be seen (Fig. 11).

13. Keeping the irrigation on, introduce the aspiration cannula; the intraocular pressure acts as a counterforce and surgeon can introduce it easily.
14. Go first for the superior cortical material so surgeons are able to see the nucleus.
15. Once surgeons can see the nuclear pieces they have fragmented, go for them. So surgeons are sure, they are keeping the cushion of the epinuclear material behind it (Fig. 12).
16. Once surgeons finish the nuclear fragments they will be able to see the epinucleus inside the capsular bag. Once they are able to see the epinuclear material, go to aspirate it, first at the opposite side of your aspirating cannula and then the rest (Fig. 13).
17. Surgeons should finish their phacoaspiration process by cleaning the cortical material. Surgeons have the advantage that they do not have to switch instrumentation and lost the anterior chamber (Fig. 14).
18. Surgeons can polish the posterior capsule with the same instrumentation, just decrease the vacuum with footpedal or change to their desired preset parameters in their phaco machine; surgeons have the advantage that they do not have to switch instrumentation (Fig. 15). Then you have a very nice, complete, and clean capsular bag (Fig. 16).

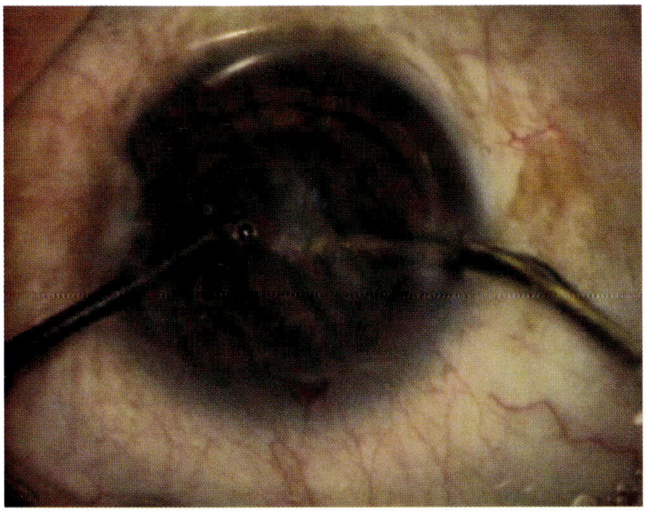

Fig. 12: Micro-biaxial nuclear pieces aspiration

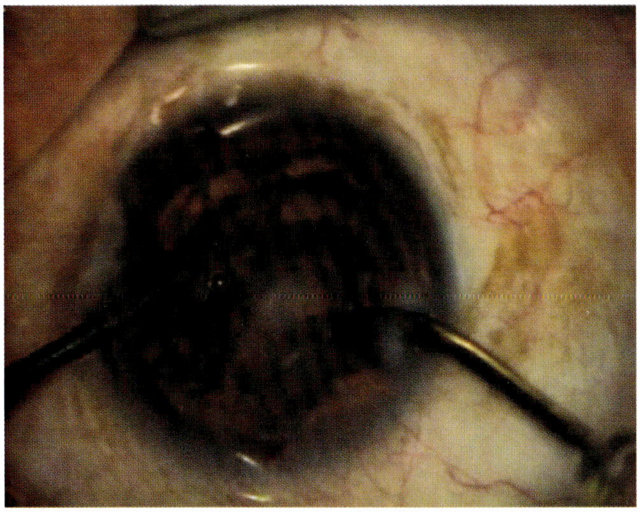

Fig. 13: Micro-biaxial epinuclear aspiration

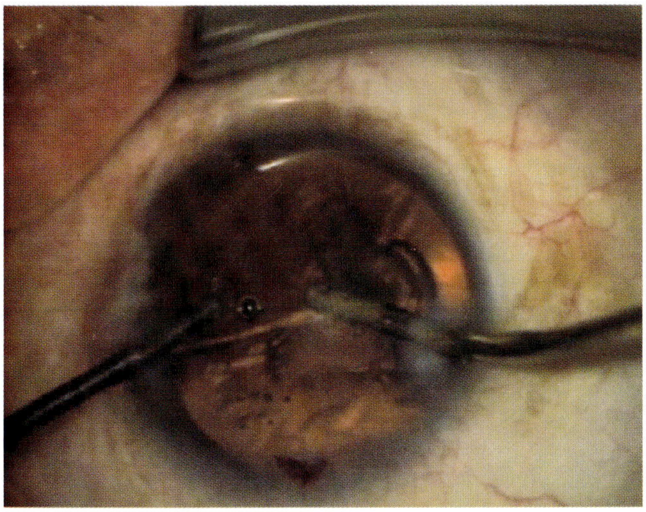

Fig. 14: Micro-biaxial cortical aspiration

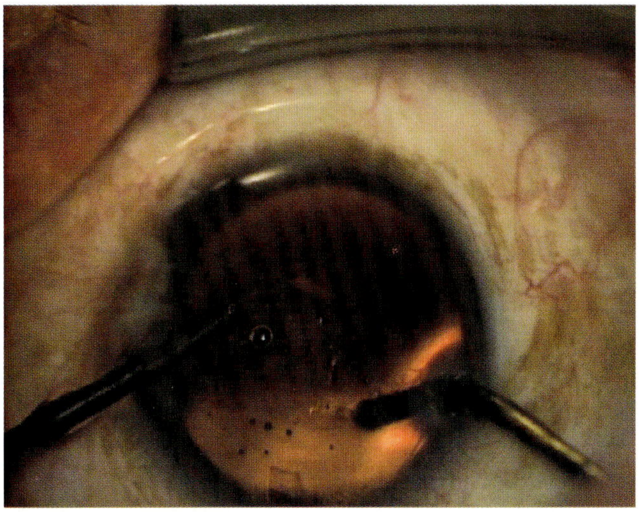

Fig. 15: Polish of the posterior capsule

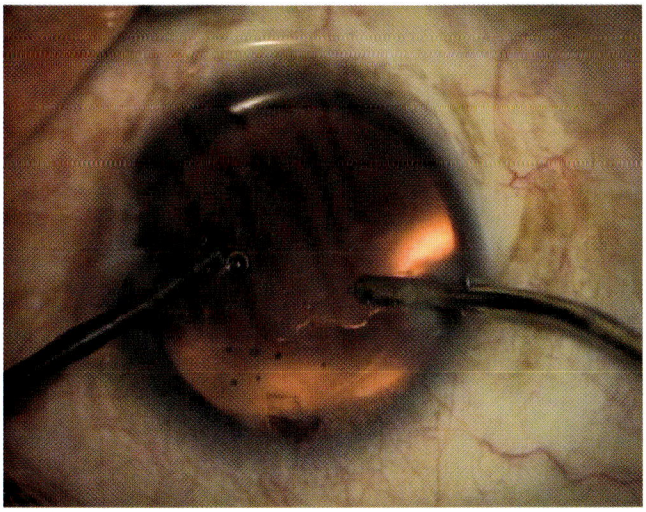

Fig. 16: Complete clean of the capsular bag

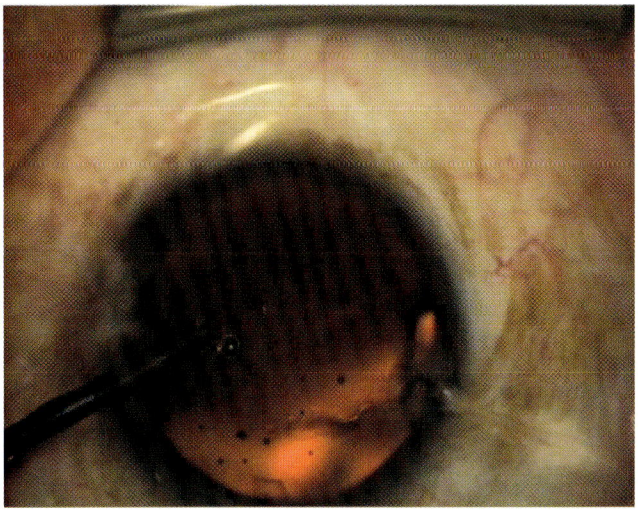

Fig. 17: Irrigating cannula maintained with irrigation inside the eye; it keeps the positive pressure

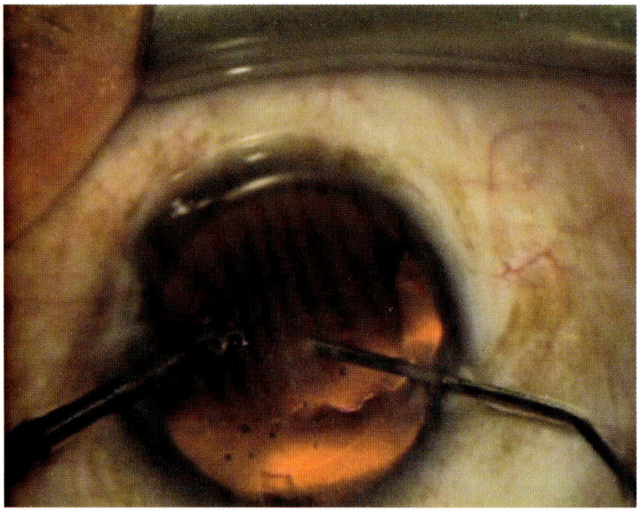

Fig. 18: Visco and irrigating cannula inside the eye

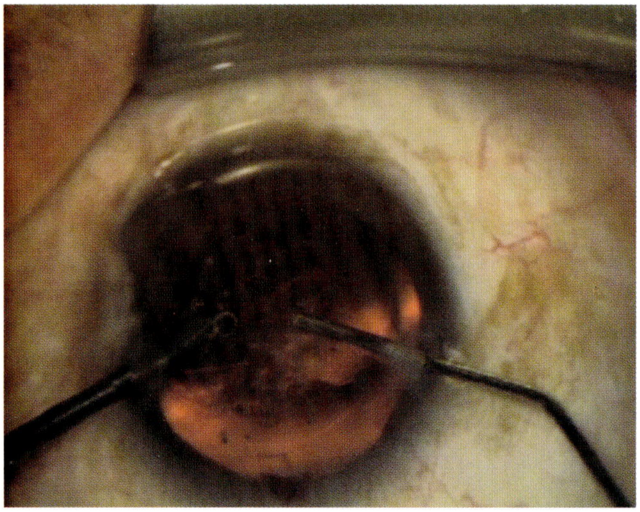

Fig. 19: Viscoelastic entering the eye

19. Do not withdraw both cannulas from the eye (Fig. 17). Remember that the positive pressure is the key in biaxial surgery; retire the aspirating cannula with the irrigation on, keep the irrigation on while switching and enter the viscoelastic cannula. Once the anterior chamber is full of visco surgeons can retire the irrigating cannula (Figs 18 to 20).
20. Remember to perform a third incision to implant the IOL, unless surgeons have a kind of IOL that doesn´t need incision enlargement.

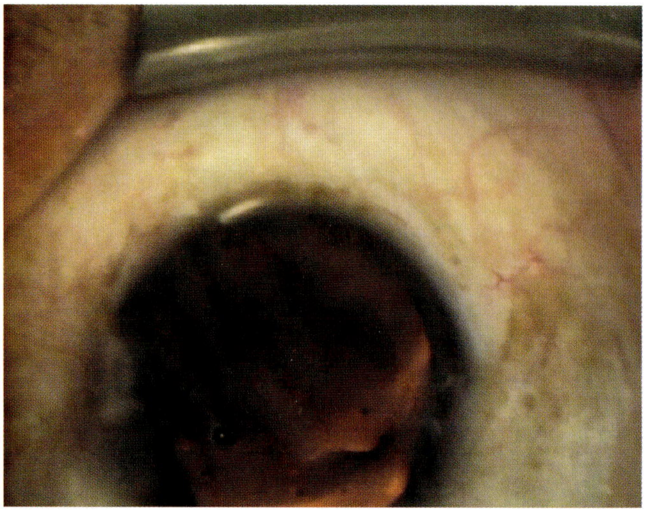

Fig. 20: Anterior chamber formed with viscoelastic

References

1. Minassian DC, Rosen P, Dart JK, et al. Extracapsular cataract extraction compared with small incision surgery by phacoemulsification: a randomized trial. Br J Ophthalmol. 2001;85:822-9.
2. Cavallini GM, Lugli N, Campi L, et al. Surgically induced astigmatism after manual extracapsular cataract extraction or after phacoemulsification procedure. Eur J Ophthalmol. 1996;6:257-63.
3. Watson A, Sunderraj P. Comparison of small-incision phacoemulsification with standard extracapsular cataract surgery: post-operative astigmatism and visual recovery. Eye. 1992;6(Pt 6):626-9.
4. Chee SP, Ti SE, Sivakumar M, et al. Postoperative inflammation: extracapsular cataract extraction versus phacoemulsification. J Cataract Refract Surg. 1999;25:1280-5.
5. Francis PJ, Morris RJ. Post-operative iris prolapse following phacoemulsification and extracapsular cataract surgery. Eye. 1997;11(Pt 1):87-90.
6. Linebarger EJ, Hardten DR, Shah GK, et al. Phacoemulsification and modern cataract surgery. Surv Ophthalmol. 1999;44:123-47.
7. Girard LJ. Ultrasonic fragmentation for cataract extraction and cataract complications. Adv Ophthalmol. 1978;37:127-35.
8. Shearing SP, Relyea RL, Loaiza A, et al. Routine phacoemulsification through a one-millimeter non-sutured incision. Cataract. 1985;2(2):6-11.
9. Agarwal A, Agarwal S, Agarwal A. Phakonit: lens removal through a 0.9 mm incision. J Cataract Refract Surg. 2001;27:1531-2.

10. Tsuneoka H, Takuya S, Takahashi Y. Feasibility of ultrasound cataract surgery with a 1.4 mm incision. J Cataract Refract Surg. 2001;27:934-40.
11. Haripriya A, Aravind S, Vadi K, et al. Bimanual microphaco for posterior polar cataracts. J Cataract Refract Surg. 2006;32(6):914-7.
12. Vasavada A, Singh R. Phacoemulsification in eyes with posterior polar cataracts. J Cataract Refract Surg. 1999;25(2):238-45.
13. Packer M, Fine IH, Hoffman RS. Refractive lens surgery. Ophthalmol Clin North Am. 2006;19(1):77-88.
14. Fernández-Vega L, Alfonso JF, Rodríguez PP, et al. Clear Lens extraction with multifocal apodized diffractive intraocular lens implantation. Ophthalmology. 2007;114(8):1491-8.
15. Braga-Mele R. Sleeveless bimanual phaco with Millennium system delivers less thermal energy to the eye. Ocular Surgery News US Edition. 2003.
16. Plager D. Pediatric cataract surgery, techniques complications, and management. Am J Ophthalmol. 2005;140(4):778.
17. Wood MG, Ogawa GSH. The challenge of pediatric cataract surgery. J AAPOS. 2000;4(5):323.
18. Wilson ME, Bartholomew LR, Trivedi RH. Pediatric cataract surgery and intraocular lens implantation: practice styles and preferences of the 2001 ASCRS and AAPOS memberships. J Cataract Refract Surg. 2003;29(9):1811-20.
19. Trivedi RH, Wilson ME, Golub RL. Incidence and risk factors for glaucoma after pediatric cataract surgery with and without intraocular lens implantation. Am J Ophthalmol. 2006;142(4):714-5.
20. Ram J, Brar GS, Kaushik S, et al. Role of posterior capsulotomy with vitrectomy and intraocular lens design and material in reducing posterior capsule opacification after pediatric cataract surgery. J Cataract Refract Surg. 2003;29(8):1579-84.
21. Pérez-Arteaga A. Step by Step in Biaxial Lens Surgery. New Delhi: Jaypee Brothers Medical Publishers; 2008.

Index

Page numbers followed by *f* refer to figure and *t* refer to table

2495